Handbook of Medic
Therapy and Child Life

The *Handbook of Medical Play Therapy and Child Life* brings together the voices and clinical experiences of dedicated clinical practitioners in the fields of play therapy and child life. This volume offers fresh insights and up-to-date research in the use of play with children, adolescents, and families in medical and health care settings. Chapters take a strength-based approach to clinical interventions across a wide range of health-related issues, including autism, trauma, routine medical care, pending surgeries both large and small, injury, immune deficiency, and more. Through its focus on the resiliency of the child, the power of play, and creative approaches to healing, this handbook makes visible the growing overlap and collaboration between the disciplines of play therapy and child life.

Lawrence C. Rubin, PhD, is a professor of counselor education at St. Thomas University in Miami, Florida, where he directs the Mental Health Counseling program. He is also an online lecturer for the counseling programs at the University of Massachusetts, Boston. Dr. Rubin is a practicing psychologist in Fort Lauderdale, where he specializes with children, teens, and their families and is the past board chair of the Association for Play Therapy.

"What a lovely collaborative book on the value of play! Child life and play therapy practitioners have worked together for the benefit of those with medical needs for years. This valuable book will further strengthen this work. The richness of the book is illuminated by the many helpful and insightful case studies. This volume will inform the work of practitioners of many disciplines and will do so to the benefit of medically involved children, adolescents, and their families."

Linda Homeyer, PhD, LPC, RPT-S, professor, Professional Counseling Program, Texas State University

"*Handbook of Medical Play Therapy and Child Life* is a timely and comprehensive volume offering professionals a unique, sure-to-be-used text! Readers will find it a rich composite filled with strength-based and resiliency-building creative approaches to healing that deal with a wide range of health-related issues. A must-have addition to any professional library!"

Athena A. Drewes, PsyD, MA, RPT-S, director of clinical training and APA-accredited doctoral internship at Astor Services for Children and Families, founder and president emeritus of the New York Association for Play Therapy

Handbook of Medical Play Therapy and Child Life

Interventions in Clinical
and Medical Settings

Edited by Lawrence C. Rubin

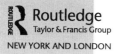
Routledge
Taylor & Francis Group

NEW YORK AND LONDON

First published 2018
by Routledge
711 Third Avenue, New York, NY 10017

and by Routledge
2 Park Square, Milton Park, Abingdon, Oxon, OX14 4RN

Routledge is an imprint of the Taylor & Francis Group, an informa business

Library of Congress Cataloging-in-Publication Data
Names: Rubin, Lawrence C., 1955– editor.
Title: Handbook of medical play therapy and child life : interventions in clinical and medical
    settings/edited by Lawrence C. Rubin.
Other titles: Medical play therapy and child life
Description: New York : Routledge, 2018. | Includes bibliographical references and index.
Identifiers: LCCN 2017034728 | ISBN 9781138690004 (hardcover : alk. paper) |
    ISBN 9781138690011 (pbk. : alk. paper) | ISBN 9781315527857 (e-book)
Subjects: MESH: Play Therapy | Pain Management | Chronic Disease—therapy | Family
    Relations | Child | Adolescent
Classification: LCC RJ505.P6 | NLM WS 350.4 | DDC 618.92/891653—dc23
LC record available at https://lccn.loc.gov/2017034728

ISBN: 978-1-138-69000-4 (hbk)
ISBN: 978-1-138-69001-1 (pbk)
ISBN: 978-1-315-52785-7 (ebk)

Typeset in Sabon and Helvetica Neue
by Apex CoVantage, LLC

Contents

[handwritten annotation: "(Using the family system as a healing tool w/i a healing modality)"]

Figures

Tables

About the Editor

Lawrence "Larry" C. Rubin, PhD, ABPP, LMHC, RPT-S, is a professor of counselor education at St. Thomas University in Miami, Florida, where he directs the Mental Health Counseling Program. He is also an adjunct professor of counselor education in the Mental Health Counseling Program at the University of Massachusetts, Boston. Dr. Rubin is the past president of the Florida Association for Play Therapy, as well as past board chair of the Association for Play Therapy. He is in private practice as psychologist, counselor, and play therapist, specializing with children, teens, and families. Dr. Rubin's research and writing interests lie at the intersection of psychology and popular culture. His textbook, *Diagnosis and Treatment Planning Skills: A Popular Culture Casebook Approach* with Dr. Alan Schwitzer is widely used in counselor education programs across the country. Other books by Dr. Rubin include *Play-Based Interventions for Children and Adolescents With Autism Spectrum Disorder* with Loretta Gallo Lopez; *Mental Illness in Popular Media: Essays on the Representation of Psychiatric Disorders; Food for Thought: Essays on Eating and Culture; Popular Culture in Counseling, Psychotherapy and Play-Based Intervention; Using Superheroes in Counseling and Play Therapy*; and *Psychotropic Drugs and Popular Culture: Medicine, Mental Health and the Media.* Dr. Rubin is on the editorial boards of the *International Journal of Play,* the *Journal of Popular Television,* and the *Journal of Child and Adolescent Counseling.* He lives in Florida with his wife Randi, two children Zachary and Rebecca, six cats, and a dog named Lilly.

About the Contributors

Mistie Barnes, LPC-S, RPT-S, was an assistant professor of counselor education at Delta State University in Cleveland, Mississippi. She was the founder and director of the Delta State University Play Therapy Training Institute and maintained a limited private practice, providing clinical consultation and supervision in counseling and play therapy. Dr. Barnes spoke nationally on play therapy and related topics, and published chapters and techniques in several books. She was the recent clinical editor for *Play Therapy* magazine, and president of the Mississippi Association for Play Therapy. She was also the 2014 award recipient of the Association for Play Therapy key award for Professional Education and Training.

Manuel H. Belver, PhD, is a professor of art education in the Complutense University of Madrid (Spain). He directs the Museum of Children's Art in this university. He has studied art and creativity in children and adolescents, and his current research is related to the applications of art in community settings (hospitals and health centers). He is author of several books about these questions.

Tanya Nathalie Beran, PhD, R Psych, is a tenured professor in medical education in the Department of Community Health Sciences at the University of Calgary. She studied at the University of British Columbia for her undergraduate degree, and the Universities of Manitoba and Calgary for her graduate education. She accepted her first academic position at the University of Calgary Werklund School of Education, where she later became director of the School and Applied Child Psychology Program. In 2008, Dr. Beran joined the Cumming School of Medicine where she teaches graduate courses in research design and statistics. With a research focus of child and adult education and health, she has published over 100 peer-reviewed papers and received tri-council funding for many years. No area of research has had such an impact on children and their families as the work with MEDi the robot.

Fraser Brown, PhD, is the first professor of playwork in the UK. He is programme leader for the BA (Hons) playwork degree at Leeds Beckett University, and specialist link tutor for the postgraduate play therapy courses run in conjunction with the Academy of Play and Child Psychotherapy. Before joining LBU, he managed a number of playwork projects in both the statutory and independent sectors. His wide-ranging research interests include the impact of deprivation on children's play behavior, the assessment of play value in children's play spaces, and the role of play in the Montessori system of education. He is well known for his research into the therapeutic effects of playwork on a group of abandoned children in a Romanian pediatric hospital. He is co-editor of the *International Journal of Play*, and his recent publications include *101 Stories of Children Playing* (2014); *Rethinking Children's Play* (2013); and *Foundations of Playwork* (2008).

Kathryn A. Cantrell, MA, CCLS, is a certified child life specialist and lecturer of undergraduate and graduate courses within the Eliot-Pearson Department of Child Study and Human Development at Tufts University. She received her BA from Austin College, her MA from Tufts University, and is currently a doctoral candidate within the Department of Counseling and School Psychology at the University of Massachusetts, Boston. Prior to her current positions, she worked as a child life specialist at St. Jude Children's Research Hospital. Currently, she is associate editor of *Child Life Focus*, the official journal of the Association of Child Life Professionals, and is completing her dissertation on online self-disclosure among young adults with HIV. Her current research interests include the intersection of technology, internalizing stigma, and disclosure in pediatrics, and her work has been published in numerous journals.

Angela M. Cavett, PhD, RPT-S, is a child and adolescent psychologist and registered play therapist–supervisor. She works in a private practice providing psychological evaluation and individual, family, and play therapy for children, adolescents, and their families. She provides face-to-face and distance consultation and supervision from mental/behavioral health professionals. Dr. Cavett is an adjunct professor at the University of North Dakota in the Department of Counseling Psychology. She is a disaster mental health volunteer for the Red Cross. Dr. Cavett is active in the Association for Play Therapy and provides workshops across the United States related to children's behavioral health.

Cindy Dell Clark, PhD, is an anthropologist who has spent her adult life conducting research that focuses on children's experiences and vantage points. She has worked both as an applied research consultant and as a scholar. Her published writings include a family-based ethnography of young children coping with severe asthma and diabetes, *In Sickness and In Play: Children Coping With Chronic Illness* (Rutgers University Press); a collected volume on the role of play in human well-being, *Play and Wellbeing* (Routledge); and many chapters and articles on topics of childhood illness, play, imagination, and ritual. Clark has been a trendsetter in methods of children's qualitative inquiry. Her book *In a Younger Voice* (Oxford University Press) has served scholars and practitioners as a methodological toolkit for learning to do child-centered ethnographic research. Clark is associate professor of anthropology at Rutgers University (Camden) and serves on the editorial board of *Medical Anthropology Quarterly*.

Meredith Cooper, MA, CCLS, LPC, is the former executive director and cofounder of Wonders & Worries, which she launched in 2001. Following 15 years of success, Meredith stepped into a founder role in 2017, where she continues providing strategic direction for national growth. Meredith has a bachelor's and a master's degree in child development. She is a certified child life specialist and a licensed professional counselor who has been involved with children's health care in the Austin community for more than 25 years, including being the first pediatric oncology child life specialist for Austin. In 2010 Meredith received the Helping Hand Home's Champion for Children Award and the Girl Scout Woman of Distinction Award in 2013. Meredith is married with one son and two daughters, and one grandson and (almost) two granddaughters.

David A. Crenshaw, PhD, ABPP, RPT-S, is clinical director of the Children's Home of Poughkeepsie, New York, and adjunct faculty at Marist College. He has also taught graduate play therapy courses at Johns Hopkins and Columbia University. He is a board certified clinical psychologist by the American Board of Professional Psychology, fellow of the American Psychological Association (APA), and fellow of APA's Division of Child and Adolescent Psychology. He is also a registered play therapist–supervisor by the Association for Play Therapy. Dr. Crenshaw is a past president of the New York Association for Play Therapy, and also the Hudson Valley Psychological Association, which honored him with its Lifetime Achievement Award in 2012. He has written or edited 15 books on child aggression, trauma, grief, resilience, and over 50 book chapters and journal articles. His latest book is *Termination Challenges in Child Psychotherapy*, co-written with Eliana Gil.

Victoria Dempsey, MS, is the research coordinator for the Pediatrics Rheumatology Department of the IWK Health Centre in Halifax, Nova Scotia. She graduated with a BSc Honours in psychology (2012) from Saint Mary's University and continued her education at Mount Saint Vincent University, where she pursued her interests around children and play. Her master's thesis, *Observations of Preschoolers' Health Care Play*, was completed as a requirement for the Master's in Child and Youth Study degree in 2015. She continues to engage in scholarship, recently as the co-author with Donna Varga on a book chapter, "Happy Captives and Monstrous Hybrids: The Flamingo in Children's Stories."

Michael E. Feeney, MA, attained his graduate degree in clinical-counseling psychology in 2015 from Radford University, and is currently a clinical psychology doctoral student at East Tennessee State University. He has previously written and/or presented on decision making and health beliefs, self-control, and group research methods. His current research interest focuses on relational and fictional influences of self-identity formation across childhood and adolescence.

Jenaya Gordon, MA, CCLS, NCC, is the child life associate clinical manager at Children's Hospital Colorado (CHCO). Her child life career began in 2001 at Children's Medical Center Dallas where she worked on the inpatient surgical/trauma and neurosurgery units. Jenaya moved to Colorado in 2004 to pursue her graduate degree in counseling psychology and was an individual/family therapist for four years. In 2008, she joined the child life team at CHCO, furthering her trauma experience by working in the inpatient surgical/trauma unit, emergency department, and pediatric intensive care unit. Jenaya presents locally and nationally on ensuring the emotional safety of pediatric patients, facilitating trauma processing, and providing trauma-informed care. She has co-presented multiple times at national child life conferences, co-facilitated a webinar, and facilitates in-person trainings throughout the country. Audiences include child life specialists, physicians, nurses, EMTs, social workers, art therapists, and therapeutic recreation specialists.

Sarah V. Grill, BS, is a master's candidate in clinical developmental health and psychology within the Eliot-Pearson Department of Child Study and Human Development at Tufts University. She received her BS in Health Psychology from MCPHS University. Sarah has held research positions at the Harvard Lab for Developmental Studies, and the Neurodevelopmental Lab for Addictions & Mental Health at McLean Hospital. In addition, she has worked as residential counselor at the Cambridge Eating Disorder Center. Currently, she is a researcher to the Adolescent Medicine division at Boston Children's Hospital & Harvard Medical School. Her current research interests include adolescent risk and resilience, anxiety and mood disorders in adolescents, and the impact of pediatric chronic illness on development.

Melissa Hicks, MS, CCLS, LPC, RPT-S, is a certified child life specialist, licensed professional counselor, and registered play therapist–supervisor. She has worked with children impacted by illness, primarily cancer and other chronic illnesses, for nearly 30 years in both hospital and community settings. Hospital settings include the Johns Hopkins Children's Center and the AFLAC Cancer Center at Children's Healthcare of Atlanta. Melissa co-founded the non-profit organization, Wonders & Worries in Austin, Texas, and was the psychosocial program director at The Camp Sunshine House in Atlanta, Georgia. Melissa has published articles and book chapters and is editor of *Child Life Beyond the Hospital*. She has served as president of the Association for Child Life Professionals and several other leadership positions within ACLP and other non-profit boards. Additionally, she received the Distinguished Service Award from the Association of Child Life Professionals and the Outstanding Alumni Award from the University of Delaware.

Kevin B. Hull, PhD, LMHC, is a private practitioner in Lakeland, Florida, where he specializes in play therapy with children, adolescents, and young adults on the autism spectrum. Dr. Hull is the author of *Play Therapy and Asperger's Syndrome* (Jason Aronson, 2011) and *Group Therapy Techniques With Children, Adolescents, and Adults on the Autism Spectrum* (Jason Aronson, 2013). In 2012 he wrote *Bridge Building* (Liberty Press) to help parents of children and adolescents with autism build closer connections with children through play techniques. In 2014 he wrote *Where There Is Despair, Hope* (Liberty Mountain Publishing). He has been an associate professor for 14 years and currently teaches practicum and internship courses for Liberty University. In his spare time Dr. Hull enjoys swimming, growing orchids, and spending time with his wife, Wendy, and their four children and one grandchild.

Jillian E. Kelly, LCSW, RPT, is a licensed clinical social worker and registered play therapist with experience working in inner-city community clinics with children and families. She is the vice president of the NYAPT, graduate of the APT's Leadership Academy, adjunct lecturer and frequent presenter on childhood trauma, and co-author of publications on resilience. Certified in trauma-focused cognitive behavioral therapy and as a registered play therapist, she is dedicated to integrating modalities to meet the unique needs of every child.

Morgan Livingstone, MA, CCLS, is a certified child life specialist, passionate about play in the lives of children and youth with serious illness, surviving trauma, experiencing loss, and facing challenges in their everyday life. In a community-based practice, Morgan has the opportunity to work closely with children and their families in their homes, hospitals, and hospices. Morgan supports and facilitates children's coping and promotes them being and feeling successful by finding and creating inspired solutions to the problems they face. Devoted to giving children a voice in their health care experience, Morgan believes it is a child's basic human right to be an active participant in all aspects of their life and death. Morgan is a strong advocate for collaboration with other professionals, and hopes to share her passion for play and spread awareness about the amazing abilities of children and youth, both locally and globally.

Jon Luongo, MS, CCLS, has worked and played in pediatric health care since 1997, first as a performer with Big Apple Circus Clown Care and since 2004 as a child life specialist. At Maimonides Medical Center in Brooklyn, New York, Jon started the sedation-free MRI program that helps children complete an entire MRI with no anesthesia. He sings, tells stories with string, and engages children in their own experience of the hospital so they can breathe and cope. Jon has presented on the benefits of using "loose parts"—artful use of what's at hand—so children can understand and construct meaning around their experience of illness and health. He makes a harmonica from two tongue depressors, rubber bands, and an index card, and plays "Pop Goes the Weasel" on a slide whistle made from a syringe. Jon taught at Bank Street College of Education and currently serves as a delegate with 1199 Healthcare Workers' Union.

Kerri Modry-Mandell, PhD, is a full-time faculty member in the Eliot-Pearson Department of Child Study and Human Development (CSHD) at Tufts University. She is the faculty-in-charge of the clinical developmental health and psychology/well-being concentration in the CSHD master of arts program and teaches both undergraduate and graduate courses. Her areas of interest include pediatric psychology, adaptation to pediatric chronic illness, pediatric health promotion, and disease prevention developmental initiatives. Her primary interests in research-practice integration focus on child health, families, and culture, psychosocial aspects of childhood cancer, and how cultural factors influence family functioning and adaptation to pediatric chronic illness.

Kristie Opiola, PhD, LPC, RPT, CCLS, is an assistant professor in the Counseling Department at the University of North Carolina at Charlotte. She has worked as a licensed professional counselor, play therapist, and certified child life specialist with children, adolescents, and families in a variety of pediatric hospitals, private practices, and agency settings for over 14 years. Kristie's clinical work specializes in children and families who are coping with acute or life-altering illness and/or interpersonal trauma.

Suzanna Paisley, MS, CCLS, began her professional career as an elementary/preschool teacher. Always knowing her passion was to work in the field of child life, she pursued her dream in New York City, receiving her master's of science in child life at Bank Street College of Education. Suzanna took the knowledge and inspiration she received at Bank Street to her role as a child life specialist at Children's Hospital Colorado. Her work focused on patients in inpatient rehabilitation and the teen hospital population. This population inspired her to focus on patients who have experienced trauma, co-presenting nationally at child life conferences, as well as a webinar on providing trauma processing interventions for patients of all ages. Suzanna now raises her two young children and provides child life services as PRN in the emergency department, urgent care, and ICUs, while continuing to educate specialists on how to support children and adolescents affected by trauma.

Jessica E. Pappagianopoulos, BA, is a master's candidate in the Eliot-Pearson Department of Child Study and Human Development. She received her BA from Stonehill College, where she was the recipient of the Psychology Department's Student of the Year Award. During that time, she worked as a research assistant on various projects (e.g., facial recognition, which was published, smoking cessation, and HIV/AIDS). Currently, she is a teaching assistant and works in the Child Health Equity Lab at Tufts University, exploring preventive health interventions and adolescent health literacy. At the Faja Lab at Boston Children's Hospital, she assists with an intervention aiming to improve executive functioning skills in children diagnosed with autism. She is completing her thesis on risk perception and smoking behavior among adolescents with asthma, and her current research interests include pediatric chronic illness and autism.

Judi Parson, PhD, MA Play Therapy, GCHE, RN, is a pediatric qualified registered nurse, registered play therapist–supervisor, lecturer in mental health, and course director for the Graduate Certificate/Diploma of Therapeutic Child Play and Master of Child Play Therapy programs at Deakin University. Her PhD, titled *Integration of Procedural Play for Children Undergoing Cystic Fibrosis Treatment: A Nursing Perspective* led her to study play therapy through the School of Psychology at Roehampton University, London. Judi is actively involved in the development of play therapy in Australia and she does this by maintaining a small private practice, presenting at conferences, providing short courses in play therapy and medical play therapy, and engaging in a range of research projects. She also offers clinical supervision as well as research supervision to candidates in the field of pediatrics and play therapy.

Michael M. Patte, PhD, is a professor of teaching and learning at Bloomsburg University of Pennsylvania where he prepares undergraduate and graduate students for careers in education. During his 25-year career he developed an interest in the fields of child development, child life, and play and has shared his scholarship through publications, international and national conference presentations, and advocacy projects. His latest co-authored/edited books include *Beyond the Classroom Walls: Developing Mindful Home, School, and Community Partnerships* (2016), *International Perspectives on Children's Play* (2015), and *Rethinking Children's Play*

(2013). Dr. Patte is a Distinguished Fulbright Scholar, co-editor of the *International Journal of Play*, past president of The Association for the Study of Play, board member of The International Council for Children's Play, and a member of the Pennsylvania Governor's Early Learning Council, responsible for planning the expansion of effective early learning and development services for Pennsylvania's young children and families.

Jacqueline Reynolds Pearson, MA, CCLS, works as a certified child life specialist at the Alberta Children's Hospital. She began her career in child life in 1992 after completing undergraduate degrees in psychology and education at the University of Calgary. In 1997, she started what is now known as the Child Health Computer Program, applying her interests in technology to child life. She completed an individualized master of arts degree in 2002 through an innovative online collaboration between Queens University and the University of Calgary. In 2015, she began her role as MEDi Project Lead, integrating humanoid robots into psychosocial care and pain management under the Vi Riddell Pain and Rehabilitation Centre. Through this position she has been extensively involved in research and quality improvement.

Dee C. Ray, PhD, LPC-S, NCC, RPT-S, is Distinguished Teaching Professor in the counseling program and director of the Child and Family Resource Clinic at the University of North Texas. Dr. Ray has published over 100 articles, chapters, and books on play therapy, specializing in research publications examining the effects of child-centered play therapy. She is author of *A Therapist's Guide to Development: The Extraordinarily Normal Years* and *Advanced Play Therapy: Essential Conditions, Knowledge, and Skills for Child Practice.*

W. George Scarlett, PhD, is senior lecturer and deputy chair of the Eliot-Pearson Department of Child Study and Human Development at Tufts University. He received a BA from Yale University, an MDiv from the Episcopal Divinity School, and a PhD (in developmental psychology) from Clark University. He has authored or co-authored six books and three major handbook chapters, and has edited or published numerous articles in journals, primarily in three areas: children's play, behavior and classroom management, and religious and spiritual development. He has been on the research teams of several internationally known leaders, including Ed Zigler at Yale and Howard Gardner at Harvard. His current writing and research focus is on children, nature, and the ecology movement.

John W. Seymour, PhD, LMFT, RPT-S, is a distinguished faculty scholar and professor at Minnesota State University, Mankato, where he teaches graduate courses in family therapy, play therapy, mental health counseling, and clinical supervision in the Department of Counseling and Student Personnel. He has been a family therapist and play therapist for over 35 years, and maintains a private practice at Journeys Toward Healing Counseling Center in Mankato. He has published and presented internationally on topics that include child and family resiliency and families with chronic illness. Current professional leadership positions include serving as a board member of both the Minnesota Board of Marriage and Family Therapy and the Association for Play Therapy.

Jason L. Steadman, PsyD, is an assistant professor of psychology at East Tennessee State University in Johnson City, Tennessee, where he runs the Childhood Anxiety, Play Therapy, and Virtual Reality Environments (CAPTVRE) research lab. He completed his doctoral studies at Baylor University, under the mentorship of Helen Benedict, PhD, RPT-S, and his predoctoral internship at The Village for Families and Children in Hartford, Connecticut. He also completed a one-year post-doctoral clinical fellowship in Community Health and Integrated Primary Care at Community Health Center, Inc. based in Middletown, Connecticut.

Joan Turner, PhD, CCLS, is an associate professor in the department of child and youth study at Mount Saint Vincent University in Halifax, Nova Scotia. Joan was the recipient of the Eleanor Blumenthal Fellowship at the University of Missouri–Columbia, Department of Human Development and Family Studies where she graduated with a doctorate degree in 2002. A child life specialist since 1987, she has contributed to the profession as a practitioner, educator, researcher, and author. As co-editor with Civita Brown, she initiated the journey of documenting the emergence of child life as a profession in North America in *The Pips of Child Life* series. Joan is dedicated to contributing to and inspiring research and scholarship emphasizing child life and child health interests. Additionally, she is engaged with early years education and early developmental intervention research and practice projects in Nova Scotia.

Ana M. Ullán, PhD, is a senior lecturer of social psychology in the University of Salamanca (Spain). She has studied the hospitalization conditions of children and adolescents and the use of play to help the children to face their health problems. She also investigates the symbolic aspects of hospital settings and the applications of art in the health area. She collaborates with hospitals and medical teams to improve the situations of children and families in health settings.

Risë VanFleet, PhD, RPT-S, CDBC, is a child and family psychologist and president of the Family Enhancement & Play Therapy Center in Boiling Springs, Pennsylvania. She is the author of dozens of books, chapters, and articles, many of which focus on the effective use of the full original version of filial therapy, which she learned from its founders. She has worked in the field for over 40 years and has been heavily involved with direct service, research, and training of professionals in empowering families living with chronic medical illness with the use of play therapy and filial therapy. She is the recipient of numerous national and international awards for her writing, training, and contributions to the field. She currently is involved in animal assisted play therapy and its many applications in mental health treatment.

Deborah B. Vilas, MS, CCLS, LMSW, is a faculty advisor and instructor in the child life program at the Bank Street College of Education in New York City, where she teaches graduate students how to provide meaningful and therapeutic play experiences for hospitalized children. Deborah has worked with children as a child life specialist, preschool teacher, and social worker. An author, blogger, and international public speaker, Deborah has presented and taught in New Zealand, the Czech Republic, Mexico, the Palestinian Territories, and Japan. In 2016, she participated in a panel presentation about child life and technology at the United Nations. In 2014, Deborah represented her profession and her country as a keynote speaker at the first global summit on pediatric psychosocial care in hospitals, addressing delegates from 46 countries on the importance of play for sick and injured children. Her blog www.pediaplay.com reaches followers in over 65 countries.

Patricia "Patty" Weiner, MS, is a mother and grandmother whose career spans over 35 years as a child life specialist and educator. With a master's degree in special education, she served as the director of child life and education services at North Shore-Long Island Jewish Medical Center. She was the founding director of the master's degree program in child life at Bank Street College of Education in New York. Patty is presently an educational and child life consultant practicing in Manhattan; an educational consultant for The Making Headway Foundation, a not-for-profit organization dedicated to children with brain and spinal cord tumors and their families; a member of the On-Going Care Team who provide post hospitalization care for these children and their families; and a graduate school student mentor in the child life program at Bank Street College. She is an expert blog contributor for Mommybites, which provides parenting resources, support, and education. Patty's work has been presented in a variety of professional forums and publications.

Crystal Wilkins, MS, LPC, RPT-S, is a licensed professional counselor and registered play therapist currently working at Austin Stone Counseling Center in Austin, Texas, providing biblically based play therapy services for children and teens. In addition, Crystal works at Wonders & Worries as a certified child life specialist, providing psychosocial support to children and teens impacted by a parent's illness. Crystal has more than 13 years of experience working with children impacted by illness and hospitalization, as both a certified child life specialist and registered play therapist. Crystal is a frequent presenter on topics such as medical play, trauma, and play therapy, and recently co-authored an article in the *Association for Play Therapy* magazine on working with children with medical anxiety. With specialized training in filial therapy and Theraplay, empowering parents in supporting their children is a passion of Crystal's and something she continues to advocate for in her clinical work.

Foreword

Kevin O'Connor

This book could not have come at a better time, as the field of integrated health care, the concurrent provision of medical and mental health services, is in the midst of a period of explosive growth. The concept of a mind–body connection and its importance in determining people's overall health has existed in Western societies since the time of the early Greeks. However, it has not always been evidenced in the practice of either medical or mental health services. As both modern medicine and psychology developed, each tended to dichotomize illness as being either medical or psychological. Patients were treated by a medical doctor or a mental health professional but not both. As medical science and practice advanced, the tendency to exclude psychological concepts increased as medicine described itself as a 'hard/real' science while psychology was pejoratively labeled a 'soft/pseudo' science. Beginning with Freud's studies of conversion disorders, physicians sometimes used psychology to dismiss complex physical problems as being "all in the patient's head." In spite of this history, the past few decades has seen a growing recognition of the impact of people's physical health on their emotional health and vice versa. For example, on the medical side of the equation, the field of psychoneuroimmunology specifically focuses on the degree to which stress and psychological issues disrupt people's immune systems, making them more susceptible to illness. The vast majority of medical and mental health professionals as well as parents recognize the degree to which medical difficulties impact children's emotional health, and emotional issues can cause medical problems to worsen and even interfere with the body's response to treatment. A comparable example of such specialization on the mental health side of the equation would be the rapid expansion of neuropsychology, which focuses the ways both normal and pathological brain functioning affect cognition and behavior. As the concept of integrated care, or the concurrent provision of medical and psychological services, has begun to take hold, many medical patients have resisted the idea, as they continue to feel as if the inclusion of a mental health provider in their medical treatment means their problems were not 'real'. Fortunately, the past decade has seen the rapid growth of the science and practice of integrated care and rapid public acceptance of the importance of enhanced psychological well-being to physical well-being and vice versa.

The inclusion of child life specialists in many pediatric settings since the early 1900s is one of the earliest examples of integrated care. Medical professionals and parents alike recognized the degree to which children were traumatized not only by their illness or injury but by the treatments designed to heal them. As a result they saw the need to provide specialized emotional support within a medical setting. In spite of this early start, children's mental health needs still tend to be seen as secondary to their medical needs. Physicians are not particularly likely to consult with a child's therapist prior to conducting a medical procedure, and children are routinely discharged from the hospital without being given the opportunity to 'terminate' their relationship with the child life specialist. Again, fortunately, these practices are changing, and there are some stellar examples of how medical and psychological services can be brought together in the best interests of the child.

As evidenced by the wide range of topics discussed in this text, integrated health care creates some amazing opportunities for mental health professionals to serve children and families in some new, exciting, and creative ways. When providing traditional mental health services, play therapists are usually in the business of helping children resolve difficulties and trauma after they have occurred. One of the most exciting things about providing play therapy and play-based activities in a medical setting, or to address medically related issues, is the degree to which the therapist can engage in not only treating trauma but actually preventing it. Although professionals use the terms somewhat differently, trauma-related interventions can be thought of as primary, secondary, tertiary and even quaternary, and all of these are reflected across the chapters in this text.

Primary prevention interventions are usually defined as those designed to prevent exposure to medical issues or trauma before they happen. Primary prevention interventions would include programs to prevent drug use or other dangerous behaviors. Good examples include teaching very young children to swim in an effort to prevent drowning or getting them to wear bicycle helmets to prevent head injuries. The development of play-based primary prevention interventions is in its infancy, and is an area with great promise for preventing major societal problems such as childhood obesity. The idea of primary prevention is best exemplified in Chapter 2 and the Appendix of this text.

Secondary prevention interventions can be defined as those that prepare children for inevitable stresses or trauma. In the context of pediatric integrated health care, some of the most important secondary prevention interventions prepare children for necessary medical procedures they may find frightening or painful such as injections, X-rays, or even cast removal. Although the use of play therapy for secondary prevention is not uncommon, it is an area with enormous growth potential. Although some elements of this type of interventions are discussed throughout this text, they are best exemplified in Chapters 16 and 18 and in the Appendix.

Tertiary prevention interventions are those designed to reduce the impact of trauma after it has occurred. These are the most common forms of mental health intervention, provided in both traditional clinical practice and integrated care settings. Tertiary prevention interventions often focus directly on the mind–body interaction. In the context of integrated care, the most common tertiary interventions usually focus on reducing the psychological impact of medical issues or treatments. This type of intervention is illustrated in Chapters 3–9 and 13–17. Tertiary interventions can also be used to facilitate stress management to reduce the symptoms of medical issues that are often exacerbated by stress such as asthma, headaches, and a wide variety of gastrointestinal disorders. This use is illustrated in Chapters 10 and 18. Lastly, tertiary interventions can also be used to increase medical compliance in disorders such as diabetes, where lifelong treatment is critical.

Quaternary prevention interventions address the trauma accompanying end of life. Although death is inevitable, the fear children and families experience as it approaches can be greatly reduced. When children are dying, each family member is likely to respond very differently, and those differences can exacerbate the stress. For example, one parent may remain in denial while the other moves on to anger; as a result, they are uncomfortable with one another and this may then interfere with their relationship with their child. Interventions are critical to maintain optimal relationships between family members through the extraordinarily difficult process of losing a child. This type of intervention is discussed in Chapters 11 and 12.

Hopefully, this text will further the development of integrated health care services for children and their families. Play therapy is an excellent way to mediate the trauma associated with medical issues and medical treatments as well as maximize the healthy interaction of mind and body. It is a great way to engage children, their siblings, and their parents in minimizing stress and maximizing health. And, maybe most important of all, it is a great way to allow children whose lives are filled with the stresses related to their medical difficulties to take a break from those difficulties and just have FUN!

Kevin O'Connor, PhD, ABPP, RPT-S
Distinguished Professor: Clinical PhD and Clinical PsyD Programs
Coordinator, Ecosystemic Clinical Child Psychology Emphasis
Director, Ecosystemic Play Therapy Training Center
California School of Professional Psychology at Alliant International University

Foreword

Jerriann Myers Wilson

"You mean they pay you to play?" Years ago (in the 1960s) when I was a new child life specialist, this was a question I or our staff heard more than once during a short elevator ride in the hospital, usually from a member of the house staff. Initially, I responded a bit defensively as my damaged ego shot back, "Yeah, I like it and it makes the kids happy." But soon I saw this as a wonderful opportunity to do a little education, and responded with a quick "Yes, and I am so lucky to have found a career that uses play and communication to make such a difference in the lives of children and their families during a hospital experience." Now I think that question doesn't happen so often, as house staff are frequently exposed to child life and the role of play even during their medical school years. And that is what this scholarly book is about: clarifying and expounding upon what play can do for children and families, and how play therapists and child life specialists and other professionals use play to create the best scenario within the realm of family-centered care.

I was pleased to be asked to write this foreword by Lawrence Rubin, who has made a positive impact on the understanding of play and play therapy and its application in hospital settings and private practice. He is a known author, counselor, and educator who has served as a clinician and teaches at the university level. Although his professional work and writings have focused primarily on play as used by Registered Play Therapists, he has a keen appreciation of the use of play by child life specialists in hospital, clinic, and non-traditional settings. He has chosen to represent the work of both of these practitioners in this book. The case studies, the medical play–related activities, the background theory and research, and the bibliographies represent both fields and are excellent.

I worked for 43 years in the child life field at the Johns Hopkins Hospital, where I directed the Child Life Department for 34 years and developed a Child Life Program at its sister hospital, the Johns Hopkins Bayview Medical Center. Our professional association (then the Child Life Council (CLC), now the Association of Child Life Professionals) has also always been an important part of my work life, and I was fortunate at the formation of the CLC to be elected as its first president. Having started in the child life field many years ago, I have seen and appreciated the many changes in the professional work and role of the child life specialist. The level of sophistication of the current specialists' knowledge of anatomy, development, research, and psychological preparation together form their approaches to providing appropriate interventions for pediatric patients and their families.

As Dr. Rubin discusses in his prologue, there are both similarities and differences in the training and the implementation of practice for play therapists and child life specialists. This book celebrates and expounds upon those aspects. Play therapists will love the play therapy descriptions, and child life specialists will also nod approvingly at the child life described cases. And because some writers have credentials in both disciplines, the applicability across both fields is marvelous. Although I understand how to use play therapeutically, as is typical in child life practice, I personally enjoyed understanding more about play therapy as a discipline. We definitely have much to share with each other. Because I am a Certified Child Life Specialist, I will concentrate on the applications to child life work. It is clear to me that child life students, new child life specialists, and even those more experienced clinicians will find these chapters helpful and interesting. I am equally sure that play therapists will gather information from the child life approach, some of which might be new and helpful.

The spectrum of patients includes all ages from infants to young adults in their twenties, plus strong recognition of providing support and therapy for siblings and families. The case studies are excellent, with vivid descriptions of a patient's problem, how an intervention was planned and carried out, and the final outcome. One chapter elaborated on the importance of self-care of clinicians as a follow-up—an area about which we all need to be reminded. The diagnoses discussed are quite varied, including many chronic diseases like cancer, cystic fibrosis, and HIV; surgical procedures; examples of trauma and post-traumatic stress disorder; and even autism spectrum disorder. The settings in which these children and youth are treated are equally varied, from hospitals to clinics to private practice offices to palliative care facilities. The book discusses providing play in a playroom, office, or at bedside. Suggestions for crafts and toys abound and include the use of puppets, the sand tray, LEGOs, video games, and so many other playthings that are familiar to us all.

One of the most intriguing parts for me was the wide variety of techniques that are named and the level of detail that is given. The descriptions of directive, non-directive, and symbolic play are expected and well-described, as well as the promotion of utilizing relaxation, mindfulness, and biofeedback as supportive services. A specialist might find helpful a list of interview questions to gain specific information, or a child-generated "learning story" and personal illness narratives, or a six-part story method developed by Israel's Mooli Lahad to identify coping styles, or using a change tree to understand the "new normal" that a child with cancer is facing, or clues on having the tough conversation about dying. There were numerous excellent descriptions of medical play, and the appendix details a process and resources for supporting families with well-care visits. It was fun to learn about the new, creative use of robots with pediatric patients, as well as two approaches called the "maker movement" and using "loose parts," which are useful in making medical play toys to increase a child's understanding and coping with medical treatments.

What a field we have all chosen, and how lucky we are to have amazing resources including this book to use in increasing our effectiveness with children, youth, and families! After digesting the work of these amazing authors and editor, no one will have difficulty explaining why it is such an honor "to be paid to play."

Jerriann Myers Wilson, M.Ed., CCLS
Associate Professor Emerita of the Johns Hopkins University School of Medicine

Prologue

At first glance, the clinical disciplines of Play Therapy and Child Life are more different than similar. These differences include the educational and clinical preparation and training as well as credentialing and licensing of their respective members. Their professionals work in overlapping, but more often non-converging ways in a wide range of venues, from freestanding mental health and medical private practices, to physicians' offices and pediatric clinics, to bustling multidisciplinary pediatric oncology units in sprawling metropolitan medical centers.

This volume, however, is not about differences that have evolved slowly in the course of social constructivist discourse or emergent clinical fiefdoms that divide professions and professionals behind great walls. Instead, it is about convergence and collaboration that over the last 100 years have brought together scholars and healers for the benefit of sick, suffering, and dying children and adolescents—and their caregivers—through the use of play.

Without attempting to invoke mystery or the mysterious, this convergence has a historical nexus in the year 1982, which saw the establishment of both the Association for Play Therapy (APT) and the Child Life Council (CLC). Neither of these watershed moments was spontaneous, however. APT, a fledgling association founded by Charles Schaefer and Kevin O'Connor, dedicated itself to the use of play in counseling and psychotherapy. It traced its origin to the early part of the 20th century and the subsequent and richly chronicled use of play in the clinical work of mental health professionals across disciplines working with children and adolescents struggling with physical health problems, among other challenges. The CLC, recently re-christened ACLP (the Association of Child Life Professionals), traces its roots to the same era, which saw the increasing use of play at children's hospitals across the country, establishment of the Child Life and Education Division of Cleveland City Hospital by Emma Plank, its evolution into the Association for the Care of Children in Hospitals (ACCH), and finally re-naming and re-visioning of the organization. And with the exponential growth in membership associated with each of these organizations came standards of training, certification, research, and publications—and reach across continents. A trove of information about each of these organizations can be found at www.a4pt.org (APT) and www.childlife.org (ACLP), respectively.

In the following pages, across 19 chapters, you will hear a number of distinct voices, those of clinicians, researchers, and educators whose work converges on the use of therapeutic play in the lives of children and adolescents in a range of medical venues. While the voices ahead speak in one language, they do so with different dialects. As a caveat, I must note that there is technically no such discipline as "medical play therapy" per se, but instead "Play Therapy." Its practitioners, depending upon their training, experience, and the vicissitudes of their professional and personal lives, practice, teach, and research at the intersections of play, childhood, and illness. Child Life, on the other hand, has grown up and is anchored primarily in the medical/health arena, where its practitioners, researchers, and educators focus almost exclusively on the use of play with children and adolescents.

In constructing this volume and in consideration of the sheer diversity of experience of the authors, I intentionally decided against a specific and formulaic chapter structure. Instead, I asked authors to consider the most current literature in the field as they thought through their case presentations, drawing upon meta-analyses, systematic reviews, and randomized control trial studies when available. I asked them to dig deeply into their clinical and subjective experiences and reflections as they put pen to paper.

* * * * *

Part I, *Medical Play in a Variety of Settings*, introduces the reader to the fields of Medical Play Therapy and Child Life through the lens of their application in a variety of medical and non-medical settings. In Chapter 1, "Therapeutic Work With Children in Diverse Settings," Fraser Brown, Cindy Dell Clark, and Michael Patte introduce us to the "continuum from playing to play therapy," as it manifests in playwork, child life, occupational therapy, and play therapy, all the while reflecting on the power of play to help children in medical crisis. In Chapter 2, "Preschoolers' Health Care Play: Children Demonstrating Their Health Literacy," Joan Turner and Victoria Dempsey qualitatively explore the health literacy of preschoolers under the developmentally oriented and watchful eye of their teacher, as they playfully investigate and begin to make sense of their bodies, the ways in which the various parts function, and the abstract concepts of health and illness. In Chapter 3, "Caring for Children With Cystic Fibrosis in a Hospital Setting in Australia: The Space Where Play and Pain Meet," Judi Parson introduces us to the varying competing discourses in the Australian hospital setting, while highlighting the particular value of play as it is brought into service with a child struggling with cystic fibrosis.

Part II, *Medical Play with Unique Health Challenges*, deepens the conversation around the utility of play-based medical interventions with children and adolescents struggling with a range of developmental and psychiatric challenges. In Chapter 4, "Play Therapy in Assisting Children With Medical Challenges," David Crenshaw and Jillian Kelly tap into the core elements of play therapy—symbolism, containment, metaphor, miniaturization, and externalization—and in so doing, take us on a journey of pain and resilience with children attempting to adapt to the often harsh realities of medical challenge. In Chapter 5, "Play Therapy With Children With ASD and Chronic Illness," Kevin Hull brings us into the painful worlds and his poignant clinical work with Angela and Stephen, two of his clients who are doubly challenged—by autism spectrum disorder and medical issues—and with whom he utilizes a variety of play therapy media and techniques in order to help them and their families to adapt. In

Chapter 6, "Children, Cancer, and Child Life: Fostering Resiliency Through Empowerment," Meredith Cooper and Melissa Hicks share their combined years of experience as child life specialists working creatively and energetically with cancer directly affecting the child, her sibling, and/or the parent in ways that utilize play and draw upon resilience. In Chapter 7, "Playing With Stigma: Medical Play for Adolescents With HIV," Kathryn Cantrell, Kerri Modry-Mandell, Jessica Pappagianopoulos, Sarah Grill, and George Scarlett utilize play, playfulness, and creativity to shine light on the painful shadowlands of teens who struggle to accept, share, and manage their HIV and its physical, social, and emotional sequelae.

Part III, *The Role of Medical Play in Childhood Medical Trauma*, focuses its gaze on youth with chronic and traumatic illnesses and injuries. In Chapter 8, "Integrative Attachment Informed Cognitive Behavioral Play Therapy (IAI-CBPT) for Children With Medical Trauma," Angela Cavett briefly reviews the trauma assessment and treatment literature with particular focus on Trauma-Focused Cognitive Behavioral Therapy, and then shares her extensive clinical experience and proposed modification of this model with an intervention program that honors the importance of relationship between therapist, parent, and child. In Chapter 9, "Trauma-Focused Medical Play," Jenaya Gordon and Suzanna Paisley discuss the importance of medical play from the perspective of child life specialists with hospitalized children who have experienced medical trauma in a way that helps us to appreciate the role of processing with and for the child and her family. In Chapter 10, "Regaining Control: Utilizing Directive Play Therapy to Help Teens With Chronic Health Conditions," Mistie Barnes introduces us to the particular clinical and developmental challenges of working with teenagers struggling with chronic health conditions, and demonstrates the applicability of directive play therapy interventions.

Part IV, *The Use of Medical Play With Terminal Illness in Children*, broaches a very painful and deeply sensitive topic of "how to help children at the end of life through play." In Chapter 11, "Child-Centered Play Therapy With Children Who Are Dying," Kristie Opiola and Dee Ray introduce us to Lina, a courageous 7-year-old terminally ill girl who, under the gentle guidance of her therapist using client centered play therapy, faces the many challenges that confront her and her family in the waning moments of her life. In Chapter 12, "It's All About the Living: Play-Based Experiences With Children Facing End of Life," Morgan Livingstone takes us to those last precious months, days, and hours of the lives of three children who, along with her serious approach to play as a child life specialist, guides and supports both them and their families.

Part V, *Medical Play Therapy Through a Systemic Lens*, helps us to understand the important role of family in understanding and intervening clinically in the lives of children impacted by illness and injury. In Chapter 13, "What About Me? Sibling Play Therapy When a Family Has a Child With Chronic Illness," John Seymour discusses the importance of the sibling bond throughout the life span, and then addresses the power and potential positive effects of that bond with the chronically ill child and the adaptive role that bond plays within the entire family system. In Chapter 14, "Family-Oriented Treatment of Childhood Chronic Medical Illness: The Power of Play in Filial Therapy," Risë VanFleet introduces us to Bernard and Louise Guerney's time-tested Filial Therapy, illustrates its applicability to children with medical conditions, and then invites us into her clinical work with Leah and her mother, who struggle against cystic fibrosis. In Chapter 15, "Play Partners: Incorporating Parents Into Medical Play Practices," Crystal Wilkins takes us on a journey from her early hospital training days to her current diversified role as both a Certified Child Life Specialist and Registered Play Therapist who shares the world of medical play with children and parents alike.

Part VI, *Expressive-Creative Research-Driven Practice*, concludes our journey by exploring how clinicians and clinical researchers bridge the gap between humanism and empiricism. In Chapter 16, "Medical Makers: Therapeutic Play Using 'Loose Parts'," Jon Luongo and Deborah Vilas introduce us to a particularly creative way of engaging playfully with children in health care settings by essentially creating hands-on, three-dimensional toys and tools that invite understanding, coping, and healing. In Chapter 17, "With Plush Toys, It Hurts Less: The Effect of a Program to Promote Play to Reduce Children's' Postsurgical Pain," Ana Ullán and Manuel Belver implement a randomized control trial study with young children on a pediatric surgery unit, successfully demonstrating that the use of parental involvement and play with a plush doctor rabbit toy are causally related to reduced postsurgical pain. In Chapter 18, "Playing With Biofeedback: A Practical, Playful Approach to Using Biofeedback in Pediatric Health," Jason Steadman and Michael Feeney bridge the ages-old divide between mind and body through the lens of biofeedback and take us on a firsthand tour of the many applications of this technology in a variety of settings, with a range of clients and with particular attention to pediatric patients struggling with a host of medically related challenges. In Chapter 19, "The Future Is Now: Using Humanoid Robots in Child Life Practice," Jacqueline Reynolds Pearson and Tanya Nathalie Beran peer into the future, so to speak, as they demonstrate the playful (and very serious) utility of MEDi, a multifaceted, programmable robot to ease children's suffering and pain as they face a range of medical conditions and challenges.

In the Appendix, "Taking Your Child to the Doctor or the Hospital: Helpful Suggestions and Practical Tips to Make Your Child's Visit More Comfortable," Patty Weiner shares her clinical experience, knowledge, and a trove of resources she has created and accumulated over years while helping parents and other caregivers to prepare their children for a range of medical and health care visits.

Lawrence C. Rubin

Acknowledgments

This book is lovingly and first dedicated to my wife, life partner, and best friend, Randi.

It is also dedicated in loving memory of my parents, Esther and Herb, who lined their shelves with my books and probably never read one, but were so proud of their son.

It is dedicated to my children, Zachary Michael and Rebecca Linn, who helped me maintain the spark of youth and play.

I thankfully acknowledge Anna Moore, my editor at Routledge, who ventured once again with me and the many fine contributors to this volume who gave of their time, passion, and energies.

And finally, this book is especially dedicated to one of its recently passed contributors, Mistie Barnes, who faithfully served children, their families, and the Association for Play Therapy.

PART I

Medical Play in a Variety of Settings

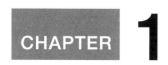

Therapeutic Work With Children in Diverse Settings

Fraser Brown, Cindy Dell Clark,
and Michael M. Patte

> *To play it out* is the most natural auto-therapeutic measure childhood affords. What-
> ever other role play may have in the child's development . . . the child uses it to make
> up for defeats, sufferings, and frustrations.
>
> —Erik Erikson (1940, p. 561)

THROUGH DIFFERENT LENSES

Playworker

He's profoundly deaf and a fluent signer. He has been removed from the family home
without signed counseling or explanation. He knows that the playground is a safe
place to explore his feelings, but our sign language skills are basic. This visit feels significant. He stands trembling in the cold and pours a bucket of dry powder paint over
his head, then goes back for another color to take outside and tip again. We watch
as layer after layer of color covers him. He stands alone, knowing he is observed. He
trusts that he will not be interrupted by playworkers. He is matted with layers of color,
pure and mixed. He has shown himself to be a mess. Layered in confusion, not knowing how to communicate this to himself, let alone anyone else. He doesn't know the
signs for the feelings he has, as hearing kids do not have the words for these concepts.
So, he paints it all over his body. When he is ready, we shower, clothe, and comfort him
as he needs (Wilson, 2014, p. 80).

Play Therapist

Charlie's teacher says he rarely speaks, often hides in the corner, can't express what's
wrong, and has little interaction with his peers; he finds it difficult to stay on task in
the classroom.

First Session: Charlie stood quietly in front of me, not knowing what to do. My natural instinct was to help him make a choice, but as a therapist I knew this would be wrong. . . . Eventually he walked over to the figures on the table, and picking up the fighter planes one by one, he examined them, shook off the sand, and took them to the sink. After washing them, he put them back on the table. This was done in silence. He then went over to the puppets, picked up the tiger, and shook its head as if saying 'no'. He whispered in its ear. He did this with all the puppets, picking them up and moving their heads from side to side—'no'. He then turned the tiger puppet to face him and nodded to it. Finally, he matched up the puppets with the same figures from the table. I felt it was important for him to do this, as was washing the planes. Was he putting things in order? Perhaps he was at last able to control a moment of his life? (Amar, 2016).

Child Life Specialist

Today a patient accidentally dislodged his breathing tube, causing extubation to occur. The Pediatric Intensive Care Unit sprang into action, and I worked with the patient and his father to provide procedural and emotional support. Throughout the procedure I held the patient's hand, as he was agitated and physically uncomfortable. I stayed by the patient's side until the procedure was complete, and he was relaxed and comfortable.

Later in the day, I stopped by to provide normative play for the patient in the form of a favorite board game and to offer information about the pet therapy program in the hospital. As I left the room, the patient's father said he really appreciated the care I provided his son throughout the day, and actually said that I had the most important job, which was to provide a sense of normalcy in the stressful medical setting. If you were to ask me at the time of the procedure whether the father even knew I was in the room, I would say probably not. He seemed distracted and distraught because his son was in pain. However, his comment holds an important lesson: no act of kindness, no matter how small or seemingly insignificant, ever goes unnoticed (Patte, 2010).

Occupational Therapist

"Oh no!" Jade (occupational therapist) exclaims loudly as >Bongk!< the shark bumps against her. The shark (i.e., ball) drifts back to Archer (boy receiving therapy for sensory integration issues) . . . he raises both hands to give it a shove. Jade hauls herself to an upright position, and being a bit more agile (when upright), twists and contorts, managing to avoid the shark as it rolls past her. Hmm, it seems Archer will have to come up with a better strategy. His grin broadens as he rolls the ball in (another) direction, taking it to the furthest reaches of the mats (in the therapy room). >Bongk!< But the ball merely snares and slows a little on the cushion beneath her feet. Archer can't seem to get the grand bump he desires. He pulls the shark (ball) back, while Jade, looking down, prepares for her next bodily contortion. Archer gives a sidelong look; but instead of reaching for the shark (ball), he tips his head, raises his arms to shoulder height in front of him, opens his jaws as wide as they can possibly go, and latches onto Jade's leg and makes the motion of taking a bite. He has her full attention (Park, 2005, p. 100).

Reflection

These vignettes, which are derived from the experience of practitioners in four different professions, are focused on the play of specific children. As such, they illustrate the complexity of children's play. They introduce us to the possibility that play can be, at one and the same time, social, physical, instructive, and creative. It may help us to build relationships and develop a deeper sense of self. In his classic text *The Ambiguity of Play*, the developmental psychologist Brian Sutton-Smith defines play as "the potentiation of adaptive variability" (1997, p. 231). Elsewhere he suggests that play serves to provide us with a "belief in the worthwhileness of merely living" (1999, p. 254).

Clearly, play means different things to different people, which is why it is so hard to define (Sherwood & Reifel, 2010). Indeed, for a definition of play to be really tenable, it would have to be inclusive of, and apply to:

- Children and adults
- Animals and humans
- Both process and product
- Positive and negative forms
- Structured and unstructured forms
- Immediate and future benefits
- Passivity and performance
- Fleeting moments and long-lasting periods.

It is unlikely that any definition can address all these things, and so it is probably more helpful to focus on generalized descriptions rather than specific definitions. This is the approach adopted by numerous authors, including Catherine Garvey (1991) and Tina Bruce (2005). Consequently, it is common in the literature to find play described as having the following characteristics. It is:

1. Freely chosen, personally directed, and intrinsically motivated
2. Associated with positive effect, pleasurable, enjoyable, egalitarian, and so forth
3. Functional, but the emphasis is on process rather than product.

Despite the popular notion that play is more about process than product, it is nevertheless clear that play has a number of developmental outcomes, albeit the player may not necessarily be aware of them. These widespread benefits of play are summarized in Table 1.1, which is an abridged version of a much larger summary of the benefits of play (see Brown, 2014, pp. 12–14).

Thus, play may be seen to be a key factor at the heart of child development. However, its cathartic and therapeutic aspects are less widely recognized. In all the vignettes at the beginning of this chapter, the professional worker is trying to help a troubled child through a difficult period in their life, so that they may eventually regain some sort of emotional equilibrium. In each case, play is being used as the therapeutic medium. It is that aspect of play that forms the focus of this chapter, and we explore its use and value via the day-to-day practice of a number of professions.

TABLE 1.1 The Benefits of Play

KEY FACTORS Contributing to development while playing	OUTCOMES In the longer term, playing helps to produce:
Fun	Happiness and the continuation of brain plasticity
Freedom	A sense of independence, and an understanding of the parameters of risk, challenge, and danger
Flexibility	Broader horizons—an understanding of the world and an open-mindedness about its true potential
Social Interaction	Friendship groups and an understanding of social networks Transmission of children's cultures
Socialization	Self-acceptance and a respect for the views and wishes of others
Physical Activity	Musculoskeletal development and physical health
Environmental Cognitive Stimulation	Knowledge and understanding, and a sense of wonder about the potential for expanding our horizons
Creativity and Problem Solving	Combinatorial flexibility leading to problem-solving skills, abstract thinking, and aesthetic appreciation
Self-Discovery	A unique individual personality; self-awareness and self-confidence

Of course, it is arguable that children's play is inherently therapeutic, and therefore children have it within themselves to cure their own ills. Freud (1900) suggested one of the functions of play was reconciliation; in other words, a process that enables children to come to terms with traumatic events. By 'playing out' the event, and possibly replaying it many times in lots of different ways, children can at one and the same time take control of the experience and gain a full understanding of it. This idea is hinted at in the opening line of the quote at the beginning of this chapter (Erikson, 1940). It is a theme taken up by Virginia Axline (1969), and applied to her professional practice, where she adopted (and promoted) a non-directive approach to play therapy. For Axline, the role of the play therapist is to create the conditions that enable the child to explore whatever has happened to them, so as to reconcile themselves to it, and hopefully have enough self-confidence to be able to move forward.

The renowned dramatherapist, Sue Jennings, in her groundbreaking book, *Healthy Attachments and Neuro-Dramatic Play*, introduces the idea of a "play to play therapy continuum, where playing can be considered a 'preventative' activity and play therapy a 'curative' activity." She goes on to say that "there is a large gap in the middle where children are able to generate their own play to help themselves; this often does not need the intervention of play therapists" (2011, p. 64). Unfortunately, contrary to that optimistic view, in the more developed industrial nations there is an increasingly "large gap in the middle" where children are *not* able to generate their own play. This is due to a combination of sociocultural circumstances; for example, increase in traffic, suspicion of strangers, excessive emphasis on academic attainment, etc. (Gill, 2007). That is where playwork comes in. Put simply, the more sociocultural changes that restrict children's freedom to play, the more we store up psychosocial problems for the future. That is why we need playworkers. In its most straightforward expression, playwork is compensatory in nature. It is about creating environments that enable children to generate their own play (Brown, 2014). Inevitably there is a therapeutic aspect to this. If Freud's analysis is correct, it follows that children will use the playwork environment in the same way as any child engaged in free play would.

Thus, in therapeutic terms we can return to Jennings "play to play therapy continuum" and suggest the following: where children are able to play freely, they will be able to use their play as a naturally therapeutic medium and reconcile themselves to minor traumatic events. Where play is restricted, children may be able to attend a playwork project, where they will be able to play freely and engage in a similar reconciliation process. Where the traumatic events are more severe, the child may need a more focused and protected environment, where a play therapist is able to offer the reassurance of a personal, one-to-one relationship to help the child come to a solution.

Child life specialists and occupational therapists are also at this end of the continuum, albeit their approaches are sometimes more structured, because they may have very specific goals in mind.

However, we should perhaps end this section with a couple of caveats. First, as Piaget (1951) tells us, a lot of children's play is actually repetition and practice of previously learned actions, so we should be very cautious when interpreting its meaning. That leads us to the second point, that is, that a child's play may not mean what we think it does. It is often the case that play is ambiguous and/or paradoxical (Sutton-Smith, 1997). The most obvious example of this is play fighting—an activity that most mammals indulge in. It is not hard to spot the difference between 'rough and tumble' and a real fight, yet adults are often quick to intervene, ostensibly so that the children don't hurt themselves. On the contrary, Sunderland (2006) suggests we should stand back, because this form of play is extremely beneficial in developmental terms, especially in relation to four of the brain's eight genetically ingrained emotional systems: caring, social bonding, playfulness, and explorative urges (the other four being rage, fear, separation distress, and lust in adults).

Therapeutic Playwork

While not being established as a full profession, the occupation of playworker is widely recognized in the UK, and there are university degree programs that qualify individuals in that line of work (e.g., Leeds Beckett University). Not only Leeds Beckett, but also the University of Gloucester offers courses in Therapeutic Playwork. The Play Therapy UK (PTUK) website defines therapeutic playwork as follows:

> Therapeutic playwork adds a therapeutic element to playwork. The prime objective is still care or work orientated, with the therapeutic element as a secondary or supporting one.
>
> (PTUK, 2016)

The implication of this is that therapeutic playwork bridges the two professions of playwork and play therapy. However, the PTUK definition is not entirely accurate, as it is based on a misunderstanding of the practice of playwork. Playwork has been defined as a generalized description of

> all those approaches that use the medium of play as a mechanism for redressing aspects of developmental imbalance caused by a deficit of play opportunities.
>
> (Brown, 2003, p. 52)

Clearly, in certain circumstances this sort of work is likely to include a therapeutic element. Indeed, it has been argued by Sturrock and Else that *all* playwork will include such an element. In their classic "Colorado Paper," they suggest that "the playworker is active at the precise point where potential neuroses are being formed" (1998, p. 5). If that is the case, then the act of playwork might be seen as potentially curative rather than merely preventative. Thus, the most significant distinction between therapeutic playwork and play therapy is probably that the former involves working with groups of children, while the latter generally takes the form of a one-to-one interaction. Consequently, it is not surprising that the two approaches share a similar underpinning philosophy and a large amount of common practice. These elements are explored in greater detail in Brown (2017).

Underpinning Philosophy

- Draws on elements from most of the major strands of psychology
- Believes in the uniqueness of every child (PPSG, 2005)
- Accepts that children may use play as a reconciliation mechanism (Freud, 1900)
- Respects the child's ability to solve their own problems through playing (Axline, 1969)
- Aims for the development of the potential inherent in all children (Bruner, 1972; Maslow, 1973; Piaget, 1951; Vygotsky, 1966).

Fundamentals of Practice

- Establishes a permissive environment of openness and honesty (Axline, 1969; Hughes, 2012)
- Works as far as possible to the child's agenda (Brown, 2008; Else, 2009), sometimes by 'joining' (Kaufman, 2016)
- Adopts an approach of Unconditional Positive Regard (Axline, 1969; Rogers, 1961)
- Internalizes negative capability as a creative approach (Fisher, 2008)
- Emphasizes the development of the child–playworker relationship (Brown, 2014; Hughes, 2012)
- Creates an atmosphere of safety and security (Brown, 2014; Hughes, 2012)
- Creates an environment characterized by fun, freedom, and flexibility (Brown, 2014)

- Encourages the development of fundamental life skills (e.g., sympathy, empathy, mimesis) (Brown, 2014; Sunderland, 2006)
- Recognizes the fundamental role of rhythm in early child development (Davy, 2008; Palmer, 2008; Trevarthen, 1996).

The following example is a series of extracts from the reflective diary of a therapeutic playworker in a Romanian pediatric hospital, working soon after the overthrow of Ceauşescu, when conditions in the state institutions were dire. The children with whom she was working ranged in age from 1 to 10 years old. They had suffered chronic neglect and abuse, and had spent most of their lives tied in cots. They were poorly fed and their nappies were rarely changed. Although able to see and hear other children, they were unable to leave their cots, and so experienced little in the way of social interaction (Webb, 2000).

> One of my aims for Virgil is really simple and more on the social side really. I want to encourage him to sit down at the table to eat his meals. Alexandru and Olympia are fine but Virgil really won't sit down! He is used to the routine of being fed standing up in his cot and must feel secure with it. I need to gradually give him opportunities to feel more comfortable sitting at the table.
>
> (Day 9)

> Nicolae is walking a lot more and doesn't get so nervous about being on his own, before long he'll definitely be more confident. I make sure that every morning I walk around the room with him several times.
>
> (Day 9)

> We got the big cuddly toys down this afternoon and the children loved it. Nicolae especially enjoyed it and I've noticed touch is very important to him.
>   He likes to feel things. When the big fluffy duck is on the floor, he lies under it for ages—really happy for the others to climb all over him.
>
> (Day 11)

> The children seem to be interacting with each other so much more already. Virgil and Olympia had a 'phone conversation' today and played together really well. They have learnt 'La' for the phone and these two particularly enjoy drawing, so I want to expand on this somehow.
>
> (Day 11)

> I found some feathers in the cupboard today and went around tickling them to observe their reactions. Virgil was really afraid at first and threw his arms up shouting, but when I tickled my own arm and showed him it was okay, he was more curious. The look on his face when he felt comfortable to feel the feather was absolutely beautiful . . . so fresh and innocent.
>
> (Day 11)

I've been watching Nicolae today. He plays a lot on his own but when he does interact with one of the others he tends to tease them. It can be quite amusing and the others (such as Virgil, Olympia and Ion) are aware of it now. He knows what he's doing, because he laughs to himself afterwards.

(Day 17)

Something else I've noticed today . . . the children are playing together more than they have done. I'm wondering if it's got something to do with them now eating together. We put the soft toys on the floor again and they just lay on them chilling out. It was lovely to watch.

(Day 17)

Ion got inside a big yellow box today, which really made us laugh. Virgil was very curious and wanted to get in with him. Whilst Ion was sitting in the big yellow box Virgil started to play a game with him, involving an imaginary object. He pretended to receive something from Edit and then took it back to Ion in the box, who took it from him and put it in his lap. The spontaneous interaction between them both was fascinating to watch. Afterwards Virgil continued playing with the yellow plastic box, by putting it on his head and walking around the room, which made me laugh and laugh. He created a sort of obstacle course out of the cots and tables. They seem to like the sensation of being under it and are not afraid any more.

(Day 19)

These extracts, which come from the early days of the therapeutic playwork project, illustrate many of the Fundamentals of Practice mentioned previously. Webb establishes a permissive environment, and works as far as possible to the child's agenda. She adopts an approach of Unconditional Positive Regard, and internalizes the non-judgmental, non-prejudicial approach that is known as negative capability. All the while the child–playworker relationship is being developed. She creates an atmosphere of safety and security, and an environment characterized by fun, freedom, and flexibility. However, perhaps more important than any of that is her acceptance that the most important aspect of her work is the fact that she is creating an environment that enables the children to learn and develop from their interactions with each other.

Child Life

Practitioners at Work

The most common way that children explore and make sense of the complex world in which they live is through play. Play in its many forms enhances whole child (cognitive, creative, emotional, physical, social) development (Patte, 2015) and should play a prominent role in all child life programs. As play is a natural modality for children, child life specialists use it to transition children into the medical environment, to help children cope with various stressors, and to ensure children thrive in the hospital setting.

Three common forms of play used by child life specialists to help children and their families cope with various medical procedures and hospital visits are normative play, medical play, and therapeutic play (Burns-Nader & Hernandez-Reif, 2016). Normative play includes activities that children relish outside of the medical setting, including soccer, board games, and drawing, to name just a few. Child life specialists provide normative play because it offers patients something familiar, helps to build trusting relationships, and allows children to pass the time in an enjoyable way. An example of normative play follows—this is an excerpt from a clinical field journal (Patte, 2010).

> Daily play experiences had a range of positive effects on the children. For some it helped to pass the time and offered a distraction, and for others it reduced anxiety and elevated their spirits. Many of the children I worked with were desperate for some type of stimulation. I provided social interaction, crafts, games, and books for them to enjoy. These activities helped the children to deflect the negative things that were happening on a daily basis and instead focus on the positive and fun things. I enjoyed alleviating their pain and filling the void with joy.

Medical play affords children the opportunity to explore basic equipment (thermometer, oxygen mask, syringe, nebulizer) used in common procedures. McCue (1988) identified four essential elements of medical play: it has a medical theme, it is child directed, it is playful in nature, and it offers mastery and control over frightening medical equipment. Children realize many benefits from medical play, including opportunities to express their fears, to clarify misconceptions, to differentiate between fantasy and reality, and to better understand the medical experience (Nabors et al., 2013). Common forms of medical play include role rehearsal, indirect medical play, and medical art (Burns-Nader & Hernandez-Reif, 2016). Role rehearsal is a form of socio-dramatic play, where children use real props to act out a medical procedure using cuddly toys as pretend patients. Allowing children to examine medical equipment in a formal manner over an extended period of time through games with a medical theme (Operation or Hospital Jeopardy) is the focus of indirect medical play. Finally, medical art immerses children and families in artistic activities (Play-Doh sculptures, finger painting, collages) with a medical theme. An example of medical play follows (Patte, 2010).

> Mary (CCLS) described the procedure to the patient and her family first, using a preparation book, and then through the exploration of medical equipment in a developmentally appropriate way. She introduced heat packs to the child as warm pillows allowing the child to squeeze each of the packs which caused them to warm up. Next, Mary described how the warm pillows when placed gently on the arms helped the nurses to locate the veins (blue lines). When the nurses found a big blue line, they will spray it with snow in a can (cold spray) she continued. The child got to spray her arms and the arms of her parents with the cold spray to experience the feeling first hand. Finally, she explained, when your arm is good and cold the nurses will poke the blue line with a tiny tube (IV) and then we will be ready for the procedure to begin. Mary provided the child with a preparation doll, an IV tube, and medical tape to practice the procedure to her heart's content.

A third type of play employed by child life specialists that enhances development, psychosocial well-being, and coping skills is therapeutic play. Recent research examining the coping strategies of hospitalized preschool children found play as their preferred method (Salmela, Salantera, Ruotsalainen, & Aronen, 2010). Therapeutic play encourages emotional expression (doll play, creative and expressive arts), instructional/educational play (prepping children for various medical experiences), and physiological play (blowing up balloons to increase lung capacity). Nabors et al. (2013) argue that when play is directly related to a child's main cause of anxiety, it has the greatest impact on their ability to cope. Although there can be overlap in the types of play used by child life specialists, they all impact the psychosocial development of children and families in medical settings. An example of therapeutic play follows (Patte, 2010).

> Outside of socio-dramatic play, when would a three-year-old get the chance to administer a shot with a pointy needle? For that matter, when is a three-year-old in control of anything? All day hospital personnel were entering Paige's room doing things that she did not enjoy. Paige's cuddly toy Gilbert was her most trusted confidant and provided comfort in this foreign environment where content and meaning were ambiguous and the outcome was uncertain. This illustrated Paige's reality within the hospital context and in her experience with cancer. Providing opportunities for Paige to play with her cuddly toys and to re-enact cherished family rituals (eating dinner with mom, dad, and siblings) offered a brief glimpse into an everyday normal life.

The Current State of Play in North American Hospitals

As part of a grant from the Walt Disney Company, the Child Life Council (CLC) conducted a survey to document play-related policies and practices of child life programs across North America in 2013. The findings of the survey are summarized in *Report on Findings of Play Practices and Innovations Survey: The State of Play in North American Hospitals* (CLC, 2014). The survey offers suggestions for expanding the role of play, highlights play-based innovations, identifies barriers to play in child life programs, and recommends potential strands for future research. Surveys were distributed to 464 program directors, with 181 responding, for an average response rate of 39%.

The CLC believes that documenting the play-based programs and services across the child life profession in North America is essential in elevating the field and the vital importance of play in health care settings (CLC, 2014). Some of its survey findings include:

- 98% of the programs had playrooms staffed mostly by volunteers
- 84% of programs reported infusing play-related innovations (child-initiated play, loose parts play, technology play) on a consistent basis
- 38% of the programs offered outdoor play areas for patients and their families; a varied assortment of play programming was identified across all programs (carnivals, celebrity visits, child-centered play, crafts, dramatic play, expressive arts, games, medical play, proms, sensory play, sports, summer camps)
- 39% of programs have a written philosophical statement on the availability, role, and value of play

- 25% of programs offered in-service training on play-related topics for child life specialists
- 20% of programs reported being influenced by a particular play theorist.

The CLC survey (2014) identified a variety of barriers impeding play across North American child life programs. For example:

- 45% of programs identified insufficient numbers of staff and lack of time as prominent barriers limiting play
- 30% reported lacking adequate space
- 18% suggested that members of the medical team do not value play
- 14% mentioned infectious control restrictions as a barrier to play.

The CLC's (2014) suggestions to overcome these barriers included:

- Providing more space for play
- Improving patient access
- Organizing additional play groups
- Offering a greater variety of play opportunities
- Improving professional training requirements
- Developing play policies
- Securing materials for play with high play values
- Revising the CLC competencies to include higher standards concerning play.

The survey also suggested future research strands that included examining the prevalence of adult-directed play at the expense of child-initiated play within the field of child life; studying the benefits of loose parts play in medical settings; exploring the impact of education, staffing, and supervision on opportunities for play in medical settings; and studying how Certified Child Life Specialists train parents about the value of play (CLC, 2014).

Since its founding at the beginning of the 20th century, play served as the cornerstone of the child life profession. Although studies previously highlighted document play's vital role in the psychosocial development of children in medical settings, this recent CLC report (2014) suggests its role in North American hospitals is mixed. While the societal and institutional barriers marginalizing play continue to spread, Certified Child Life Specialists must remain vigilant advocates for play, as it embodies the very essence of our beautiful profession.

Occupational Therapy

The century-old profession of occupational therapy traces its name to what occupies human beings in the context of their lives, including play, work, and self-care. Occupational therapy has been closely aligned with medical systems of care since the 1920s, although occupational therapists also work in non-medical settings. Contemporary occupational therapists use play as a means to achieve therapeutic goals. Play leverages a child client's engagement and motivation, thereby enhancing therapeutic progress. Moreover, occupational therapists believe that playfulness is a capacity that is itself a worthy therapeutic goal. For an occupational therapist, play serves two essential roles:

1. It is a medium of care for physical, social, cognitive, or sensory processing difficulties
2. It is a crucial mode of human flexibility in and of itself.

Therapeutic play within occupational therapy is highly child-focused. Children are active play partners who have directing influence on a session. Occupational therapists are trained to reflect back to each child, responding in reflective, artful, improvisational ways to what children say and do.

Take, for example, how Emma (pseudonym for an occupational therapist) dealt with Dillon, a boy receiving therapy for sensory integration issues including deficits in visual perception, visual-motor integration, bilateral coordination, and proximal stability. Emma and Dillon had been moving about a room full of therapeutic apparatus, pretending that they were carrying small plush toys (Beanie Babies) to a nature museum; Dillon often visited natural history museums with his family, so the choice of theme reflected Dillon's interests.

As illustrated by the following excerpt, the therapist facilitated Dillon's active role through the course of ongoing play. First, she invited him to influence the play ("Who's going first?"). Then she reiterated his suggestion of a play topic ("There's a twister coming?"). And finally, she embraced his novel suggestion that rather than pretending to seek safety from the tornado, he intended to inhabit the non-human role of the whirlwind storm (Park, 2005, pp. 190–194).

Emma: Who's going first?

Dillon: Heeeyy! Hey!

Emma looks up slightly and drags the hound dog [toy] with her left hand . . . She puts the hound dog directly on [Dillon's] stomach so that it peers at him directly.

Dillon: Uhhhh—there's a twister.

Emma: There's a twister coming?

Emma nods, then points to the hammock swing [in the therapy room]. "Then you'd better get on the car, so you can be safe."

"Argh," grunts Dillon in half-dismay. How can he put what is so obvious? "No a tor-," he stops and interrupts himself as if trying to figure out how to make Emma understand the situation. "No a car will get [pointing his right forefinger toward the ceiling] up." . . . "How are you," asks Emma, leaning over him and gathering up his hands, "going to get safe?" "If you go in the house will you be safe?"

Dillon: I want to be the twister.

Emma gently tugs once more on his hands, "you want to be the twister?" . . . "Yeah okay." In one fluid movement, Emma gently continues the steady pull on his hands until he is sitting and then let's go.

Dillon turns over onto his hands and knees, "I'm going to take this—," grabs the hound and begins spinning with both arms outstretched while making a "hoooo" sound.

He revolves several times, grinning wide, before letting loose! And the hound flies off and >THUD< hits the far wall. "Oh no!" adds Emma appreciatively . . . Dillon [is] already on to the next victim. Without stopping, he revolves, his right arm extended and horizontal to the ground. He slows just a bit to bend and fluidly pick up the koala. "Get them all," chimes Emma as koala flies from his hand and [goes] >SPLAT< on the mat. "Oh my gosh!" exclaims Emma, "they're going all over." Dillon giggles [while] wildly spinning [and] grabs raccoon, as Emma with worried tone asks "How are they going to get"—>SPLAT< raccoon hits the floor—"to the museum?" . . . "Oooooweeee," hums the Twister-Dillon as it [he] lifts a frog to shoulder height and . . . >SPLAT< against the brick wall. Emma, in a hushed tone, plays her part well, "Oh my gosh! Now no-one gets to go to the museum!"

Emma's response to Dillon's role as a tornado shows her commitment to maintaining intersubjective connection by being an active, responsive listener to his intentions. She contributed by expressing amazement and by helping to narrate the pandemonium of Dillon's pretending. During a session, occupational therapists make the most of unforeseen suggestions and situations, working in dialogue with a child to creatively incorporate his or her direction.

Still, occupational therapy also requires advance planning and analysis. Prior to beginning therapy, occupational therapists conduct an assessment that considers a child's needs and issues. Therapists ascertain what children play at (outside therapy), how supportive the child's everyday environment is for play, and what drives a child's interest in particular activities. When working with hospitalized children, therapists take into account how hospitalization itself disrupts play through its hard and fast routines. A test of playfulness known as the 'ToP' is a structured instrument sometimes used systematically to measure a child's predilection to be playful (Skard & Bundy, 2008). This test considers that children, in play, must feel free to suspend reality, to engage their own intrinsic motivations, and to give and receive cues indicating an act is framed as playful.

Within occupational therapy, children's idiosyncratic interests from life experiences, media, or books are accommodated to boost a child's motivation for therapy. Often, kids readily engage with characters in therapeutic play that exhibit a poetic relevance to personal challenges. In research by Mattingly (2003), an 8-year-old girl with severe spina bifida was fascinated with the Disney character Little Mermaid, a character who (parallel to the girl) lacked workable legs. A boy with severe facial burns, who had to wear a medical mask 24 hours a day for a year, was attracted to the character Buzz Lightyear (from the movie *Toy Story*), an astronaut who perennially wore a space helmet covering his face. Cooperating with a child in acting out a child's favored figures and themes introduces a way for occupational therapists to meet boys or girls on their own ground, deepening the intersubjective connection between child and occupational therapist (Mattingly, 2008).

While apparatus is prepared prior to therapy, the use to which that equipment is put goes beyond the literal. For a regimen of therapy for a girl with vestibular problems (Mattingly & Garro, 2000), equipment was tailored to her particular challenges in touching, swinging, whirling, and jumping. At the girl's instigation, the apparatus was taken up in play as the site of a pretend Olympic event, in which the girl 'athlete' scored points and, ultimately, won a gold medal.

In this way, play fulfills three goals of occupational therapy. First, the activity addresses specified goals, based on a particular disability. Second, the client finds the treatment approach engaging and relevant. Third, the therapy becomes a co-acted, social event that bonds therapist and client.

Play during occupational therapy not only aids the child, but also is intrinsically revealing of occupational therapists' shared professional paradigm. Occupational therapists use a form of clinical logic that is by and large different from physicians' reasoning. Relative to physicians, occupational therapists are more committed to a dialogical process of "partnering up" (Lawlor, 2012). Occupational therapists do not limit their materials to patent medical evidence, but consider it beneficial to employ personally relevant, imagined, and subjective resources. The client's view, in short, is more deeply embedded into pediatric occupational therapy than it is in contemporary pediatrics.

CONCLUSION

Playworkers, play therapists, child life specialists, and occupational therapists agree that play is therapeutically valuable as well as relationship enhancing. When children have the freedom to play as they wish, they play in non-clinical settings to better cope with stresses or illness (Clark, 2003). But in contemporary contexts, full freedom to play is not always afforded to children; traumas can also exceed children's capacity to 'play it out' without support. As the clinical examples in this chapter corroborate, professionals trained in disparate fields act to catalyze, direct, compensate, and amplify playfulness, a testament to play's robust, resilience-enhancing potential.

REFERENCES

Amar, S. (2016). *Notes from a play therapy session*. Unpublished.

Axline, V. (1969). *Play therapy* (rev. ed.). New York: Ballantine Books.

Brown, F. (Ed.). (2003). *Playwork theory and practice*. Buckingham: Open University Press.

Brown, F. (2008). The fundamentals of playwork. In F. Brown & C. Taylor (Eds.), *Foundations of playwork* (pp. 7–13). Maidenhead: Open University Press.

Brown, F. (2014). *Play and playwork: 101 stories of children playing*. Maidenhead: Open University Press.

Brown, F. (2017). Therapeutic playwork: Theory and practice. In F. Brown & B. Hughes (Eds.), *Aspects of playwork, play and culture studies* (Volume 14, in press). Lanham, MD: University Press of America.

Bruce, T. (2005). Play, the universe and everything! In J. Moyles (Ed.), *The excellence of play* (2nd ed., pp. 255–267). Maidenhead: Open University.

Bruner, J. (1972). Nature and uses of immaturity. In J.S. Bruner, A. Jolly & K. Sylva (Eds.), *Play: Its role in development and evolution* (pp. 28–64). New York: Basic Books.

Burns-Nader, S., & Hernandez-Reif, M. (2016). Facilitating play for hospitalized children through child life services. *Children's Health Care, 45*(1), 1–21.

Child Life Council. (2014). *Report on findings of play practices and innovations survey: The state of play in North American hospitals*. Rockville, MD: Child Life Council.

Clark, C.D. (2003). *In sickness and in play: Children coping with chronic illness*. New Brunswick, NJ: Rutgers University Press.

Davy, A. (2008). Exploring rhythm in playwork. In F. Brown & C. Taylor (Eds.), *Foundations of playwork* (pp. 154–157). Maidenhead: Open University Press.

Else, P. (2009). *The value of play*. London: Continuum.

Erikson, E.H. (1940). Studies in the interpretation of play: Clinical observations of play disruption in young children. *Genetic Psychology Monographs*, 22, 561.

Fisher, K. (2008). Playwork in the early years: Working in a parallel profession. In F. Brown & C. Taylor (Eds.), *Foundations of playwork* (pp. 174–178). Maidenhead: Open University Press.

Freud, S. (1900). The interpretation of dreams. In S. Freud (Ed.), *The standard edition of the complete psychological works of Sigmund Freud* (24 volumes), translated from German under the general editorship of James Strachey, in collaboration with Anna Freud; assisted by Alix Strachey and Alan Tyson. London: Hogarth Press, Institute of Psycho-Analysis.

Garvey, C. (1991). *Play* (2nd ed.). London: Fontana.

Gill, T. (2007). *No fear: Growing up in a risk averse society*. London: Calouste Gulbenkian Foundation.

Hughes, B. (2012). *Evolutionary playwork*. London: Routledge.

Jennings, S. (2011). *Healthy attachments and neuro-dramatic play*. London: Jessica Kingsley.

Kaufman, R. (2016). *The Son-Rise Program versus ABA*. The Option Institute. [Internet]. Retrieved November 12, 2016 from: www.autismtreatmentcenter.org/contents/other_sections/aba-vs-son-rise-program.php

Kuhaneck, H.M., Spitzer, S.L., & Miller, E. (2010). *Activity analysis, creativity, and playfulness in pediatric occupational therapy*. Burlington, MA: Jones & Bartlett Learning.

Lawlor, M.C. (2012). The particularities of engagement: Intersubjectivity in occupational therapy practice. *OTJR: Occupation, Participation, and Health*, 32(4), 151–159.

Maslow, A. (1973). *The farther reaches of human nature*. Harmondsworth: Pelican Books.

Mattingly, C. (2003). Becoming Buzz Lightyear and other clinical tales: Indigenizing Disney in a world of disability. *Folk*, 45, 9–32.

Mattingly, C. (2008). Pocahontas goes to the clinic: Popular culture as lingua franca in a cultural borderland. *American Anthropologist*, 108(3), 494–501.

Mattingly, C., & Garro, L.C. (2000). *Narrative and the cultural construction of illness and healing*. Berkeley: University of California Press.

McCue, K. (1988). Medical play: An expanded perspective. *Children's Health Care*, 16(3), 75–85.

Nabors, L., Bartz, J., Kichler, J., Sievers, R., Elkins, R., & Pangallo, J. (2013). Play as a mechanism of working through medical trauma for children with medical illnesses and their siblings. *Issues in Comprehensive Pediatric Nursing*, 36(3), 212–224.

Palmer, M. (2008). The place we are meant to be: Play, playwork, and the natural rhythms of communities. In F. Brown & C. Taylor (Eds.), *Foundations of playwork* (pp. 132–136). Maidenhead: Open University.

Park, M.M. (2005). *Narrative practices of intersubjectivity: An ethnography of children with autism in a sensory integration based occupational therapy clinic*. Doctor of Philosophy, University of Southern California, Los Angeles.

Patte, M. (2010). *Field notes taken during a child life internship*. Unpublished.

Patte, M. (2015). *The evolution of school recess and corresponding implications for the next generation of children*. White paper for Playworld, Playworld, Lewisburg, PA.

Piaget, J. (1951). *Play, dreams and imitation in childhood*. London: Routledge and Kegan Paul.

PPSG. (2005). *Playwork principles*, held in trust as honest brokers for the profession by the Playwork Principles Scrutiny Group. [Internet]. Retrieved November 14, 2016 from: www.playwales.org.uk/page.asp?id=50

PTUK. (2016). *Definition of therapeutic playwork*. [Internet]. Retrieved December 8, 2016 from: http://playtherapy.org.uk/ChildrensEmotionalWellBeing/AboutPlayTherapy/MainPrinciples/TheraPWDefinition

Rogers, C. (1961). *On becoming a person*. Boston: Houghton Mifflin.

Salmela, M., Salantera, S., Ruotsalainen, T., & Aronen, E. (2010). Coping strategies for hospital-related fears in pre-school-aged children. *Journal of Pediatrics and Child Health*, 46(3), 108–114.

Sherwood, S., & Reifel, S. (2010). The multiple meanings of play: Exploring preservice teachers' beliefs about a central element of early childhood education. *Journal of Early Childhood Teacher Education*, 31(4), 322–343.

Skard, G., & Bundy, A.C. (2008). Test of playfulness. In L.D. Parham & L.S. Fazio (Eds.), *Play in occupational therapy for children* (pp. 55–70). London: Mosby Elsevier.

Sturrock, G., & Else, P. (June 1998). The playground as therapeutic space: Playwork as healing. In: Guddemi, M., Jambor, T. & Skrupskelis, A. *Proceedings of the IPA/USA Triennial National Conference, Play in a changing society: Research, design and application*. Longmont, CO, June 17–21. Little Rock, AR: Southern Early Childhood Association.

Sunderland, M. (2006). *What every parent needs to know*. London: Dorling Kindersley.

Sutton-Smith, B. (1997). *The ambiguity of play*. New York, NY: Harvard University Press.

Sutton-Smith, B. (1999). Evolving a consilience of play definitions: Playfully. In S. Reifel (Ed.), *Play and culture studies, play contexts revisited* (Volume 2, pp. 239–256). Stamford: Ablex.

Trevarthen, C. (November 1996). *How a young child investigates people and things: Why play helps development*. Keynote speech to TACTYC Conference 'A Celebration of Play', London.

Vygotsky, L. (1966). Play and its role in the mental development of the child. *Voprosi Psikhologii*, No. 6, originally published 1933, translated by Catherine Mullholland. [Internet]. Retrieved August 14, 2016 from: www.marxists.org/archive/vygotsky/works/1933/play.htm

Webb, S. (2000). Therapeutic playwork project: Extracts from a reflective diary. In F. Brown (Ed.), *Play and playwork: 101 stories of children playing*. Maidenhead: Open University Press.

Wilson, P. (2014). The painted boy. In F. Brown (Ed.), *Play & playwork: 101 stories of children playing* (p. 8). Maidenhead: Open University Press.

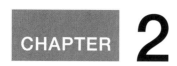
Preschoolers' Health Care Play

Children Demonstrating Their Health Literacy

Joan Turner and Victoria Dempsey

> Shouldn't we be doing something more important than playing? No, just keep doing what you are doing, you will understand it as you go along.
>
> —McCue (1995)

INTRODUCTION

> Dr. Germs was treating Vicky using the stethoscope. He had the earpieces in and the chest piece in place. "Your heart isn't bumping" he said, "Let me check your blood." Wrapping the blood pressure cuff around Vicky's arm, he squeezed the bulb. "Nope, not flowing." He put the tools down on the table, wrinkling his brow—not sure he had the answer for this one. He looked back at Vicky and asked, "Have you been eating a lot of cake?" "I have" she responded. "Well, that's what it is. This is why you have a cold. You can't eat a lot of cake or sugary things. You can have cake once a year."

The roots of organized hospital play for children go way back to the days when volunteers introduced play activities in convalescent homes and children's hospitals as early as 1910 (Turner & Grissim, 2014). However, the shift in attitudes toward children and play in hospitals did not occur until well into the second half of the 20th century, when the progression of interest in the well-being of children and recognition of play as a method to promote learning in early childhood occurred in tandem (Turner & Grissim, 2014). Back then, the options available to women with aspirations for higher educational achievements often related to interests around the care, development, and education of children. Mary McLeod Brooks (1911–2007), for example, often played 'hospital' as a child with her brothers and her dolls (Brown, 2014). Subsequently, both brothers became physicians; likewise, Mary found a pathway into the hospital. One of the original 'play ladies,' her discovery of the nursery school at Smith College synced with the establishment of the experimental play program at Children's Memorial Hospital of Chicago in 1932 (Turner, 2014). Children's interest in hospital-themed play was also recognized and tapped in these early days. In fact, the availability of manufactured play doctor kits dates back to the 1940s when the educational supply company, Hasbro, moved into the toy industry. To this day, children continue to play doctor with or without props, often as an expression of their construction of health care knowledge.

Framework

Play activities of children have undergone a vast amount of scientific study since *The Psychology of Play Activities* was first published (Lehman & Witty, 1927). Indeed, changes in the amount of time spent in play, the location of play, and the marketing of play and play materials have been well-documented as Western society, in particular, has become more achievement-focused. Today, play in its normative and unstructured form is less prevalent, even less valued than it once was in both education (Bergen, 2016) and health care (Bolig, in press). Unfortunately, the study of normative play that intersects the edges of early childhood education and health care practice is rare. Even more so, children's knowledge of health and illness is most often examined in isolation from the environments through which knowledge is constructed. Little time has been taken to pause and observe the unique qualities of children's play around health-related themes afforded in the early childhood setting. For that reason, an observational study in an early childhood classroom was designed to capture ways in which children demonstrate knowledge and behaviors around health-related themes during episodes of pretend play—to essentially explore the question, *what does health literacy look like in young children?*

The observation of play by caring adults offers an opportunity to see the world through the child's eyes. The American Academy of Pediatrics clinical report (Milteer, Ginsburg, the Council on Communications and Media, & Committee on Psychosocial Aspects of Child and Family Health, 2012) reminds us, "Even small children use imaginative play and fantasy to take on their fears and create or explore a world they can master" (p. e206). In addition to contributing to physical health, healthy brain development, and developing social emotional ties, play allows children to practice adult roles. Young Dr. Germs created a fantasy role that allowed him to demonstrate knowledge, competency, confidence, and his beliefs while engaging in health care role-play with an adult. For pediatric health care professionals, observation of the interest, involvement, ideas, knowledge, and feelings that children hold around health and wellness topics can provide valuable insight for the advancement of child health literacy. Within the context of patient- and family-centered care, interest in improving health literacy of younger patients to become empowered with health related knowledge and skills is growing (Borzekowski, 2009). This chapter encourages pediatric health care practitioners to take a good look at children's health care play for evidence of developing concepts around health and health care.

Recently an emerging researcher did just that. Interested in the ways in which preschool children engage in different forms of health care play using both non-health care–related and health care–related materials, Dempsey (2015) conducted a participant observation study in an early childhood classroom. Observations of children's play activities were documented and later developed into learning stories informed by the child life and early childhood education literature. Learning stories offer an approach for understanding what is occurring as a child is engaged in play activities through enhanced perspectives, because children are given a voice in the process (Nyland & Alfayez, 2012).

Excerpts from play scenarios are presented throughout this chapter to illustrate elements of children's play of interest to child health care practitioners and educators. Pretend play, or make-believe play, and health care play observed in the preschool environment offer insight into developmental and health-specific concepts relevant to understanding child health literacy. This cross-discipline perspective is unique, for the context of child health care play has yet to be documented as a vantage point for the appraisal of children's advancing health literacy.

Child Health Literacy

Children are exposed to health-related themes everywhere as they go through their daily activities. They learn about everyday life through norms and routines within the family and through interaction with social, educational, and media messages present in the environment. However, the future health outcomes of young children are mostly dependent on proximal adults providing and supporting their emerging sense of health and wellness as expressed through interactions in varying day-to-day situations. This parallels the concept of health literacy as it relates to adults: "the capacity to acquire, understand and use information in ways which promote and maintain good health" (Nutbeam, 2009, p. 304). Nutbeam rightly points out, however, that the content and context of health literacy is different for adults than for children. Yet attention is most often paid to the health literacy of parents and care providers as a proxy for child health literacy. One comprehensive test of adult health literacy, the Health Activity Literacy Scale (HALS), delineates five competency domains (health promotion, health protection, disease prevention, health care and maintenance, and systems navigation) as well as literacy tasks and skills (Nutbeam). However, a parallel approach to the assessment of child health literacy has yet to be developed. Indeed, little attention has been given to the examination of developing health literacy in children. This opens the door for the exploration of the question, *what does health literacy look like in young children?* as a reasonable place to start an inquiry.

Prior to the establishment of reading, writing, and numeracy skills and the cognitive capacities required to maintain and promote good health, young children demonstrate competence in unique ways. Just as literacy is established as a foundation of health literacy for adults, for children "health literacy involves abilities of how to use the provided information in an age- and developmentally appropriate way and thereby be involved in health issues of its own" (Stålberg, Sandberg, & Söderbäck, 2016, p. 460). Almqvist, Hellnas Stefansson, and Granlund (2006) provide support for this idea. Findings emphasize that simple experience-based facts, often expressing engagement and participation with desired activities such as play, are important to 4- to 5-year-old children in response to questions about health-related concepts. Understanding health perceptions from the point of view of the child is important for early childhood educators and health care practitioners looking to promote health literacy in the early years. Following a critical review of the impact of pretend play on children's development, Lillard et al. (2013) concluded that the most positive means to help young children's development is seen in hands-on, child-driven play. From this perspective, the provision of child-directed play is not only essential for healthy cognitive, physical, social, and emotional development of children, but also a potential context for the construction of health literacy in the early years (Ginsburg the Committee on Communications & the Committee on Psychosocial Aspects of Child and Family Health, 2007). Indeed, Borzekowski (2009) asserts that through developmentally appropriate approaches, young children have the capacity to gain the necessary knowledge and skills for the ongoing development of health literacy.

The importance of identifying ways in which children are distinct from adults regarding issues of health literacy is exposed through the exploration of ways in which children are also a part of the larger health literacy picture. In general, health literacy refers to the ability to access, understand, evaluate, and communicate health care information across the life span (Nutbeam, 2009). This is necessary as a means of promoting, maintaining, and improving health in a variety of settings throughout one's lifetime. For children, adults are the primary source for the development of knowledge, attitudes, and behaviors that support healthy development and the foundation for a healthy future. But in a media-saturated world, it is also necessary to consider the sway of messages potentially influencing the ability of adults and children to explore and make informed choices about their health and well-being. Adult health literacy can be demonstrated in a variety of behaviors, such as seeking out medical information, understanding dosage directions on a prescription bottle, and having a conversation with one's family doctor about health questions and concerns. Although research using experiments and interviews has documented children's conceptual understanding of health and illness, ways in which young children *demonstrate* their construction of related concepts may best be found during the observation of children in health- or medical-related play scenarios.

Early research studies on children's understanding of health and illness focus on developmental changes in children's concepts. Bruhn, Cordova, Williams, and Fuentes (1977) viewed wellness as an active process of development and learning that continues in time. At each level of development, age-appropriate knowledge and behaviors referred to as wellness tasks are suggested to become established. Posited as aligned with Erickson's eight developmental stages, minimal wellness tasks for the early years suggest behaviors to be supported during each developmental stage (e.g., learning about foods, exercise, and sleep). In line with Piaget's stage theory, early studies by Bibace and Walsh (1981), Burbach and Peterson (1986), Kalish (1996a, 1996b), and Solomon and Cassimatis (1999) describe children's development of concepts of illness causality, explanations of types of illness, and children's known facts as linked to their understanding of germs, symptoms, and contamination. Although children learn an abundance of facts as they mature, Solomon and Cassimatis conclude that young children often limit their explanations of illness to contagion (placing illness causation on the proximity of objects or people). Almqvist et al. (2006) framed their deductive content analysis of children's interviews around the International Classification of Functioning, Disability and Health (ICF). In contrast to Solomon and Cassimatis, evidence of children's multidimensional perception of health was found, with responses corresponding with ICF dimensions such as positive body functioning, ability, participation and engagement in activities, and environmental factors. This body of research provides an important foundation for understanding children's perceptions of health, but the documentation of the *behaviors* of children as they construct an understanding of health and illness is absent.

Later, Borzekowski (2009) added to the narrative by compelling health care professionals to play an active role in children's health literacy through encouraging and enabling health literacy skills at a young age. Framing the discussion within a developmental perspective, Borzekowski encouraged consideration for the abilities of even the youngest children to gain the necessary knowledge, attitudes, and behaviors to develop health literacy. A decade earlier, Rushforth (1999) suggested that patient education programs should focus on what children can achieve rather than on developmental limitations. However, documentation of variations in the achievement of child health knowledge, attitudes, and behaviors supporting health literacy across stages of development has still not been documented.

Of course, children experience episodes of illness and recovery frequently during the early years. Parents play a large role in illness prevention by avoiding infections, responding to symptoms, and accessing health services and providers. The caregiving behaviors of parents, as well as health care providers, vary in the degree that communication references illness causation, symptoms, care, and consequences. However, during related interactions, the influence of caring adults on the development of children's understanding of the physical, social, and emotional aspects of illness can be powerful, for example what to expect from others, how to feel about themselves, and ways to get better. We often see this in children's picture books featuring a health-related theme; indeed, Turner (2006) found an emphasis on social-emotional aspects of care and recovery with a focus on caregivers, health care professionals, and positive consequences of experiencing an illness such as returning to typical activities, interactions with others, and special care or treats. What remains absent from this body of literature is the voice of the child as illustrated through observation and documentation of their behavior, interactions, and dialogue around health-related themes. For this, we look to the work of child life specialists and early childhood educators.

Medical Play

The concept of medical play is most likely familiar to pediatric care providers, specifically child life specialists. However, medical play is also provided in early childhood settings where it is often referred to as health care play. Child life pioneer Kathleen McCue (1988) asserts, "Most theorists would concur that there is value and meaning for the player in the process of play" (p. 158). She explains that medical play, a distinct concept within the phenomenon of play, should be made available to any child who may enjoy or need it because positive and comprehensive play can occur with even the most basic medical materials. Regardless of setting, this self-directed play can provide children opportunities to demonstrate their understanding of health care topics through the uses of materials and language, and also provide opportunities to explore, create, and discover outside the health care environment.

Four specific characteristics define medical play as distinct in the realm of general play behaviors (McCue, 1988). First, medical play is said to always have a medical theme as a component of the play. Second, although it may be initiated by an adult, medical play is motivated and maintained by the child. Third, a range of emotions may be demonstrated by the child: often enjoyable, it may be observed with laughter and relaxation, or it may reveal intense feelings such as aggression. Finally, medical play is emphatically stated to be separate from preparation for medical procedures. This final element, reinforcing the child-directed focus of the play, lends support to the proposition that the observation of children in play-based early childhood settings may be ideal for the documentation of children's construction of health literacy.

The term 'medical play' conjures an image of a child using medical equipment to act out a pretend medical procedure, such as using a stethoscope to listen to a heartbeat on a toy bear. However, this illustrates just one of four categories of medical play originally described by McCue (1988) as she began the process of documenting the work of child life specialists in health care settings. Child life specialists provide a context whereby a child is provided with opportunities to gain mastery and control in the medical setting, where emotional expression and learning co-occur with pretend play. Medical play also creates a context for the observation and documentation of children's understanding of health-related materials, experiences, and emotions behind the experiences that children may bring to their play. Providing common medical supplies such as bandages, cotton balls, tongue depressors, syringes, and thermometers can encourage health care–related play; however, symbolic objects, including specific health care equipment, as well as the presence of a parent or child life specialist, are more likely to elicit unique expressions of feelings and experiences than typical toys and games (Bolig, in press).

McCue describes the following categories of medical play involving both common play and symbolic materials (1988). These categories offer a practical scheme for the organization of observed play behaviors in children, as illustrated with excerpts from the observation study (Dempsey, 2015).

1. **Role rehearsal/role reversal**. This type of play involves children taking on the role of a health care professional and re-enacting medical events on models, such as dolls, puppets, or stuffed animals, using real medical equipment as well as commercially made materials specifically intended for medical play. For example, a doctor or nurse kit is used by a 4-year-old girl:

    Lilly cared for her patient during a check-up. She picked up the toy syringe and placed the tip of it up to the top of Vicky's shoulder. Lilly said, "You need a needle.

It's a flu shot." After she pressed the top of the syringe she removed it and picked up a Band-Aid, gently placing it over the area.

2. **Medical fantasy play** features children's role play with elements of pretend play. Medical themes are enacted, but without the use of medical equipment. For example, children may assign functions to everyday toys and materials as seen in Noah's play:

> Noah picked up a pencil and the notebook and began to draw. He made many lines covering a large portion of the paper. He explained it was a picture of all the scars that needed treatment. He turned the page and continued to draw more into what he called "The book of scars." Noah said, "You have so many scars you will have them forever and never get better."

3. **Indirect medical play** involves a variety of opportunities for exploration and information around medical content, but without the elements of health-related role-play themes. The availability of hospital-themed puzzles or games, for example, may bring a health-related topic to the forefront through either medical or non-medical equipment. This play provides opportunities for children to engage with health care content in their play and express experiences and beliefs relative to their interest as well as their comfort level. The play scenarios derived from these materials vary; a syringe may become a microphone, or a toy pager may be used as a phone to call a friend:

> When the puzzle was complete the girl held it up and said, "His body is now put back together." Rose and Will passed it back and forth as they smiled and looked over both sides of the body. Rose noticed that the skeleton puzzle had two sides: "This side looks different."

4. **Medically related art** is less structured, providing children with potential opportunities to express their understanding of, and reaction to, their medical experiences. Art activities range from direct painting and drawing to three-dimensional creations using medical materials, like med cups and cotton balls:

> Ben shouted, "Let's build a rocket ship." But once he got the glue bottle in his hands the plan changed. He glued two med cups face-down and filled the bottom rim of the cup with glue. He shouted, "This is a volcano" as he added a cotton ball on top. He continued to squeeze the glue on the top of the cotton ball until it began to pour down the sides.

Medical play is frequently offered as a child-directed exploratory activity; however, it is also initiated by child life specialists supporting specific psychosocial goals. Additionally, observations made by child life specialists are used to inform activities and interventions. Using play as a therapeutic modality, child life specialists direct play as a means to support the achievement of positive therapeutic or educational outcomes (Turner, in press). Insight gained through the observation of children's exploration and communication of health-related themes can also result in the identification of a child's ongoing coping and learning. For example, *Fern sat and rocked the doll back and forth for a while. Then she pulled the Band-Aid from the doll's leg. She said, "Elle doesn't need it anymore. We can throw it out. It's old."*

The availability of simple materials, such as Band-Aids and baby dolls, can allow children like Fern to take control of their play and regain a sense of autonomy lost during prior experiences. Approaches to the presentation of medical play vary depending on context. Individual, group, playroom, and classroom medical play activities may be introduced by child life specialists and others interested in facilitating play through the provision of props that allow children to express curiosity and engage with materials directly. Each approach affords a different type of provocation resulting in unique responses as individuals or groups of children react, explore experiences, share knowledge, experiment, and ask questions.

Social patterns of interaction and activity observed in children's play are informative relative to a child's prior experiences with play, social skill development, peer relationships, cognitive and physical strengths and limitations, and competence with social and health care–related situations (Turner, in press). Just as child life specialists present a variety of play-based activities, so too do early childhood educators. The purpose, however, is different. Child life specialists approach play as a context for addressing children's potential risk of adverse outcomes during experiences of illness and health care. Early childhood educators, on the other hand, have an interest in supporting children's learning across domains of development. While there is little documentation specific to children's health care play in the early childhood literature, examples of children playing doctor, dentist, veterinarian, caregiver, and related themes are often provided in discussions of children's dramatic or pretend play. Play-based learning settings offer a context where play occupies a large amount of time for children to demonstrate behaviors through experiential, hands-on learning with peers and adults, supported with a range of materials to stimulate their interest, involvement, engagement, and emotions.

Preschoolers' Health Care Play

A qualitative participant observation study by Dempsey (2015) of preschool children's play with health care–related materials resulted in the compilation of learning stories presented here to answer the question, *what does child health literacy look like?* The goals of the study were twofold. The first goal was to use an assessment process known as *Learning Stories* to document the health care play of 4- and 5-year-old children over a 10-day period in a play-based learning setting. The second goal was to motivate reflection on the question, *what can learning stories tell us about children's prior understandings and new knowledge about health and health care?* One reason for seeking children's perspectives about their learning is that it allows children to be viewed as social learners with their own opinions and views. While introducing the health care play materials into the preschool environment, Dempsey documented the children's play through field notes, photographs, and audio recording, while at the same time attempting to remain minimally intrusive in the children's play. Through documentation with an intense focus on children's experiences, memories, and thoughts in the course of their play, as well as an understanding of what is going on in the work of the children, the researcher attempted *to make the children's learning visible* (Kline, 2008).

An understanding of what is occurring as a child is engaged in play activities is largely improved when the perspectives of the child are given a voice and included in the documentation process. Nyland and Alfayez (2012) described the use of narrative accounts of children's learning situations enriched with photographs and artifacts illustrating and offering insight regarding the learning that has occurred during the experience. Nyland and Alfayez presented the concept of *learning dispositions* to be used as a framework for understanding what is occurring during play activities. The learning dispositions (taking an interest, being involved, persisting with difficulty, expressing an idea or feeling, and taking responsibility) illustrate what a child brings to the play. The learning story, representing an event that has taken place, consists of four parts: the narrative, the learning dispositions, a discussion of the learning, and an exploration of what is next.

"learning dispositions"

Three learning stories are now presented. Each learning story is segmented to highlight the children's learning dispositions followed by discussion of the learning story relative to the question, *what does child health literacy look like in children?* For child health practitioners and educators, the awareness gained through learning stories about the interest, involvement, ideas, and feelings children hold around health–related topics can motivate practices designed to acknowledge, encourage, and enable child health literacy in the early years.

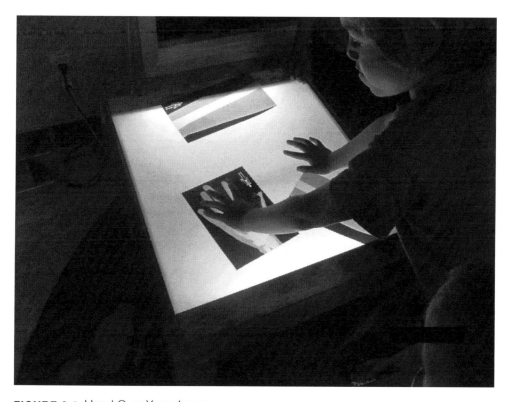

FIGURE 2.1 Hand Over X-ray Image

LEARNING STORY: X-RAYS ARE COOL!

Showing an interest: Bobby noticed something new in the health care play corner: a chest X-ray with light shining through the film, highlighting an image on the light table. Bobby looked and said, "Cool!" He could see the ribcage and shadows in the chest cavity.

Being involved: Picking up the X-ray film, he placed it against his body, pressing it over the top of his chest. He held the X-ray in place as he presented his discovery to the teachers and children. Walking back over to the light table, he removed the chest X-ray and began looking at the other images. Seeing an image of a hand, he placed his own hand over top of the image (see Figure 2.1).

Expressing an emotion: It aligned with his own: "Look, it's my hand!"

Taking responsibility: Colin, who had been playing nearby, approached the light table. He flipped through the different X-ray images. Looking at Bobby, who still had his hand over the X-ray, Colin pointed to one of the X-ray images and quietly said, "Leg bone." Almost immediately, Bobby responded, "No, that is actually a picture of an arm bone." Bobby ran his finger over the top of the image, tracing along the ulna and radius making up the lower part of the arm and said, "This picture has to be of the arm bones."

As Bobby picked up the additional X-ray images, he named each one. He labeled the leg bones, arm bones, hands, and the skull appropriate to each image. He picked up one of the arm X-rays and placed it over the top of his arm, calling out "I need a hand one, too, to make my whole arm." The teacher, who was watching the boy's X-ray investigation, asked, "Can I help you with the hand?" Bobby gave her the hand X-ray. She positioned it on Bobby's hand with his fingers spread out. The lower arm X-ray and the hand X-ray completely covered as he matched up the bones. Bobby smiled as he looked down at his arm.

Persisting with difficulty: His attention was then drawn to a different part of this image. Bobby noticed there was a small image of the entire human skeleton on this X-ray, with a frame highlighting the area represented in the image. He pointed to this small legend that now had Colin's attention as well. They chatted back and forth about where this highlighted section would be on a human skeleton. They pointed to each other's body parts to explore where the image was focused. Back and forth, each boy looked at the image and then at the other boy. Pointing to the arm, they agreed that the framed image was highlighting the arm.

Analysis of Learning Dispositions: Both Bobby and Colin participated with interest, demonstrating a foundation knowledge of the human skeleton over the duration of the play. Through cooperative, hands-on engagement with the materials, the boys showed knowledge and recognition of the images of bones through words (it's my hand) and behavior (he placed the X-ray on his body). Additionally, they were challenged to discern the relationship of images in the legend with their own body in a process of jointly creating a new level of understanding of the relationship of parts (bones) to the whole (skeleton). The positive emotions demonstrated during moments of discovery reinforce the learning resulting from the exploration.

What's next? The introduction of resources related to the human skeleton in the play area to inspire further exploration and learning (e.g., puzzles, books, open-ended art, and health care materials) will build on the interest and activity demonstrated by Bobby and Colin. Teachers can listen closely to the learners and be prepared to provide additional resources to enhance the depth of exploration and learning, for example building a skeleton with tongue depressors.

What Does Child Health Literacy Look Like?

Knowledge of the human body is but one of the components of health literacy. Both boys revealed a lot about their knowledge and emerging understanding of the human body through their indirect medical play. Bobby's recognition and interest in the materials expressed through his behavior, emotion, and language is evidence supporting the notion that children have the ability to learn about health-related subjects through developmentally appropriate approaches. Bobby's actions with the chest X-ray show us that he not only recognized the chest cavity but also recognized it as a representation of his

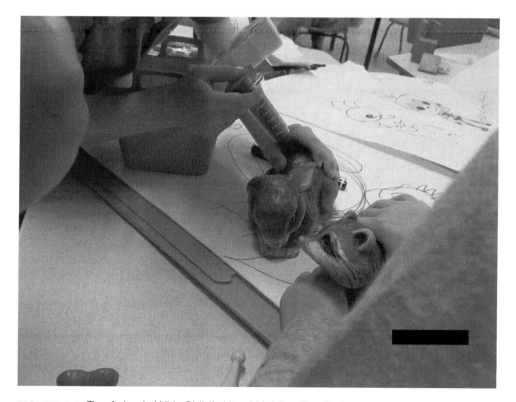

FIGURE 2.2 Toy Animals With Child's Hand Holding Toy Syringe

own body. This was repeated with the images of the hand and forearm. The emotions expressed by Bobby not only attracted Colin but indicated both boys' capacity for learning as it was driven by curiosity. The opportunity for the two boys to carry on a conversation about specific elements of the materials (e.g., relating the legend of the skeleton to the larger image) allowed for observation of the spontaneous expression of their knowledge and understanding. Each child's existing knowledge was observed to be expanded during the interaction. The labeling of body parts demonstrated knowledge on one level (facts); the matching of the abstract image to the human body demonstrates an emerging understanding of the body as a system composed of multiple, interrelated parts.

LEARNING STORY: GOOD DOCTOR/BAD DOCTOR

Showing an interest: A small group of children gathered in the health care play area. Animal toys from the classroom had been moved into the medical play area inspiring a shift in the play. Jasmine was giving care to a bunny. She applied bandages, 'cream,' and an ice bag to the back of the bunny. Using the thermometer, she flipped it upside down, pressed the tip, and applied the cream (see Figure 2.2).

Being involved: Noah and Aiden watched Jasmine for a few moments before Noah picked up the otoscope and began aiming it at Vicky's mouth. Cards displaying body parts were spread on the table. Noah held up the image of the leg and said, "I am checking for scars," he said, "And there is a lot!" He handed Aiden a cotton ball and said, "Take this." Using this image, Noah held it next to Vicky's leg: "Your leg is broken." He added, "I gave you germs. I am Dr. Germs! Aiden is Dr. Badness."

Expressing an idea or emotion: Jasmine quickly comforted Vicky: "I am a good doctor. I can help you with my good pills and fairy dust." She pressed down on the top of an empty bottle, spraying her fairy dust all over Vicky and the boys. "This can make you better and you will be good doctors."

"Everything I have given her was bad. The pills all had germs to make her sick and the good pills will never work," replied Dr. Germs (Noah). Dr. Goodness (Jasmine) continued to treat Vicky, giving her good pills, insisting they will work.

Dr. Germs picked up the otoscope, stuffed a cotton ball into the back of it, and aimed it at Vicky's mouth. "This is a germ shooter." Next he placed a cotton glove on his head: "Blasts germs right inside of you!" he explained. He told Dr. Badness (Aiden) to put 'bad feelings' inside the patient using the stethoscope placed on the patient.

Persisting with difficulty: "That won't work," responded the boys. Jasmine raised one hand in the air and placed the other on her hip and said, "Well, I am Dr. Goodness and I can make her all better!" Dr. Goodness continued spraying fairy dust and gave good pills to the patient to help fight the germs.

Taking responsibility: As the play was winding down, Noah told Jasmine that her fairy dust would never work until he ran out of germs. "And I still have lots left. Ten hundred thousand and forty!" As the boys walked away, Dr. Goodness waited until they were out of sight and continued to spray. Vicky said, "I am feeling better."

Analysis of Learning Dispositions: Initially begun as two play scenarios, the children's interest in the health care theme merged in the form of a mix of role-play and fantasy play scenario. Jasmine shared her interest and knowledge around care giving as a positive social interaction. Noah and Aiden revealed through fantasy play a general understanding around germs as bad and a sense of the potential of medicine for having both positive and negative qualities. As well, Noah showed some understanding of internalization, an association of sickness with bad feelings, and the absence of germs as relevant to the effectiveness of medicine.

What's next? The association of illness, germs, and medicine revealed in the children's play suggests an interest to further explore these concepts. Opportunities to engage with topics such as hygiene, contamination, and internalization through messy play and games could apply concepts beyond the fantasy play observed.

What Does Health Literacy Look Like?

The dynamics of the surfacing of health- and illness-related concepts can be seen as the role rehearsal/role reversal play of Jasmine, Noah, and Aiden converge. The dominant role of providing treatment observed in Jasmine's play demonstrates her feelings around the promotion of good health through care. Observations of Jasmine's play suggest an association of positive emotion, with caregiving perhaps reflecting her experience as a receiver of care. In contrast, the boys' play exhibited the emerging development of their understanding of illness causality, explanations for illness, and known facts. They incorporated ideas around germs, broken bones, and scars in an extended scenario that allowed them to act out roles such as those often seen in non-health care–related play (i.e., good guy/bad guy roles). The theme of germs captured in this one observation signals the boys' level of understanding of germs as a causation of illness. Noah's play further indicates an emerging understanding of the presence of germs internally as a cause of sickness. The incidental mention of bad feelings suggests a connection made between physical sickness and not feeling well. As previously advised, symbolic objects are more likely to elicit play that is informative of a child's prior experience and/or competence around health-related topics and medical equipment. The provision of the bandages, thermometer, cotton balls, and otoscope allows children to use their health-related knowledge and to build the play scenarios (see Figure 2.3). As the play unfolded over time, the health care play scenarios merged with the fantasy play scenarios to reveal the children's assorted understandings of complex associations among concepts such as medicine, germs, and health and illness.

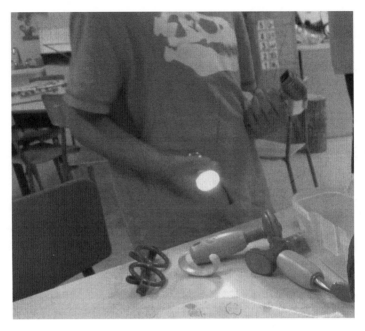

FIGURE 2.3 Child's Arm/Hand Holding a Flashlight Directed at Toy Medical Kit Contents

LEARNING STORY: TERMITES IN MY MOUTH!

Showing an interest: Ben picked up the plastic Band-Aids and placed them on Vicky's arms and shoulders. Vicky asked, "Why do I need the big Band-Aid?" and he told her, "Your arm is broken."

Being involved: Ben had brought a small flashlight to school that day and used it with a toy otoscope to look at Vicky's eyes and mouth. He turned away to pick up the thermometer, then directed his attention to her forehead. Vicky asked, "Am I okay?"

Expressing an idea or emotion: Ben responded, "Not really, you're cold." He went back and forth using the flashlight/otoscope and the dentist mirror to examine her.

Treatment continued as he picked up the syringe, pushed the plunger, and said, "You need to take this medicine." Vicky responded, "Am I all better now?" Ben replied, "No, now you are too hot." Ben continued to use the dentist mirror, flashlight, and otoscope while looking inside Vicky's mouth.

Persisting with difficulty: After a few minutes, she asked Ben if he could see anything. He quietly checked inside her mouth. Nicolas, watching Ben, began looking inside Vicky's mouth as well. Again, Vicky asked Ben, "Do you see anything?" This time Ben responded, he said, "I am looking for little bugs." Pausing for a movement, he continued, "Termites."

Taking responsibility: Ben explained that termites were little bugs that live inside the mouth and were living inside her teeth, and that Vicky had gotten them from not brushing her teeth. Over and over again, he asked her to open her mouth so he could look with the mirror and then again with the flashlight/otoscope.

Analysis of Learning Dispositions: The flow of ideas in this play scenario moved from a basic health care examination incorporating ideas around Band-Aids, bones, and body temperature toward a specific theme of the dental examination. Ben is demonstrating his understanding of what happens when you go to a dental office using the materials at hand. The flashlight is an interesting addition to the medical play kit, as it appears to invite a level of exploration above what can be pursued with basic materials. As the actions of a dentist present somewhat of a mystery from a child perspective, the behaviors of Ben and the interest of Nicolas suggest a shift toward understanding the perspective of the doctor and the construction of ideas around what the doctor may be looking for during an examination (broken bones, temperature, bugs). Perhaps Ben was indeed looking for bugs!

What's next? Interest in the dentist office, examination, and dental hygiene are linked and can be extended with a variety of additional materials, including dental equipment such as models, mirrors, and lights, as well as storybooks with themes such as visiting the dentist, brushing your teeth, and dental cavities. A dentist office play corner could be introduced as a provocation for deeper exploration of related roles and knowledge supportive of children's future dental care experiences. Creative approaches to distinguishing germs and bugs through playful activities indoors and outdoors may also be explored.

What Does Child Health Literacy Look Like?

The elements of child health literacy observed in Ben's play relate to his knowledge and understanding around the use of health care equipment, diagnosis, and illness causation. Through his role play as a doctor, Ben demonstrates his competence relative to the appropriate use of the Band-Aids, syringe, otoscope, dentist mirror, flashlight, and thermometer. The manner in which he uses these materials indicates an awareness of specific medical tools used by the doctor—some to provide treatment and others used to help make a diagnosis. His familiarity with the examination–diagnosis sequence of a procedure is supported through the use of the medical props and communicated particularly around the idea that the diagnosis is a definitive element of the process. By acting out roles, children show their interpretation of what happens in a doctor's office, conversations that take place between a doctor and patient, and ways that doctors may help. A glimpse into the beginnings of health literacy is captured through observation of children's exploration of health promotion, protection, care, and maintenance, as well as system navigation in their play scenarios.

Personal Reflections *Play is a window into a child's world.*

The observation of play offers an opportunity to see the world through the child's eyes. Children's interest in health care play goes back a long way. It is possible that many child health care practitioners relate well to this type of play—perhaps as a sentimental diversion. But it is also likely that the play would be offered for its value as a context for the accomplishment of assessment, intervention, or education-centered goals relevant to their profession. To observe children's play strictly through our professional lens may result in missing some of the nuances of the expressions of knowledge and competence that arise when children are 'just playing.' We think Kathleen McCue would agree. When adults are able to take a secondary role and observe quietly while children play for a period of time, the value and meaning of the child's play from the child's perspective can be discovered.

"*What's on the health table today?*" Play-based learning environments are ideal contexts outside the family where children construct their understanding of health-related concepts and processes contributing to health literacy. The environments in many play-based early childhood settings are set up to respond to the early interests of children rather than to impose a set curriculum for teachers and children to follow. The health care play materials provided in the observation study clearly sparked the interest of a number of children over the course of two weeks. Although consent was obtained for all the children in the program, a steady group of 11 children regularly entered into the health care play for extended periods of time. Learning stories were created daily and posted in the morning for the children to review, discuss, and respond to in their subsequent play. Seeing the enthusiasm of the children, program teachers also got involved by adding health care–related materials to the classroom and building on the interests of the children during regular activities. Through the astute observation and documentation practice of learning stories, the interest, participation, engagement, and abilities of children were acknowledged. Additionally, learning outcomes of interest were documented and the children's interactions in the physical and social environment were made visible.

The learning stories presented in this chapter support the assertion that children can demonstrate their capacity for health literacy when given open-ended and symbolic materials, uninterrupted time, and the permission to explore, discover, and inquire. By focusing attention on children's abilities to gain knowledge, attitudes, and behaviors that support their developing health literacy, our perspectives on professional roles can change. A shift toward thinking of play spaces in health care facilities as learning environments affording opportunities for observation and innovative documentation approaches can contribute to a better understanding of health literacy from the perspective of the child. In fact, we see this observation of preschool health care play as a starting point for health care professionals to consider health literacy as an area of early learning that is valued as a foundation of future health and well-being.

SUMMARY

The health care play scenarios presented in the chapter characterize a simple and innovative context for the exploration of children's developing health literacy. Through pretend play with health care materials, children aged 4–5 years express their interest, engagement, ideas, feelings, and understanding around related themes. The play setting provides a naturalistic environment for children to *demonstrate* their competence with health-related themes. The health care play scenarios often reveal behaviors children have previously engaged in, or seen adults engage in, supported through interactions with peers. For example, knowledge of the human body, behaviors associated with a medical visit, feelings around care, and attitudes toward health and illness were illustrated in the learning stories. Observations of children's health care play, supported by the documentation of children's learning, contribute to an understanding of what health literacy looks like in young children. The children's play scenarios presented as learning stories in this chapter provide insights into children's understanding of their social environment related to health and health care.

Future practice directions for child health practitioners and educators can include consideration of the approaches used in early childhood settings to support child-directed play and to include children's voices in the documentation process. As evidenced in the learning stories, young children have the capacity and ability to develop health literacy from an early age. Although no one is likely to dispute this, indications of the documentation of children's health literacy are not evident in the extant literature. The growing interest in determining children's understanding of health literacy is driven partly through current initiatives directing resources to the early years of child and family life. For pediatric health care professionals, observation of the interest, involvement, ideas, knowledge, and feelings that children hold around health and wellness topics can provide valuable insight for the advancement of child health literacy in their practice.

The presentation of observational data collected in an early childhood classroom was designed to capture the attention of health care professionals interested in ways to envision children's emerging sense of health literacy. By illustrating elements of children's play of interest to child health care practitioners and educators, we hope to motivate activities designed to acknowledge, encourage, and enable child health literacy in the early years.

Future research initiatives dedicated to examining child health literacy in the early years should consider ways in which children demonstrate their knowledge and understanding of health and health-related concepts. Mixed methods proposals can be designed to include qualitative indicators of children's learning in addition to objective measures of, for example, stress and coping. Child health researchers looking for ways to expand beyond quantitative measures may find qualitative approaches that capture children's learning processes will strengthen a research design. The use of learning stories as a method for the documentation of children's developing health literacy has yet to be explored in empirical research; however, the potential to feature children as social learners with their own opinions and views around health and health care may be appealing to medical play therapists and child life practitioners in particular.

REFERENCES

Almqvist, L., Hellnas, P., Stefansson, M., & Granlund, M. (2006). 'I can play!' Young children's perceptions of health. *Pediatric Rehabilitation*, 9(3), 275–284.

Bergen, D. (2016). Play, toys, learning, and understanding. *American Journal of Play*, 8(2), 145–156.

Bibace, R., & Walsh, M. (1981). Children's concepts of illness. In R. Bibace & M. Walsh (Eds.), *Children's conceptions of health, illness, and bodily functions* (pp. 31–48). San Francisco: Jossey-Bass.

Bolig, R. (in press). Play in children's health-care settings. In J. Rollins, R. Bolig & C. Mahan (Eds.), *Meeting children's psychosocial needs across the health-care continuum* (2nd ed.). Austin, TX: ProEd.

Borzekowski, D.L.G. (2009). Considering children and health literacy: A theoretical approach. *Pediatrics, 124*, 282–288.

Brown, C. (2014). Play and professionalism: The legacy of Mary McLeod Brooks (1911–2007). In J. Turner & C. Brown (Eds.), *The pips of child life: Early play programs in hospitals* (pp. 57–64). Dubuque, IA: Kendall Hunt.

Bruhn, J.G., Cordova, F.D., Williams, J.A., & Fuentes, R.G. (1977). The wellness process. *Journal of Community Health, 2*(3), 209–221.

Burbach, D., & Peterson, L. (1986). Children's concepts of physical illness: A review and critique of the cognitive-developmental literature. *Health Psychology, 5*, 307–325.

Dempsey, V. (2015). *Observations of preschoolers' health care play*. Unpublished Master's Thesis, Mount Saint Vincent University, Halifax, Nova Scotia.

Ginsburg, K.R., the Committee on Communications, & the Committee on Psychosocial Aspects of Child and Family Health. (2007). The importance of play in promoting healthy child development and maintaining strong parent-child bonds. *Pediatrics, 119*(1), 182–191.

Kalish, C. (1996a). Causes and symptoms in preschoolers' conceptions of illness. *Child Development, 67*, 1647–1670.

Kalish, C. (1996b). Preschoolers' understanding of germs as invisible mechanisms. *Cognitive Development, 11*, 83–106.

Kline, L. (2008). Documentation panel: The 'making learning visible' project. *Journal of Early Childhood Teacher Education, 29*, 70–80.

Lehman, H.C., & Witty, P.A. (1927). *The psychology of play activities*. New York: A.S. Barnes.

Lillard, A.S., Lerner, M.D., Hopkins, E.J., Dore, R.A., Smith, E.D., & Palmquist, C.M. (2013). The impact of pretend play on children's development: A review of the evidence. *Psychological Bulletin, 139*(1), 1–34.

McCue, K. (1988). Medical play: An expanded perspective. *Journal of the Association for the Care of Children's Health, 16*(3), 157–161.

McCue, K. (1995). Oral history DVD. *Child life council archives*. Utica, NY.

Milteer, R.M., Ginsburg K.R., the Council on Communications and Media, & Committee on Psychosocial Aspects of Child and Family Health. (2012). The importance of play in promoting healthy child development and maintaining strong parent-child bond: Focus on children in poverty. *Pediatrics, 129*(1), e204–13.

Nutbeam, D. (2009). Defining and measuring health literacy: What can we learn from literacy studies? *International Journal of Public Health, 54*, 303–305.

Nyland, B., & Alfayez, S. (2012). Learning stories-crossing borders: Introducing qualitative early childhood observation techniques to early childhood practitioners in Saudi Arabia. *International Journal of Early Years Education, 20*(4), 392–404.

Rushforth, H. (1999). Practitioner review: Communicating with hospitalised children: Review and application of research pertaining to children's understanding of health and illness. *Journal of Child Psychology, 40*(5), 683–691.

Solomon, G.E.A., & Cassimatis, N.L. (1999). On facts and conceptual systems: Young children's integration of their understandings of germs and contagion. *Developmental Psychology, 35*(1), 113–126.

Stålberg, A., Sandberg, A., & Söderbäck, M. (2016). Younger children's (three to five years) perceptions of being in a health-care situation. *Early Child Development and Care, 186*(5), 832–844.

Turner, J. (2006). Representations of illness, inquiry, and health in children's picture books. *Children's Health Care*, 35(2), 179–189.

Turner, J. (2014). A new attitude in using play: Anne Smith. In J. Turner & C. Brown (Eds.), *The pips of child life: Early play programs in hospitals* (pp. 37–46). Dubuque, IA: Kendall Hunt.

Turner, J. (in press). Theoretical foundations of child life. In R. H. Thompson (Ed.), *Handbook of child life* (2nd ed.). IL: C. C. Thomas.

Turner, J., & Grissim, L. (2014). Care and conditions of children in hospitals circa 1930. In J. Turner & C. Brown (Eds.), *The pips of child life: Early play programs in hospitals* (pp. 13–24). Dubuque, IA: Kendall Hunt.

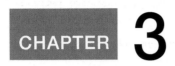

CHAPTER 3

Caring for Children With Cystic Fibrosis in a Hospital Setting in Australia

The Space Where Play and Pain Meet

Judi Parson

> If I never had CF, I'd be a little taller, my lungs a little fuller, my skin a tad less salty. If I never had CF, I'd take my sweet time, take it all for granted, be terrified of doctors and hate the smell of hospitals.
>
> —Lauren Bombardier (2010)

To explore the lifeworld of a child with cystic fibrosis (CF), Jaime, an 11-year-old boy, will be introduced, along with a range of health care professionals who care for him, within the context of an Australian hospital setting. Drawing on doctoral studies, professional knowledge, and clinical experience, this chapter explores the complex relationships found in medical environments through the lens of discourse theory. This is because discourse theory offers a way to understand the lifeworld of the child within the hospital setting from different positions. For example, the discourse of play is often marginalized in favor of the dominant biomedical discourse (Parson, 2008). However, the techniques and skills found in humanistic play therapy may be integrated into health care practice either before, during, or after medical procedures or when a child is suffering chronic or acute pain and as such provides a voice for the child.

The roles of the medical play therapist and/or child life specialist are particularly important to communicate to the child in and through play and to model and interpret therapeutic play interventions to others. Therapists are able to translate play-based assessments and behaviors to health care professionals such as medical doctors, nurses, and other allied health care providers, which in turn helps to expand the psychotherapeutic space needed for hospitalized children. The quality of the relationship establishes the foundation on which therapeutic play with child patients is based. And using a holistic humanistic approach to child-centered and family-focused health care practice is core to 'being with' the sick child. Thus, humanistic play therapy will be explored and linked to medical play therapy in this chapter to bridge discourse theory with clinical practice in the context of the hospital setting.

The lifeworld concept is based upon one's life experiences, events, or incidences and how these are perceived at a given point in time. Children admitted to hospital come into the medical world with their own health history and experiences. Sometimes children have experienced multiple admissions and have a sophisticated understanding of the hospital system and medical terminology. Children may speak in ways that make them sound older than their chronological age. When this happens, health care professionals could lose sight of the child's developmental need for play. Therefore, evaluating the child's development holistically is important when considering play-based therapeutic interventions. The inclusion of assessments, such as Mooli Lahad's (1992) six-part story method, may be useful to therapists to facilitate psychotherapy that focuses on the child's strengths and coping capacity. This chapter includes one of Jaime's stories to introduce this method. First, an overview of discourse theory sets the theoretical scene.

THEORETICAL ORIENTATION

The concepts that guide this chapter focus on the social construction of 'reality' through discourse. Specifically, discourse constructs relate to both the child with CF and the health care professionals' perception of 'reality' or 'truth', which are *experienced* within the context of an acute pediatric ward within a hospital in Australia. The sociological context considers relationships found in the medical environment. Tension is created at the site of multiple discourses that construct the child's reality within the hospital ward. The informal relationships of the community, family, and lifeworld of the sick child intersects with the formal relationships found in an acute pediatric ward, professional, and hospital culture, and the world of biomedicine (Parson, 2008).

Emerging from postmodernism, discourse theory typically aims to provide a lens to observe symbolic aspects of human and social life from a sociological viewpoint (Wodak, Maingueneau, & Angermuller, 2014), and as such is useful to examine the positions found in hospital environments as a social construct. Discourse is all about the way language is used within a specific field, and as a way of speaking that in turn gives meaning to experiences from a particular perspective (Danaher, Schirato, & Webb, 2000). Discourse represents what people do, think, and act, and at the same time portrays the relationship of power and subjectivity (Wodak et al., 2014). Thus, the relationship between people and experiences, the place in which they dwell, encompasses a specific 'field', be it the field of science, sport, or pediatric care in a hospital.

The Complexity of Discourse

Meaning is constructed from experiencing ourselves in the world, and meaning is communicated as representations (Larkin, 2004), such as perceptions and language, maps and traffic signs, artwork and play. While this appears simple, it becomes complicated by multiple and sometimes opposing discourses. Foucault's idea that power and knowledge are interrelated is a complex conceptual construct. Discourse is a medium for and an effect of power, privileging a point of view and silencing opposing points of view (Foucault, 1981). This is particularly important in relation to play, which is a marginalized discourse in relation to the hegemonic discourse of biomedicine (Parson, 2008).

Biomedicine: The Hegemonic Discourse

It is extensively documented that the dominant biomedical model influences Western health care practice (Haralambos, van Krieken, Smith, & Holborn, 1996; Jenkins, 2014; Turner, 1987). Biomedicine bases its knowledge on the scientific method of research to understand and cure illness. To do this, an objective, mechanistic, positivistic, biologic, scientific approach is used (Grbich, 2004). While medicine has indeed made some remarkable advances in the last few decades, "these scientific and technological advances have contributed to the shift away from models of person-centred medical care to models which may depersonalize the patient" (Clifton-Soderstrom, 2003, p. 447). Thus, as Jenkins (2014) states, biomedical hegemony continues to be an ethical problem. If, in the acute pediatric ward environment, the focus is fixed on the biological aspects of illness, then other aspects may not be seen, such as the importance of play in the lifeworld of the child. Discourse theory provides a way to consider the hegemonic discourse together with other socially constructed discourses.

Descriptions of phenomena may be drawn from several available discourses. Examples of other competing discourses in hospital environment include hospital and organizational discourse, multidisciplinary team discourse, nursing discourse, family discourse, play discourse, and procedural play discourse (Parson, 2008). Play is represented in the literature as the child's way of communicating what he or she knows about the world and is an essential aspect of the child's physical, emotional, cognitive, and social world. Procedural play may be integrated into the child's hospitalization experience and becomes a medium to help assess, plan, implement, evaluate, and reflect upon the child's thoughts and feelings about their medical treatment and pediatric care. However, Parson (2008) found that procedural play was a silenced discourse in hospital settings due to lack of knowledge, understanding, and skills to integrate or action procedural play. In the context of an acute pediatric ward environment, discourses could also include child-centered or family-centered care (Ahmann, 1998), evidence-based practice (Foster, 2004), together with organizational, economic, or political discourses to articulate, or position, discussion regarding the facilitation or inhibition of integrating a specific clinical practice including play therapy. Drawing on discourse theory to construct the meaning of caring for a child with CF may be considered according to subject positioning.

Discourse theory asserts that language positions people, and therefore discourse creates subject positions (Wetherell, 2001). Subject positioning is the flexibility to move within and between available discourses, and the factors that facilitate or inhibit flexibility depend on power relationships and the context where interactions occur (Hardin, 2001; Sundin-Huard, 2001). The transitory nature of subject positioning provides the richness to view context and culture through discourse. The clinician can then consider and analyze a variety of subject positions as a point of entry into the discourse. This is the important point that showcases the role of the therapist in being able to move between subject positions to translate and communicate play as a language and to promote the voice of the child. One such subject position is the therapeutic language and stance that therapists use to engage the child through play.

Therapeutic Positioning

Play therapists are mindful of the lifeworld of the whole child. This means that they are cognizant of the child's past and present, and how the medical condition has impacted on all domains of the child's life, including physiological, psychological, emotional, social, and spiritual health and well-being. Consideration is given to whether or not the medical condition is a source of concern for mental health or if psychopathology impacts on the medical condition. This is an important point of difference, as some health care professionals may prioritize the physical body, attend to activities of daily living, such as feeding, toileting, and providing medical care, and have limited time to prioritize and 'be present' to the child's psychosocial health care and need to play. However, all hospital personnel could develop and model relational skills by adopting a humanistic stance. Play therapists develop and integrate a therapeutic approach by communicating through their skills in providing the core conditions: unconditional positive regard, empathy, and congruence as described by Rogers (1961). Axline (1947) provided an extension of Rogers's work by developing the Eight Basic Principles, which include that the therapist:

1. Develops a warm, friendly relationship with the child
2. Accepts the child exactly as they are
3. Establishes a feeling of permissiveness within the relationship so the child can fully express their thoughts and feelings
4. Attunes to the child's feelings and reflects these back to help the child gain insight into their behavior
5. Respects the child's ability to solve their own problems, leaving responsibility to make choices
6. Tries not to direct the child's behavior or conversation, but rather the therapist follows the child's lead
7. Tries not to attempt to rush therapy and recognizes that therapy may be a gradual therapeutic process
8. Sets only limits that anchor the child to reality or make the child aware of responsibilities in the relations.

While it is not always possible to employ all eight principles in short-term hospital admissions, it is possible to generate the attitudinal approach that facilitates the humanistic stance. Medical play therapists must quickly establish a therapeutic relationship and be mindful of the lifeworld of the child and the support systems around the child in the hospital setting. Nursing and medical play therapist literature seem to align to support the child using a humanistic approach.

MEDICAL PLAY THERAPY

Medical play therapy is similar to the humanistic approach to play therapy, with the added dimension of an acute or chronic medical ailment/diagnosis. In medical play therapy, the focus is always on the child first and how the diagnosis may impact on the child's physical condition and in relation to the child's mental health and well-being. The physical condition may either exacerbate the child's emotional responses or may be the source of distress. Therefore, therapists need to understand the child's interpretation of what this means to them and how they will respond to medical treatment.

To do this, the same play therapy skills and techniques are used to develop a secure and trusting relationship. The child cannot play if he or she is scared. Play is the child's voice! This is particularly important in the care of the child patient with CF, because the relationship is established from the very first admission to hospital and built upon with every subsequent hospitalization encounter over the years. As Parson (2008) identified, nurses who integrate procedural play into their clinical practice may quickly observe the short-term benefits to the child patient and may even witness the long-term benefits. It needs to be acknowledged that

> every moment creates the context in which the next moment will take place. And the immediate context is crucial in determining the direction and final form of what will happen. In other words, each present moment influences the destiny of where things will go next. And the next moment will serve as the context for the moment that follows, and so on.
>
> (Stern, 2004, p. 367)

The nursing and family discourses become visible at the site of interpersonal interaction before, during, and after medical treatment. Within the social milieu of the play relationship, Parson (2008) listed a number of facilitating factors that influenced successful integration of procedural play. These findings centered on positive relationship values of trust, honesty, understanding, acceptance, and friendship. Nurses understood the importance of gaining the child's trust and the negative impact caused by losing the child's trust in their relationship with the child and the child's family.

Crole and Smith (2002) identified four phases of nursing care of the hospitalized child, namely, the introductory phase, the building trusting relationship phase, the decision-making phase, and the comfort and reassurance phase. While play and trust are featured in all phases, in the second phase of building a trusting relationship, play is strongly encouraged, for both the child and the nurse.

> Building trusting relationships with children is achieved through a nurse's use of appropriate language, games and play, adequate preparation of a child for procedures, and providing explanations and encouragement . . . A child will be more trusting of nurses who are willing to get down on their level and play on their terms. Play has many benefits for both children and nurses. Play can be a normalising experience for children in hospital. It may enhance development and prevent regression resulting from stressful experiences.
>
> (Crole & Smith, 2002, p. 30)

Crole and Smith (2002) state that if trust is not established or is impeded, it becomes more difficult to obtain the child's cooperation. The potential for losing trust occurs when the child's sense of autonomy is damaged, for example by being physically or chemically restrained for treatment (McGrath, Irving, & Rawson-Huff, 2000). This issue is also raised in another Australian study. Bricher (1999) identifies a dilemma in the child–nurse trust relationship, whereby trust is seen as particularly important by nurses, but breaking trust was seen as essential for completing clinical procedures. She goes on to state that little is known about the types of strategies used to develop trust or how they repair damaged relationships (Bricher, 1999). Parson (2008) identified that nurses were aware that play strategies facilitated the establishment of trust and that nurses were aware of the link between general play and procedural play for establishing and repairing trust in the child–nurse relationship. Preventing the loss of trust is the ideal, but if trust is lost, then post-procedural play may also help to re-create and preserve the relationship. More research into the complexity of these play interactions is warranted to understand the short-term and long-term development of the establishment and maintenance of the child–nurse or child–therapist trust relationship.

All health care professionals should, therefore, be aware that for every clinical decision made and acted upon, consequences will follow. If the child is offered procedural play within a trusting relationship, subsequent procedural experiences will be anticipated according to the child's prior experiences. During an invasive procedure, decision making occurs rapidly and highlights the importance of developing the trusting relationship through procedural play. If at any stage trust is lost during a procedure, it is important to allow time to re-establish the trust relationship (Crole & Smith, 2002).

> A person [parent] cannot be committed to a child unless other people [nurses] are committed to that person's commitment to children.
>
> (Bronfenbrenner cited in Grille, 2005, p. 361)

This statement acknowledges and positions the lifeworld of the child as dependent not only on the child's family, but also on the people supporting the family in caring for the child. In terms of procedural play, parents depend on their own abilities and previous experiences to support their child through the current procedural experience. The health care professionals should act as the support people to work with the child through this family-focused framework.

> Family-centred care can be literally defined as placing the needs of the child, in the context of their family and community, at the centre of care and devising an individualized and dynamic model of care in collaboration with the child and family that will best meet these needs.
>
> (MacKean, Thurston, & Scott, 2005, p. 75)

Modern parents are more participatory in the care of their children when compared with previous generations. The literature indicates that parental participation and involvement is central to their child's hospitalization experience. Early work stemming from the Platt Report of 1959 into the Welfare of Children in Hospital (United Kingdom) indicates that parental presence is vital for children to cope with hospitalization (Darbyshire,

1994; Harvey, 1980; Livesley, 2005; Shields, 2000). Since expanding visiting hours to include parental living-in, further demands have been placed on parents to become more involved in the care of their children. This transition has increased from parental access, to participation in the usual parent–child tasks such as bathing and feeding, to more technical nursing roles such as assisting with invasive procedures in hospitals (Melnyk, 1994; Piira, Sugiura, Champion, Donnelly, & Cole, 2005), to operating complex machinery in the home (Jamieson & Wilson, 1997). Parents now share the tasks of preparing and treating their children with the nursing staff and hospital-based play therapists. Parents know their children intimately and are the most appropriate human resource to help staff assess and plan for their child's needs.

Recommendations have previously been documented to include the concept of the child–parent dyad as a singular patient unit during any interaction with a health care service (Shields & Nixon, 2004). However, not all parents are able to be physically and/or emotionally present for their children in hospital (Livesley, 2005). It is important to acknowledge that sharing of roles within the care triad has added additional burdens to both parents, as co-workers, and nurses, in providing parental support and education to parents as co-clients (Callery, 1997). Health care professionals should not expect that parents have the skills to independently prepare their children. In an Australian study, Goodenough, Thomas, Champion, Perrott, Taplin, von Baeyer, and Ziegler (1999) identified that in one-quarter of children requiring venipuncture, the child had not been told by their parent that they were about to have a blood test. During the assessment phase of preparing a child for an invasive procedure, nurses ought to identify and build on the information, if any, which has already been imparted to the child. Parents also require sound education regarding their role in assisting with their child's procedures. The literature also states that some parents are not always able to assist their child in coping because of their heightened anxiety, which can be transmitted to the child (Barrera, 2000). Hence, part of the pre-procedural planning must incorporate assessing the parents' abilities and desire to assist in providing procedural care.

To further enhance the effectiveness of procedural preparation, it has been suggested that making the child and parent more active participants in the learning process might lead to more clinically significant outcomes (Peterson & Shigetomi, 1981). Leblanc and Ritchie (2001) demonstrate that parental participation and involvement in play therapy do indeed provide a significantly higher predictor of a positive outcome. However, this participation has taken longer to be integrated into acute health care encounters. One concern that health care professionals expressed was that parental presence would reduce procedural efficiency and increase parental distress. However, Bauchner, Vinci, Bac, Pearson, and Corwin (1996) conducted a randomized controlled trial to determine the effect of a parent-focused intervention on pain and performance of an invasive procedure, anxiety of parents and clinicians, and parental satisfaction with care. While this study did not reveal a reduction in pain during procedures, it did indicate that parental presence did not negatively affect performance of the procedure or increase clinician anxiety. In fact, this study demonstrated that parents who were present were less anxious than parents who were absent. This is further supported in a systematic review of the literature, when Piira et al. (2005) found that there are potential advantages for parents, that is, less parental distress and parents more satis-fied due to being present during medical procedures, however the benefits to the child remain unclear.

Parson (2008) found that nurses' awareness of the child's developmental attri-butes and an ability to assess the child's individual attributes positively influenced the integration of procedural play within the care triad. This may be because chil-dren cope better with adult guidance. A significant increase in both parent and child coping was demonstrated when parents were supplied with information about the child's procedure (Melnyk, 1994). However, the majority of children undergo-ing painful, invasive procedures do not engage in effective coping strategies unless prompted to do so by an adult (Barrera, 2000; Broome, 2000). Children require an understanding of what is happening to them and an ability to be distracted so that pain perception is reduced (Broome, 2000). One study examined the efficacy of training children to cope with immunization pain with or without the assistance of a breathing technique and positive self-statements (Cohen, Bernard, Greco, & McClellan, 2002). In this study children demonstrated an understanding of the tech-niques, but they did not use the coping skills during the procedure. The authors offered several reasons for this outcome, but supported the understanding that chil-dren need the guidance of adults to cope with procedural experiences. This indi-cates that nurses and parents are in a position to plan developmentally appropriate pre-procedural educational play, as well as individualized strategies from the child's perspective to cope with the procedure.

While family-centered care is a valued, collaborative and respectful model of care in pediatrics conceptually, interpretation and implementation of family-centered care differs among individuals and institutions (Regan, Curtin, & Vorderer, 2006). The lit-erature identifies that the practice of family-centered care is not routinely safeguarded by policy and procedures within the National Health Service in Britain (Walker, 1999) or in the United States (Regan et al., 2006). Peden-McAlpine, Tomlinson, Forneris, Genck, and Meiers (2005) found one way to integrate family-centered care philosophy into pediatric wards was to use a family-focused, reflective practice intervention. The researchers found that nurses who participated in the intervention:

- Acknowledged and re-framed preconceived ideas about families
- Recognized the meaning of family stress
- Began to incorporate the family into nursing care.

This led to change in the nurses' attitudes about family, enhanced their communication skills and their ability to build trusting relationships with families, and brought about a new appreciation of the uniqueness of family stress (Peden-McAlpine et al., 2005).

Acknowledging that parents are co-workers within a care triad has demonstrated a shift in the power relationship of caring for hospitalized children. Parents are an impor-tant human resource that health care professionals ought to utilize for assessing and preparing children for medical procedures. Parents should also have the choice to be involved (or not) in preparing and assisting with procedural play with the aim of pro-viding family-centered care. This has highlighted the great importance of developing a trusting relationship with the child patient and his or her family, and one way this can be achieved is through a successful procedural play interaction.

It is important to understand the discourse of play in relation to other discourses found within the hospital environment. The powerful biomedical discourse needs to acknowledge general play and procedural play. Parson (2008) states that play is a fragile, unspoken discourse in hospital settings. It is explicitly understood that play is difficult to define due to the many complex and varied definitions available, and may be one reason why procedural play is silenced. However, the benefits of play have been well-established in educational literature (Honig, 2006). It forms the basis of learning, creative thinking, problem solving, the ability to cope with tensions and anxieties, acquiring new understandings, the ability to use tools, and the development of language (Christie & Johnsen, 1983; Piaget, 1972; Rothleim & Brett, 1987). Play offers children the opportunity to express, both verbally and non-verbally, their thoughts and feelings (Wittenborn, Faber, Harvey, & Thomas, 2006). However, and most importantly, the value of play in hospital has been clearly recognized over the past century (Murphy, 1910).

Children with CF are vulnerable to emotional distress, pain, anxiety, fear, and procedural trauma, and therefore these factors highlight the need for therapeutic play interventions through procedural play. It is from this position that the potential positive integration of play and specific procedural play may be built. As stated earlier, the clinician may consider and analyze a variety of subject positions as a point of entry into the discourse. In practice, this means the entry point is based on the lifeworld of the child and how the child is presenting in real time. To do this, the following case describes one assessment to help facilitate an entry point to commence therapeutic engagement.

JAIME: A CASE DISCUSSION

The pediatric ward manager notifies me that Jaime, an 11-year-old boy, is about to be admitted. Jaime is well-known to staff, with his charismatic personality and incredibly brave persona due to his routine visits to the CF clinic since his birth and recurring admissions to the pediatric ward in the general hospital in regional Australia. He is familiar with the ward environment and is able to navigate his way through admission to an awaiting bed. He knows he is being hospitalized for elective surgery "to have a port put in." An implanted port, or port-a-cath, is a device that is inserted to allow for frequent and long-term access to the bloodstream (Cystic Fibrosis Foundation, 2016). Because Jaime has to have an upcoming extensive medication treatment, the port will allow for repeated antibiotics, IV nutrition, and other IV fluids. When he gets his port placed, he will not need repeated peripheral IV catheters put in; instead the port is accessed. Thus, while it may be initially more painful than a regular IV catheter, it is anticipated that the pain will be reduced for a year or two.

CF affects 1 in every 2,500 births and is one of the most serious genetic diseases in Australian children today (Lai, Cheng & Farrell, 2005). It is an autosomal recessive genetic disease that affects the exocrine glands of the body, and is characterized by abnormal airway secretions, chronic endobronchial infection, and progressive airway obstruction (Mogayzel et al., 2013). This means that people with CF produce thick mucus, which eventually clogs the lungs and may lead to a variety of lung infections. It also affects the exocrine glands in the pancreas, which deactivates the digestive enzymes to break down and absorb food. However, the most common reason children are admitted into hospital is for the administration of intravenous antibiotics and intensive physiotherapy to treat respiratory exacerbations of CF, commonly referred to as a 'tune-up' (Parson, 2014). For more information about CF, visit https://cysticfibrosisnewstoday.com.

Jaime's first admission to the ward was when he was 2 years old, and since then he averaged one or two admissions per year. He lives with his mother, Margaret, and father, Robert, and two younger sisters, Beth (7 years) and Sarah (5 years). Neither of his sisters has CF, but each has a 50% chance of being a carrier of the CF gene. Jaime's parents must manage their time very carefully to meet the needs of all family members. However, Margaret assumes most of the parenting responsibilities and is the primary carer for Jamie and his sisters. Robert works full-time as a lawyer and often stays at work late into the evening. Developmentally, like most children, Jaime was advanced in some areas and lagged behind in others. Academically, his teacher reported that Jaime was a fairly bright student, he was more of a visual learner and preferred electronic media compared to reading or writing. He likes to create, draw, and paint, and engage in a range of art activities, but he said that "I don't think I am very good at it." Physically, he is thinner and shorter than his peers. He does not enjoy sport, because as soon as he starts to play he would often cough, and cough, and cough, and he didn't like it when other children looked at him. Recently, he discovered that he liked surfing, which had the added bonus of helping him to breathe in the fresh, salty air. Margaret said that she was so pleased that he liked it, and it was a sport that would help him in the long term.

According to the Cystic Fibrosis Foundation, it seems that surfing can extend the life of people suffering from CF. Australian doctors observed that young surfers with cystic fibrosis had significantly healthier lungs. He had been introduced to surfing through a school friend, Frank, who had another friend with CF. Frank had been upset to hear that Jaime had CF because his other friend had died. According to Margaret, Jaime seemed preoccupied with death since he had heard about the other boy with CF who had died because of a bad respiratory infection.

While the admission focus was on inserting the port, an assessment was required to ascertain the most appropriate educational procedural play plan. So in order to understand Jaime's coping strengths, it was suggested to draw a six-part story, based on Mooli Lahad's (1992) BASIC Ph method. I asked him to draw a story that had six pictures; this prompted him to divide the page into six boxes, and he was guided to draw as follows (see Figure 3.1):

1. A main character hero or heroine
2. Identify a task or mission
3. Who or what helps the main character
4. Who or what are obstacles to prevent the task or mission being accomplished
5. How does the main character deal with the obstacle
6. Then what happens next.

Jaime then drew from top left to right in relation to the numbers 1, 2, and 3 and bottom left to right as numbers 4, 5, and 6.

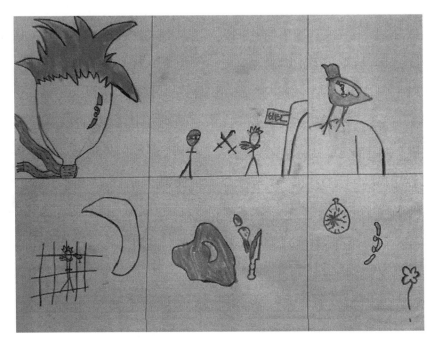

FIGURE 3.1 Jaime's Cartoon

Once he completed the drawings without interruption, Jaime then described each drawing based on the six aspects in the list and stated:

> Once upon a time there was a boy named Frisk and he has blonde hair and a vibrant red scarf and a blue tattoo on his face. The tattoo was given to him at birth. He lived for over 100 years in the form of a 14 year old. Frisk feels like a caged bird, he appears happy enough but on the inside, he is truly emotionless. His mission is to protect and do jobs for the village. The village is called Tatakai.
>
> Frisk's companion is a brightly colored red bird with a black collar and she has the same tattoo on her wing that Frisk has on his cheek. The bird is called Chiara, pronounced Cara. Chiara is part of Frisk and contains Frisk's emotions and is like his soul. She is not able to fly. Because of the tattoo, Frisk cannot leave the village at night. To stop this from happening he carved off the skin that had the tattoo on it. The tattoo, whilst it keeps him inside the village at night, it also prevented him from dying. He wanted to experience what night-time was like and he had lived a very long time and he thought it was time to do so. When this happened Chiara could fly. But after he carved off the tattoo he knew that in three years' time, Frisk would finally die.

Additional clarifying information was provided by Jaime after the story was narrated.

> Frisk's mother gave him the scarf which she sewed herself and soon afterward she had given it to him she died in a war. The village was always at war. Frisk's father was a warrior too and he died in the same war. The village chief, Puro, raised Frisk to be a protector of the village.

The BASIC Ph is an acronym that emerged from the various aspects that the six-part story method assessment measures, which represent the following: Belief, Affect, Social, Imagination, Cognition, and Physical (see Table 3.1). Each domain has particular strengths and is useful to inform the therapist how the child's coping strategies may be enhanced. The story is scored based on the contents of the story. For Jaime's story, a lot of information (cognition) is given in the details about the main character Frisk and his companion Chiara. In this case, it can be hypothesized that his coping strength focused on cognition and social, then to a lesser degree drawing on beliefs and physical elements, and finally with

TABLE 3.1 The Integrative Model References

Domain	Theorist	Domain	Skills & Subskills
Belief (B)	Frankl (1963) Maslow (1962)	Self, ideology	Attitudes Beliefs Life span Value clarification Meaning
Affect (A)	Freud (1933) Rogers (1951)	Emotions	Listening skills Emotions Ventilation Acceptance Expression of feelings (verbal and non-verbal)
Social (S)	Adler (1956) Erikson (1963)	Roles, others, organizations	Social role systems Social skills Assertiveness Groups role-play Simulations
Imagination (I)	De Bono (1992) Jung (1977)	Intuition, humor	Creativity Play Psychodrama 'As if' symbols Guided imagery/fantasy
Cognition (C)	Ellis (1994) Lazarus and Folkman (1984)	Reality, knowledge	Information Order of preference Problem solving Self-navigation Self-talk
Physical (Ph)	Pavlov (1927) Watson (1924)	Action, practical	Activities Games Exercise Relaxation Eating Work

Source: Adapted from Lahad and Leykin (2013)

limited or silenced affect. This final aspect is interesting as it is also reflected in the story as well. This first phase of the assessment process is useful to provide an understanding of the child's coping style. For more information about scoring and the full and subsequent assessment steps, read Ayalon, Lahad, and Shacham (2013).

Therefore, in order to engage Jaime in play-based interventions, a cognitive approach would be the most aligned. Psychoeducational information giving and open discussion would be of benefit to explore the concepts of death and dying. Using a humanistic approach to acknowledge Jamie's concern and worries about death and dying, he subsequently led to an open discussion. He revealed that he didn't want to talk to his Mum or Dad because he didn't want to upset them, and wanted to protect his parents because they would think it was their fault. He said he felt all alone. This discussion led to providing some of the facts about the life expectancy of people living with CF. The life expectancy of individuals with CF has increased in the last few decades, and since 2014 for the first time in Australia there are more adults with CF than children (CF Foundation, 2016). Acknowledging that no one really knows when they will die, I could provide some hope, and informed Jaime about other children and young people living with CF, including a man I personally knew who at the time was 65 years old, and that although he had to have a lung transplant, he was happily living in a regional part of Australia. This conversation then led to a discussion about Jaime's newfound love of surfing and how doctors were looking into how surfing has been noted to help people with CF have healthier lungs. Finally, procedural play in the form of psychoeducation was provided to prepare Jaime for his port insertion.

Personal Reflections

I believe that children have a right to health care treatment that is genuinely child- and family-centered. Children have the right to be informed in a developmentally sensitive and age-appropriate manner about any procedures that may be performed on them while in hospital. As a registered nurse, I had to find ways to help children cope with their experiences. To do this, I often asked the child or their family how I could best help him or her. While the child did not always have the words to be able to tell me, and sometimes the parent could not either, I closely observed their body language, appearance, expressions, and non-verbal communications. I intuitively knew that if the child could eat, drink, and breathe, they always strived to play. Play became my ally, my go-to point of entry to engage the child. Jaime was able to draw a story, then find words to project onto the drawing, real-time thoughts and feelings about Frisk and Chiara. He was working in the metaphor, and what a creative and heart-wrenching metaphor was communicated. I hypothesized that Jaime too felt alone in his thoughts and feelings about death and dying. However, by being present to the needs of Jaime's emotional pain, in the context of his lifeworld, provided an entry point through the BASIC Ph assessment. I understood it was more important at that time to facilitate the discussion of death and dying, otherwise the procedural education would not be heard. Jaime had developed many relationships with hospital staff, including myself, and found a safe space through the creative expression of play to explore his thoughts and feelings about death and dying.

SUMMARY

Discourse theory provides a lens to review and reflect on the dominant biomedical model at the site of the marginalized and silenced discourse of play and procedural play in the hospital setting. The inclusion of assessments, such as Mooli Lahad's (1992) six-part story method, may be useful for therapists to facilitate psychoeducational and therapeutic play because it focuses on the child's strengths and coping capacity. This chapter included one of Jaime's stories to introduce the first phase of this method. Even though Jaime had already experienced multiple admissions to the regional hospital and had an understanding of the system, use of the six-part story method (BASIC Ph) provided an entry point into the lifeworld of Jaime. He was able to explore death through the metaphor, which had been worrying him. Once this was acknowledged, he was able to hear the preparatory information being given to him about his port insertion. This demonstrates that holistically evaluating the child's development is important when considering implementation of play-based therapeutic interventions.

REFERENCES

Ahmann, E. (1998). Examining assumptions underlying nursing practice with children and families. *Paediatric Nursing, 24,* 467–469.

Axline, V. (1947). *Play therapy.* New York: Ballantine.

Ayalon, O., Lahad, M., & Shacham, M. (2013). *The "BASIC Ph" model of coping and resiliency: Theory, research and cross-cultural application.* London: Jessica Kingsley.

Barrera, M. (2000). Procedural pain and anxiety management with mother and sibling as co-therapists. *Journal of Pediatric Psychology, 25*(2), 117–121.

Bauchner, H., Vinci, R., Bac, S., Pearson, C., & Corwin, M. (1996). Parents and procedures: A randomised control trial. *Pediatrics, 98*(5), 861–868.

Bombardier, Lauren. (2010). *If I never had CF.* Retrieved December 2016 from: https://cysticlife.org/BlogProfile.php?id=488

Bricher, G. (1999). Paediatric nurses, children and the development of trust. *Journal of Clinical Nursing, 8,* 451–458.

Broome, M. (2000). Helping parents support their child in pain. *Pediatric Nursing, 26*(3), 315–317.

Callery, P. (1997). Caring for parents of hospitalized children: A hidden area of nursing work. *Journal of Advanced Nursing, 26,* 992–1008.

Christie, J., & Johnsen, E. (1983). The role of play in social-intellectual development. *Review of Educational Research, 53*(1), 93–115.

Clifton-Soderstrom, M. (2003). Levinas and the patient as other: The ethical foundation of Medicine. *Journal of Medicine and Philosophy, 28*(4), 447–460.

Cohen, L. L., Bernard, R. S., Greco, L. A., & McClellan, C. B. (2002). A child-focused intervention for coping with procedural pain: Are parent and nurse coaches necessary? *Journal of Pediatric Psychology, 27*(8), 749–757.

Crole, N., & Smith, L. (2002). Examining the phases of nursing care of the hospitalised child. *Australian Nursing Journal, 9*(8), 30–31.

Cystic Fibrosis Foundation. (2016). *Vascular access devices: PICCs and ports.* Retrieved December 2016 from: www.cff.org/Life-With-CF/Treatments-and-Therapies/Medications/Vascular-Access-Devices-PICCs-and-Ports

Danaher, G., Schirato, T., & Webb, J. (2000). *Understanding Foucault*. Sydney: Allen & Unwin.

Darbyshire, P. (1994). *Living with a sick child in hospital: The experiences of parents and nurses* (1st ed.). London: Chapman & Hall.

Foster, R.L. (2004). Partnering with children and families for evidence-based practice. *Journal for Specialists in Pediatric Nursing, 9*(1), 3–5.

Foucault, M. (1981). The order of discourse. In R. Young (Ed.), *Untying the text: A post structuralist reader* (pp. 48–78). Boston: Routledge & Kegan Paul.

Gee, J. (2014). *An introduction to discourse analysis: Theory and method*. Abingdon, Oxon and New York: Routledge.

Geller, S.M. (2013). Therapeutic presence: An essential way of being. In M. Cooper, P.F. Schmid, M. O'Hara & A.C. Bohart (Eds.), *The handbook of person-centered psychotherapy and counselling* (2nd ed., pp. 209–222). Basingstoke: Palgrave.

Goodenough, B., Thomas, W., Champion, G.D., Perrott, D., Taplin, J.E., von Baeyer, C.L., & Ziegler, J.B. (1999). Unravelling age effects and sex differences in needle pain: Ratings of sensory intensity and unpleasantness of venipuncture pain by children and their parents. *Pain, 80*(1–2), 179–190.

Grbich, C.F. (2004). *Health in Australia: Sociological concepts and issues*. Sydney: Pearson Longman.

Grille, R. (2005). *Parenting for a peaceful world*. Alexandria, NSW: Longueville Media.

Haralambos, M., Krieken, R.V., Smith, P., & Holborn, M. (1996). *Sociology themes and perspectives: Australian edition*. Melbourne: Addison Wesley Longman.

Hardin, P.K. (2001). Theory and language: Locating agency between free will and discursive marionettes. *Nursing Inquiry, 8*(1), 11–18.

Harvey, S. (1980). The value of play therapy in hospital. *Paediatrician, 9*(3–4), 191–198.

Honig, A. (2006). What infants, toddlers, and pre-schoolers learn from play: 12 ideas. *Montessori Life, 18*(1), 16–21.

Jamieson, S., & Wilson, S. (1997). *Responding to children with complex health-related care needs: The homecare program*. Paper presented at the AWCH National Conference, October 9–10.

Jenkins, E.K. (2014). The politics of knowledge: Implications for understanding and addressing mental health and illness. *Nursing Inquiry, 21*(1), 3–10.

Lahad, M. (1992). Story-making and assessment method for coping with stress: Six-piece story and BASIC Ph. In S. Jennings (Ed.), *Dramatherapy and practice* (Volume 2, pp. 150–163). London: Routledge.

Lahad, M., & Leykin, D. (2013). Introduction: the integrative model of resiliency The BASIC Ph model of what do we know about survival. *The BASIC Ph model of coping and resiliency—Theory, research and cross-cultural application*, 9–303.

Lahiri, T., Hempstead, S.E., Brady, C. et al. (2016). Clinical practice guidelines from the Cystic Fibrosis Foundation for preschoolers with Cystic Fibrosis. *Pediatrics, 137*(4), e20151784.

Lai, H.J., Cheng, Y., & Farrell, P.M. (2005). The survival advantage of patients with cystic fibrosis diagnosed through neonatal screening: evidence from the United States Cystic Fibrosis Foundation registry data. *Journal of Pediatrics, 147*(3), S57-S63.

Landreth, G. (2012). *Play therapy: The art of the relationship* (3rd ed.). New York: Routledge.

Larkin, M. (2004). *What is social construction?* Retrieved May 24, 2005 from: www.psy.dmu.ac.uk/michael/soc_con_disc.htm

Leblanc, M., & Ritchie, M. (2001). A meta-analysis of play therapy outcomes. *Counselling Psychology Quarterly, 14*(2), 149–163.

Livesley, J. (2005). Telling tales: A qualitative exploration of how children's nurses interpret work with unaccompanied hospitalized children. *Journal of Clinical Nursing, 14*(1), 43–50.

MacKean, G. L., Thurston, W. E., & Scott, C. M. (2005). Bridging the divide between families and health professionals' perspectives on family-centred care. *Health Expectations, 8*(1), 74–85.

McGrath, P., Irving, H., & Rawson-Huff, N. (2000). The preferred option: General anaesthetic for paediatric lumbar puncture. *Cancer Strategy, 2*, 69–75.

Melnyk, B. (1994). Coping with unplanned childhood hospitalization: Effects of informational interventions on mothers and children. *Nursing Research, 43*(1), 50–55.

Mogayzel, P., Naureckas, E., Robinson, K., Mueller, G., Hadjiliadis, D., Hoag, J., . . . Marshall, B. (2013). Cystic Fibrosis pulmonary guidelines chronic medications for maintenance of lung health. *American Journal of Respiratory and Critical Care Medicine, 187*(7), 680–689.

Moustakas, C. (1997). *Relationship play therapy.* Lanham, MD: Jason Aronson.

Murphy, L. M. (1910). Entertaining sick children. *American Journal of Nursing*, 734–736.

Nabors, L., Bartz, J., Kichler, J., Sievers, R., Elkins, R., & Pangallo, J. (2013). Play as a mechanism of working through medical trauma for children with medical illnesses and their siblings. *Issues in Comprehensive Pediatric Nursing, 36*(3), 212–224. https://doi.org/10.3109/01460862.2013.812692

Parson, J. (2008). *Integration of procedural play for children undergoing cystic fibrosis treatment: A nursing perspective.* Doctor of Philosophy, Central Queensland University, Rockhampton.

Parson, J. (2009). Play in the hospital environment. In K. Stagnitti & R. Cooper (Eds.), *Play as therapy: Assessment and therapeutic interventions* (pp. 132–144). London: Jessica Kingsley.

Parson, J. (2014). Holistic mental health care and play therapy for hospitalized, chronically ill children. In E. Green & A. Myrick (Eds.), *Play therapy with vulnerable populations: No child forgotten* (pp. 124–136). Lanham: Rowman & Littlefield.

Peden-McAlpine, C., Tomlinson, P. S., Forneris, S. G., Genck, G., & Meiers, S. J. (2005). Evaluation of a reflective practice intervention to enhance family care. *Journal of Advanced Nursing, 49*(5), 494–501.

Peterson, L., & Shigetomi, C. (1981). The use of coping techniques to minimize anxiety in hospitalized children. *Behavior Therapy, 12*(1), 1–14.

Piaget, J. (1972). *Play, dreams and imitation in childhood* (C. Gattegno & F. M. Hodgson, Trans. 3rd ed.). London: Routledge & Kegan Paul Ltd.

Piira, T., Sugiura, T., Champion, G. D., Donnelly, N., & Cole, A. S. J. (2005). The role of parental presence in the context of children's medical procedures: A systematic review. *Child: Care, Health and Development, 31*(2), 233–243.

Ray, D. C., & Jayne, K. M. (2016). Humanistic psychotherapy with children. In D. J. Cail, K. Keenan & S. Rubin (Eds.), *Humanistic psychotherapies: Handbook of research and practice* (2nd ed.). Washington, DC: American Psychological Association.

Regan, K. M., Curtin, C., & Vorderer, L. (2006). Paradigm shifts in inpatient psychiatric care of children: Approaching child- and family-centered care. *Journal of Child and Adolescent Psychiatric Nursing, 19*(1), 29–40.

Roehrer, E., Cummings, E., Beggs, S., Turner, P., Hauser, J., Micallef, N., . . . Reid, D. (2013). Pilot evaluation of web enabled symptom monitoring in cystic fibrosis. *Informatics for Health and Social Care, 38*(4), 354–365.

Rogers, C. R. (1961). *On becoming a person.* Boston: Houghton Mifflin.

Rothleim, L., & Brett, A. (1987). Children's, teacher's and parent's perceptions of play. *Early Childhood Research Quarterly, 2*, 45–53.

Shields, L. (2000). *The delivery of family-centred care in hospitals in Iceland, Sweden and England: A report for the Winston Churchill Memorial Trust.* Brisbane: Winston Churchill Trust.

Shields, L., & Nixon, J. (2004). Hospital care of children in four countries. *Journal of Advanced Nursing, 45*(5), 475–486.

Shields, L., Munns, A., Taylor, M., Priddis, L., Park, J., & Douglas, T. (2013). Scoping review of the literature about family-centred care with caregivers of children with cystic fibrosis. *Neonatal, Paediatric & Child Health Nursing, 16*(3), 21.

Stern, D.N. (2004). The present moment as a critical moment. *Negotiation Journal, 20*(2), 365.

Sundin-Huard, D. (2001). Subject positions theory—its application to understanding collaboration (and confrontation) in critical care. *Journal of Advanced Nursing, 34*(3), 376–382.

Turner, B.S. (1987). *Medical power and social knowledge.* London: Sage.

Walker, J. (1999). *The culture of healthcare.* Retrieved November 1, 2003 from: www.nahps.org.uk/Milestones.htm

Wetherell, M. (2001). Themes in discourse research: The case of Diana. In M. Wetherell, S. Taylor & S.J. Yates (Eds.), *Discourse theory and practice: A reader.* London: Sage.

Wittenborn, A., Faber, A., Harvey, A., & Thomas, V. (2006). Emotionally focused family therapy and play therapy techniques. *American Journal of Family Therapy, 34*(4), 333–342.

Wodak, R., Maingueneau, D., & Angermuller, J. (2014). *The discourse studies reader: Main currents in theory and analysis.* Amsterdam: John Benjamins.

PART II

Medical Play With Unique Health Challenges

CHAPTER 4

Play Therapy in Assisting Children With Medical Challenges

David A. Crenshaw and Jillian E. Kelly

> And above all, watch with glittering eyes the whole world around you because the greatest secrets are always hidden in the most unlikely places. Those who don't believe in magic will never find it.
>
> —Roald Dahl, *The Minpins*

This chapter will focus on the authors' experience with treating a range of serious and chronic illnesses in children drawing from a range of cases and conditions. Some of the conditions treated include cancer, obesity, asthma, renal conditions, seizure disorders, and cardiac abnormalities. Play therapy offers some unique advantages in enabling these children to cope with their experiences of painful medical tests and procedures, the disruption to family life, and the confusions and fears about health and well-being. The essential features of play therapy, which include symbolism, containment, metaphor, miniaturization, and externalization, will be addressed throughout the chapter. The authors of this chapter reject the current overemphasis on techniques and wish to focus instead on the rich clinical process created in the play therapy room, notably the therapeutic relationship that provides a corrective relational and developmental experience. This rich therapeutic work is truly an intricately woven tapestry of compassion, warmth, and understanding through play.

The unique features of play therapy combine to create a safe space that allows a child to work with threatening and sensitive material within their window of affect tolerance (Siegel, 2012). In no other form of therapy can the child so effectively regulate the pace of the therapy, giving a vitally needed sense of personal control. This is especially the case with seriously or chronically ill children whose sense of personal control (vital to the mental health of any person) has been shattered.

IMPACT ON CHILD AND FAMILY: INTRODUCTION

When a family member is seriously and/or chronically ill, the resources of the family are monopolized by that ill member, and even more so in the case of a child. A serious and/or chronic illness of a child can challenge the stability of functioning in even the closest knit and loving families. Families that are high functioning prior to the illness can be disrupted and destabilized even when the parents aspire to remain strong and keep the family together, not only for the ill child but for any other children in the family whose needs can only be set aside for a limited period. Of course, in the case of serious illness like childhood cancer, trips back and forth to the hospital can span years in the development of children and may dominate the family story. Although a chronic illness in a child can preoccupy a family and challenge their resources to an extreme degree, we should not overlook the other side of the equation and forget about the amazing resilience seen sometimes in children and families that enable them to overcome even the worst struggles and hardships, and consequently grow stronger.

Research literature is far more abundant in reviewing the consequences of illness in adults, but there is a growing research base in recent years on the consequences of childhood serious medical illness and invasive medical procedures. One important study concluded that the younger the child, the more serious the illness, and the more invasive the procedures, the more likely the child will suffer ongoing adverse effects and post-traumatic stress disorder (Rennick, Johnston, Dougherty, Platt, & Ritchie, 2002). A study of 43 children ages 5–12 undergoing cardiac surgery were at risk of post-traumatic stress disorder, particularly if the intensive care unit (ICU) stay was prolonged (Connolly, McClowry, Hayman, Mahony, & Artman, 2004). In addition, a life-threatening illness has a major impact on the parents of the child. The emotional trauma for the parent may interfere with their ability to nurture and to be attuned in an empathetic way with their sick child. In some cases, the parents may unwittingly distance from the child in a self-protective way (Santacroce, 2003). The crisis created by having a child diagnosed with cancer diminished the capacity of mothers to take care of their other children (Young, Dixon-Woods, Findly, & Heney, 2002). A study of parents of children following the diagnosis of leukemia in their child revealed that 68% of the mothers and 57% of the fathers had moderate to severe post-traumatic stress disorder (Kazak, Boeving, Alderfer, Hwang, & Reilly, 2005). A more recent study with Iranian mothers with a child diagnosed with leukemia found the same level of elevated anxiety, but found that supportive Rogerian psychotherapy was helpful in reducing the anxiety symptoms (Nazari, Moradi, & Sadeghi-Koupaei, 2014). Not surprising was the finding in one study that a primary and urgent need of parents, in addition to emotional support, is information to help the parents understand their child's disease (Fischer, 2001).

Approximately 10%–20% of medically ill children meet criteria for post-traumatic stress disorder, while 25%–30% of medically ill children will develop post-traumatic stress symptoms. Parents of medically ill children manifest even greater frequency of post-traumatic stress symptoms (Forgey & Bursch, 2013). In working with a medically ill child, often the first step is assessment, and typically both the child and family are interviewed separately. It is essential that interviewers in medical settings, typically nurses and medical assistants, are trained in developmentally sensitive methods of asking questions. A guide to conducting such interviews with sensitivity to both developmental and emotional issues of children (Caplan & Bursch, 2013) is recommended to those unfamiliar with interviewing children. Child therapists across many disciplines have learned that the fewer questions asked, the more the child typically shares. When doing an assessment, however, the interviewer must ask questions, but they can do so in a developmentally appropriate format. Play is inherently disarming and allays anxiety, enabling children to engage. Highly anxious children or severely traumatized children often do not play. What we hurried adults tend to forget, including parents, but especially the myriad health professionals swirling about the child, is that even the tone of the medical setting can impact a child's inner experience. What do our facial expressions convey? Are we concurrently documenting at the expense of eye contact and true connectedness? It matters. All of it. The use of 'co-interviewers' such as puppets and other child-friendly adaptations with toys and props will be addressed later in the chapter.

While the interventions in this chapter are centered on individual play therapy and family therapy, including family play therapy, it is important to recognize that play therapy groups are often used in hospitals by child life specialists to enable children to allay their anxieties and fears about their illness, surgery, or other medical procedures (Nabors, Bartz, Kichler, Sievers, Elkins, & Pangallo, 2013). The play therapy is often offered in the larger theoretical frame of family systems theory because the suffering pervades and occupies a central role in the lives of all the family members. Like the findings of Santacroce (2003), Wijnberg-Williams, Kamps, Klip, and Hoekstra-Weebers (2006) found that anxiety was high for parents of children newly diagnosed with cancer. Family systems theory considers the impact of the change in one part of the system affecting the rest of the system. Family systems that have destabilized strongly seek to return to homeostasis. When the destabilization is the result of a serious and/or chronic illness of the child, it is expected that the process of returning to homeostasis will be lengthy and marked by recurrent crises and setbacks. Play therapy offers many compelling advantages in working with the individual child who is ill.

IMPACT ON CHILD AND FAMILY: GUILT, FEAR, ANGER

Normalizing the inevitable guilt, fear, and anger of family members can be a helpful first step. When parents and siblings understand that their fear, anger, and guilt are expected as a fully human response to such a devastating experience of a suffering child, the feelings of shame, loneliness, and isolation may be relieved to some degree. The family members may also feel less alone when parents and children together can share feelings that are kept hidden out of embarrassment and shame. The same is true, of course, of the ill child, who may be included in some family sessions regarding the feelings of each member as they go through such a difficult journey together. The ill child may want to share her/his feelings of being treated 'differently' and the impact this treatment has on their sense of self.

Fear, of course, is a typical feeling of family members that when expressed and shared tends to diminish in comparison to unexpressed emotions that are borne alone by each person. Fear because their child or sibling is ill, and for what is going to happen to the child and their family, and perhaps fear for their own health and mortality. The chronically ill member particularly may benefit from opportunities to share her/his worries, fears about the illness, and the agony of uncertainty when no one knows for sure what comes next or what the long-term future holds. The ill child and other children in the family may fear the unraveling of the family due to the stresses of a seriously or chronically ill child on the parents, especially the mother. High levels of anxiety may be experienced by the children as well as the parents when there is confusion and uncertainty about the diagnosis and prognosis. Parents are in constant search for answers that are sometimes elusive.

Anger is another typical feeling of family members because the life of the family is organized around the sickness of the child that consumes the time, energy, and often finances of the family. The siblings will invariably feel left out and marginalized. Guilt feelings may arise because family members feel angry, while knowing full well it is not the fault of their suffering sibling or in the case of the parents, their child. This would especially be the case if a sibling is suffering from a genetically-linked disease. In the future, play therapists may be working with more families who become aware of their risk for genetic diseases. Mapping the human genome has enabled clinicians to find out who is genetically at risk for some illnesses (McDaniel, 2005). The impact on an individual or family upon learning their genetic vulnerability will vary among individuals and families, of course, and by disease. Diseases like Huntington, a single gene disorder with no known effective treatment, would be devastating in most cases and may be reflected in the low rates of family members seeking testing for the disease (McDaniel, 2005).

IMPACT ON THE FAMILY: PLAY IN FAMILY THERAPY

When families are hurting beyond words, introducing playfulness into a family therapy session can be restorative. This is especially so when one pauses to consider both the tangible and intangibles losses the child and family experiences. When a family member is ill, playfulness may be a remote memory, overshadowed by the gravity and urgency of the current or ongoing health crisis. The ability to laugh, enjoy, and have fun together strengthens the bonds of family, and during illness, the family may simply regard family fun as a luxury they cannot afford to devote such time to. The authors have walked into family sessions when the tension, pain, and grief of the family was unspeakable. In such situations, bringing a balloon in the room (in one instance transforming a medical glove into a turkey balloon) and asking the family to join us in keeping the balloon in the air can momentarily break the grip of the tension, pain, and immobilization of the family.

While it might seem absurd to introduce playfulness in such dire circumstances, when the room is filled with laughter and joyous sounds, we have not found it necessary to explain why we brought the balloon into the session. The therapeutic value of fun and laughter is self-evident. One caution is that we would never want families to feel that we are making light of their grief and pain. Rather we are simply offering them a brief respite from their suffering so that they might be able to approach their grim situation with more imagination and creativity, qualities that tend to be inhibited during times of suffering.

[handwritten: ↘ Discussion board #2 on painting act. a Ronald McD house]

CASE VIGNETTES: INTRODUCTION

My (JEK) interest in play therapy was cultivated while stumbling upon an internship at a children's hospital in Ireland. Curious about how to better support families from rural settings who passed long days, weeks, and months in a city hospital due to medical treatments for their young children, I had ventured to Ireland for the summer with the goal of conducting research in the nursing department. But it was on the standard-issue guided tour of the hospital that I found the most magical of places: the play room. Being part of that magical space became my primary goal. It was there that I marveled at the therapeutic powers of play in aiding children's ability to cope, heal, and smile during incredibly challenging life experience. What a remarkable experience it was to find that the innocence and beauty of childhood continued within the confines of a hospital and among all the unknowns brought about by chronic or serious illness.

Each play room had its own unique design and specific toy selection based on the unit's specialty (e.g., oncology, burns, cardiology), but the purpose of each room was the same: to give children and their families a moment of spontaneous, non-demanding, and untethered joy. And to invite children to pick and choose what they wanted to play with and how they wanted to play with it, and for the parents to watch in delight *[handwritten: normalize]* as their child smiled a bright smile during times of otherwise great despair was inspiring. The play rooms were large and bright. And although most of the children were limited in their mobility, their imaginations were boundless. They could, and did, go anywhere. Were they pirates on a ship? Of course! A penguin on an iceberg? You bet. A princess escaping a dragon? Sure thing! They were patients on journeys full of painful symptoms and arduous medical treatments. They were patients who, if only for a few moments, were magically transformed into bold pirates, brave penguins, heroic princesses, and fire-breathing dragons. In listing the key unique features of play therapy here, the authors wish to credit the wisdom and teaching of Dr. Eliana Gil, who has spoken frequently about the rich process variables in play therapy in her many writings and teachings.

Symbolic Play

Children seek mastery through play when experiences or emotions are overwhelming. *[handwritten: The physical movement to the playroom in and of itself was a mood boost]* The symbolism may be disguised to the degree necessary to allow a child to safely engage in repeated attempts at mastery without getting overwhelmed or disrupted in the play. Using stuffed animals, puppets, and miniatures can serve to aid in a child's understanding of what will happen to his or her body during specific treatments or surgeries. Family puppet play is a favorite of the authors as it engages the family in meaningful dialogue often kept at a distance. The Family Puppet Interview (FPI), initially created by Irwin and Mallory (1974) and adapted by Gil (1994), asks each family member to choose a puppet, and then instructs the family to make up an original story with a beginning, middle, and end. The family members can be encouraged to perform a puppet show, a poem, or even a rap song! During this time, the therapist observes the family members' level of enjoyment and engagement, communication patterns, structural issues, and leadership styles (Gil & Sobol, 2000). Staying within the metaphor, the therapist may directly question each puppet or perhaps observe how the puppets work together and solve problems big and small.

Containment

Containment within symbolic play provides a framework for playing out traumatic events or particularly painful experiences such as grief in a way that does not overwhelm. There is no need to protect others, such as family members whose own pain might inhibit the child's expression of their pain and distress. That which is created through play and art orders and communicates the child's experience of illness in a way that is honest, creative, and safe. Charles Sarnoff was a pioneer in studying latency-aged (school-age) children and understanding the play of children from a psychodynamic framework. In the classic book, *Latency* (Sarnoff, 1976), the issue of containment with symbolism in play was discussed in depth. Sarnoff recommended that play therapists monitor the play closely for signs of what he termed "affect porous symbols." Affect porous symbols such as fires, earthquakes, floods, blood, violence, and other catastrophes were signs that the anxiety of the child was breaking through and the therapist may need to shore up the child's defenses, or in the language common today, to build and reinforce the coping resources of the child.

Metaphor

Metaphor is a symbolized form of condensed but precise communication. Play and art therapists are taught to stay with the metaphors created rather than making jarring verbal interpretations of similarities between the metaphors and real life. The magical and wise teachings inherent in metaphor provide gentle guidance and protection during hard times when the search for meaning is challenging for the child, family, and the treatment team. Children often connect to the journey of the caterpillar as it becomes a butterfly through the experience of being in an unknown and frightening darkness before taking shape through a new journey. A lyrical, informative, and tender book by Joyce Mills (2003), *Gentle Willow: A Story for Children About Dying* uses metaphor to describe the stages of illness and death for children who are ill or who have friends who are ill and may not recover from their illness. In the *Pain Getting Better Book* by Mills and Crowley (1986, pp. 174–179), children learn a guided healing process for their suffering with chronic pain. The visual and kinesthetic nature of this tool provides an opportunity for painful sensations to be objectified while also exploring inner resources that are awaiting being accessed. The dissociation that happens while drawing helps alter the physiology of the pain due to its effects on the endorphin system (Mills, 2014).

A clinician can implement this by asking the child to imagine first "how the pain looks right now," then "how the pain looks all better," and finally "what will help picture one change into picture two?" Children can be encouraged to make a notebook and take this to medical visits. When given the opportunity to share a tangible depiction of the pain, the child is moving from the unknown to the known. A child can gain some distance from the pain and imagine it differently. The child's inner resources are actualized. Psychiatrist and medical anthropologist Arthur Kleinman (1988) writes, "The experience when ill need not be self-defeating; it can be—even if it often isn't—an occasion for growth, a point of departure for something deeper and finer, a model of and for what is good" (p. 144). Opportunities abound for play therapists to creatively relate a story line to meet the fears or symptoms the child and family is facing.

Miniaturization *→ pop. of sand trays*

Play therapy offers opportunities for children to work with their "big problems." The very act of working with puppets, putting miniatures in the sand to make a picture, or drawing people or scenes 'shrinks' the problem down to manageable level for children, enabling them to gain mastery. In the community health center settings where I (JEK) have practiced, counseling services are co-located with the medical services. Children, regardless of medical condition, routinely visit for exams and checkups. Having items such as a toy medical kit, bottles of 'medicine,' and similarly frightened puppets allows the child to shrink this big fear down enough to gain mastery of this frightening experience.

Externalization

When children externalize thoughts, feelings, and images that reside internally, some- *and when they "act out" behaviorally* thing important happens in terms of understanding and mastery. Children externalize compelling facets of their inner world when they play. What gets externalized is experienced as more manageable than that which remains internalized. Externalization is particularly important when considering the confusion a child experiences regarding illness and disease.

Case Vignette: Leila

Leila was diagnosed with chronic medical illnesses including intractable epilepsy and right hemiparesis during childhood. She took upwards of 15 pills per day, which produced side effects such as lethargy, bloating, and coarse hair growth. These illnesses caused erratic twitching and shaking and cognitive deterioration, and made fine motor skills like holding a pencil quite difficult. For several days each month, she and her parents would go to the hospital for inpatient procedures and monitoring. Other days she would return to the hospital's outpatient clinic for various scans and checkups. Leila disliked this new medical attention and the many procedures required of her. She was especially oppositional toward her mother and medical staff, and fiercely defiant of the adjustments that had to be made. Leila's problematic behaviors were the visible wounds of inner grief she was experiencing, having lost the ability to participate in the normal activities of childhood because of the need for ongoing medical appointments and procedures. In therapy sessions, she gravitated toward a stuffed bear with wings named Angie. After several sessions of play with Angie, Leila decided it would be a good idea for Angie to take field trips out of the office as support during her medical visits. Leila and her therapist spent some time deciding what Angie would be permitted to do. This discussion allowed for exploration of the rationale for certain expectations of patients—in both child and angel categories—during medical visits, and it enabled Leila to develop insights into her own behavior that would re-define how she presented during medical visits. The therapist asked Leila how she envisioned Angie helping her, and she decided that Angie would be responsible for containing intense feelings during medical visits, and on days Leila was capable of doing that herself, Angie would switch roles to that of a watch-guard for signs of magic. The following session, Leila confidently entered the room. She sat down and asked to use the medical kit. Gathering the kit along with some rubber bands and gauze, Leila intently began repairing the body of Angie, whose arm had fallen off after a heated protest between Leila and medical staff. Leila empathized with the hurt Angie experienced. Using the toy medical kit and various props, she tenderly repaired Angie's wounds. While observing Leila's gentle demeanor, placing Band-Aids and ointment on her fluffy patient, the therapist was struck by the care she took in describing complex medical terminology to her fearful patient. An internal repair process was unfolding as she engaged in this powerful external repair process (Goodyear-Brown, 2010).

Case Vignette: Caitlin

Children who suffer serious medical illness from birth and are expected to have a shortened life span face formidable challenges both physically and psychologically. In addition, families of such a child faced with the chronic stress of life-threatening illness in that child, experience frequent medical follow-ups, ongoing hospitalizations, surgeries, mounting medical bills, and the always present worry of losing a child. Caitlin was born with a serious congenital heart defect that required frequent medical intervention and multiple surgeries, and the strain on her and her family was enormous. Caitlin was angry and demanding, and as a result didn't have many friends, and she often alienated her siblings who alternated between anger and guilt. The strain on her mother resulted in a psychiatric collapse and hospitalization. Her father, although loving and concerned, was a salesperson who traveled often, so he was somewhat buffered from the daily struggles at home. Caitlin, like many chronically ill children, was emotionally functioning at a much younger age than her chronological age of 12. She was prone to quite dramatic temper tantrums when she did not get her way, and became more and more self-focused as her illness resulted in continuing hospitalizations and medical crises. Caitlin had an intuition that the end was coming closer, which she expressed in a picture of a bridge that "led to a better place." She drew herself on the bridge and placed herself about one-third of the way on the bridge in the direction of a better place.

Caitlin frequently drew pictures of hearts expressing love for her mother and her therapist, realizing that she had put a great strain on both but most especially her mother. The price of her congenital heart defect far exceeded the physical pain of her multiple

[handwritten margin note: externalizing anger]

operations and the frequent insertion of needles for IVs that became increasingly difficult and painful due to collapsing veins in her arms. Her therapist saw her during her hospital days as well as for regular outpatient therapy. Often she would rage at her therapist because he was unable to fix the medical problems that had devastated her life. The therapist understood and did his best to validate and contain her rage—after all, where else could she possibly express this degree of anger and disappointment? Close collaboration with her primary physician, a pediatrician, was essential due to the extent of the medical challenges. The therapist received a call from the pediatrician one evening that Caitlin had died and asked that he come to the hospital to console the family. Upon arrival at the hospital, the mother insisted on taking the therapist into the room at the emergency room to view Caitlin's body. No training or graduate course had prepared the therapist for the difficulty of holding a grieving mother as she viewed the lifeless body of her 12-year-old daughter. While the family realized that Caitlin's life could be cut short and the odds of her reaching adult life were slim, still the shock of her sudden death was incredibly difficult. While the family's life was immeasurably less stressful when they no longer were burdened with the care and frequent medical crises with their daughter, her death left a hole in their hearts that is felt keenly and is likely to be felt throughout their lives. The same can be said for her therapist.

[handwritten margin note: boundaries ?]

Case Vignette: Arturo

Six-year-old Arturo was referred for therapy by his pediatrician after reporting symptoms of anxiety secondary to his medical diagnoses of asthma and sleep apnea. Arturo was one of many children in an inner-city community facing a similar combination of medical conditions due to air quality in the area. He used inhalers daily and wore a mask that supplied oxygen nightly. Arturo considered whether he could participate in gym class, the proximity of his inhaler at recess, and whether he could accept an invitation to a sleepover at his friend's home with all his equipment. In addition to his difficulty breathing, one can see how a child might develop somatic and emotional expressions of anxiety about the health and well-being of his body. Asthma is the leading chronic pediatric disease in the United States, with a tremendously high rate in inner-city communities (CDC's National Asthma Control Program). Asthma can be triggered by mold and rodent infestations, a combination found all too frequently in public housing within low income communities. Arturo was drawn to the superheroes within the office, creating scenes of both despair and triumph (Rubin, 2006). During the final stage of treatment, Arturo was encouraged to create his own version of a superhero self. Approaching this directive with a tentativeness initially, Arturo began to construct and re-construct an artistic representation of his own superhero. This superhero representation now resides with and within Arturo, and he often returned to the clinic to share his superhero story with other children newly diagnosed with these conditions.

Case Vignette: Selia

Selia had just turned 10 years old when she was diagnosed with a chronic renal condition, which caused recurrent urinary tract infections and constipation. She experienced great pain urinating and defecating. Selia presented for short-term therapy at our community health center to address feelings of helplessness, shame, sadness, and worry. In school, she experienced frequent accidents, having partially numbed herself from the pain of the physical sensations in her bladder and bowels signaling that it was time to release. Her peers teased her due to the odor that she carried throughout the day. Using dolls and a particularly goofy looking vest with organs affixed to it, she and her therapist playfully explored the magic of the human body. Her therapist wore the vest, which immediately stirred belly laughs from both therapist and child. The intervention helped to externalize, explore confusion, and provide concrete information about the body. The intervention also enabled Selia to visualize her organs as a team, with corresponding names (i.e., Buddy the Bladder and Kaylie the Kidney). Therapy served in the coping with her daily experience of illness, and in developing an understanding of the complex way in which our bodies delicately interact.

PERSONAL REFLECTIONS/COUNTERTRANSFERENCE

The authors share a concern of trivializing the experience of disease and illness through a desire for meaning-making. While meaning-making is surely important during our journey through life, it is not to be forced and is only truly to be found when the fullness and richness of each child and family's story is shared and honored. It is especially important that we honor the suffering of the children and the families we treat. As Maya Angelou tenderly writes, "We delight in the beauty of the butterfly, but rarely admit the changes it has gone through to achieve that beauty." If we do not validate their suffering or show sensitivity to the journey they have taken, they may feel that we simply do not understand. It is also important to be sensitive to the fact that many low-income families embrace a religious faith that they rely on to help them get through hard times. They may express such beliefs such as "the dear Lord doesn't give us more than we can handle." Some well-meaning therapists trained primarily in a cognitive therapy approach might be tempted to challenge the logic of such a belief. This would not only be insensitive but overlooks the robust protective value of spiritual faith in coping with adversity (Miller, 2015). In fact, the research by Miller indicates that in enhancing resilience there is no more powerful factor than spirituality, especially shared spirituality such as spiritual beliefs shared by mothers and children, and grandparents and children. Low-income families also express the belief that they are being tested by their suffering, and take pride in their ability to bear their suffering. If this and similar beliefs were disputed by the therapist based on logic, it could undermine one of the key resources that such families rely on to cope with the harsh realities of their lives.

CONCLUSION

Families facing the challenge of a sick child tend to be acutely stressed. The stress and accompanying symptoms of anxiety, depression, and post-traumatic stress disorder are increased geometrically when more than one family member is ill, when the *acute stress* of illness + other stressors = anxiety dep. PTSD for "any family member

illness of the child(ren) is chronic or life-threatening, and when the family is besieged by other stressors such as financial problems, separation or divorce, substance abuse, and school-related problems in one or more of the children, to name just a few of the problems that families commonly encounter. Not only the ill child but the whole family needs emotional support through the difficult journey. Play therapy offers some unique advantages when combined with family therapy or family play therapy in coping with these severe stresses. Play allows symbolization and metaphor to create safe distance from events too overwhelming to confront directly, along with externalization, playfulness, miniaturization, and containment of affect safely within the confines of the play and family therapy setting. While the child suffering chronic or devastating illness has intense needs that deserve intense focus, the needs and well-being of the rest of the family cannot be ignored. Family therapy and family play therapy expands the focus to include not only the highly stressed parents, but also siblings who may suffer greatly due to the necessary monopolization of the family resources due to illness. It is not unusual for siblings to alternate between anger, guilt, and fear when their brother or sister is dealing with a major illness, and these feelings can be confusing and anguishing at a time when their parent's energy and focus is devoted to their sick child. The work is demanding of the play and family therapist, and close monitoring of countertransference and careful attention to adequate self-care cannot be overemphasized. While professionalism and maintaining proper boundaries per ethical standards of our professions will always be essential, it also critical in the minds of the authors that therapists never lose their humanity. To maintain their humanism while doing what is sometimes heart-wrenching work, the importance of adequate self-care cannot be overemphasized. Everyone doing this work needs to have their own self-care package—one that works for them. While healthy habits of life such as good nutrition, adequate rest and sleep, regular exercise, and nourishing relationships with family and friends are basic ingredients for such a plan, each therapist will need to decide what works for them. We hope that the plan for our readers is full of play, fun, and laughter.

whole family system

REFERENCES

Caplan, R., & Bursch, B. (2013). *"How many more questions?": Techniques for clinical interviews of young medically ill children*. New York: Oxford University Press.

Connolly, D., McClowry, S., Hayman, L., Mahony, L., & Artman, M. (2004). Posttraumatic stress disorder in children after cardiac surgery. *Journal of Pediatrics*, 144(4), 480–484.

Fischer, H.R. (2001). The need of parents with chronically sick children: A literature review. *Journal of Advanced Nursing*, 36(4), 600–607.

Forgey, M., & Bursch, B. (2013). Assessment and management of iatrogenic pediatric medical trauma. *Current Psychiatric Reports*, 15, 340–349.

Gil, E. (1994). *Play in family therapy*. New York: Guilford Press.

Gil, E., & Sobol, B. (2000). Engaging families in therapeutic play. In C.E. Bailey (Ed.), *Children in therapy: Using the family as a resource* (pp. 353–357). New York: W.W. Norton.

Goodyear-Brown, P. (2010). *The worry wars: An anxiety workbook for kids and their helpful adults*. USA: Paris Goodyear-Brown.

Irwin, E.C., & Mallory, E.S. (1974). Family puppet interviews. *Family Process*, 14, 170–191.

Kazak, A., Boeving, A., Alderfer, M., Hwang, W.T., & Reilly, A. (2005). Posttraumatic stress symptoms during treatment in parents of children with cancer. *Journal of Clinical Oncology, 23*(30), 7405–7410.

Kleinman, A. (1988). *The illness narratives: Suffering, healing, & the human condition.* New York: Basic Books.

McDaniel, S.H. (2005). The psychotherapy of genetics. *Family Process, 44,* 25–44.

Miller, L. (2015). *The spiritual child: The new science on parenting for health and lifelong thriving.* New York: St. Martin's Press.

Mills, J. (2003). *Gentle Willow: A story for children about dying.* Washington, DC: Imagination Press.

Mills, J. (2014). *Reconnecting to the magic of life.* USA: Imaginal Press.

Mills, J., & Crowley, R. (1986, 2014). *Therapeutic metaphors for children and the child within* (2nd ed.). New York: Routledge.

Nabors, L., Bartz, J., Kichler, J., Sievers, R., Elkins, R., & Pangallo, J. (2013). Play as a mechanism for working through medical trauma for children with medical illnesses and their siblings. *Issues in Comprehensive Pediatric Nursing, 36*(3), 212–224.

Nazari, S.H., Moradi, N., & Sadeghi-Koupaei, M.T. (2014). Evaluation of the effects of psychotherapy on anxiety among mothers of children with leukemia. *Iran Journal of Child Neurology, 8*(1), 52–57.

Rennick, J.E., Johnston, C.C., Dougherty, G., Platt, R., & Ritchie, J. (2002). Children's psychological responses after critical illness and exposure to invasive technology. *Journal of Developmental and Behavioral Pediatrics, 23*(3), 133–144.

Rubin, L.C. (2006). *Use of superheroes in counseling and play therapy.* New York: Springer.

Santacroce, S.J. (2003). Parental uncertainty and post-traumatic stress in serious childhood illness. *Journal of Nursing Scholarship, 35*(1), 45–51.

Sarnoff, C. (1976). *Latency: Classical psychoanalysis and its applications.* Lanham, MD: Jason Aronson.

Siegel, D. (2012). *The developing mind (2nd ed.): How relationships and the brain interact to shape who we are.* New York: Guilford Press.

Wijnberg-Williams, B.J., Kamps, W.A., Klip, E.C., & Hoekstra-Weebers, J.E. (2006). Psychological distress and the impact of social support on fathers and mothers of pediatric cancer patients: Long-term prospective results. *Journal of Pediatric Psychology, 31*(8), 785–792.

Young, B., Dixon-Woods, M., Findly, M., & Heney, D. (2002). Parenting in a crisis: Conceptualizing of mothers of children with cancer. *Social Science Medicine, 10,* 1835–1847.

Play Therapy With Children With ASD and Chronic Illness

Kevin B. Hull

> Even if my vital spark should be blown out, I believe that I should behave with courageous dignity in the presence of fate, and strive to be a worthy companion of the beautiful, the good, and the true.
>
> —Helen Keller, "The Light of a Brighter Day"

INTRODUCTION

Imagine you are walking in suction cup shoes. It takes all your strength to move just one step because you must reach down and pull your other leg up to take the next step. Your vision is blurred and it is hard to see. People and things are moving past you at very high rates of speed and sometimes they knock into you. You are invisible to them and they are oblivious to you. No one stops to talk to you. Then the pain comes. It slices through your brain and stomach like a chainsaw. It is scary. No one understands. Everyone's voices sound like they are yelling. If someone does talk to you, they just tell you to get out of the way. My mom is sad all the time. She says it is not my fault but I feel like it is. I can't go to school anymore and I miss my friend. I feel like I'm in a castle like a prisoner but I put myself here. This is what it is like to have autism and ulcerative colitis. It is terrible and I hate it (Steven, age 10, describing his life with autism and ulcerative colitis).

The Centers for Disease Control and Prevention (CDC, 2014) state that about 1 in 68 children has been identified with autism spectrum disorder (ASD). Many are unaware of the fact that ASD often co-occurs with other "developmental, psychiatric, neurologic, or medical diagnoses" (Levy et al., 2010, p. 267), and that the co-occurrence of one or more non-ASD developmental diagnoses is an alarming 83% (CDC, 2014). Children who fall into this category are not only struggling with the challenges of ASD, but also with the complications of other diagnoses that cause even more problems for themselves and caregivers. Therapists who are working with children with ASD should be aware of the possibility of a co-occurring disability, which can increase the negative symptoms of ASD and cause significant developmental delays. Also, families of children with ASD and a co-occurring non-ASD diagnosis will experience a significantly higher amount of stress that will affect the family system. Working with families who fall into this category requires extra support and understanding from the therapist.

The purpose of this chapter is twofold. First, to help the reader grasp the magnitude of the challenges associated with being a child living with ASD and a co-occurring psychiatric, neurological, or medical condition, and to understand the stress that is placed on the caregivers and the families of these children. Second, to provide the reader with play therapy techniques that increase the coping skills of the child so that she can move up the developmental ladder as unencumbered as possible. Due to the high percentage of co-occurring diagnoses with autism, it is imperative that play therapists be prepared to work with this unique population. The chapter will present foundational literature and several case examples to demonstrate a picture of the difficulties these children and their families face and how the techniques can be applied in practical ways.

THEORETICAL DISCUSSION

Clinical and Behavioral Features of ASD

ASD is, in and of itself, a baffling bundle of nebulous characteristics. 'Spectrum,' the current term given in the diagnostic and scientific literature, does little to help define ASD or narrow down a specific description. The term does imply that the symptoms of ASD are broad and have much variation among the general population. Some children may appear 'autistic' and have symptoms that seem to stand out to the casual observer, while other children, whose symptoms are just as restricting, may go undetected and undiagnosed. The *Diagnostic and Statistical Manual of Mental Disorders* (5th ed.; *DSM-5*; American Psychiatric Association, 2013) specifies that for an individual to be diagnosed, the person's day-to-day functioning must be impaired due to the condition and the symptoms have been present since early childhood. In addition, all three of the following characteristics must be present:

- *Problems reciprocating social or emotional interaction.* The child tends to live life in a 'one-way' manner, meaning that he only sees a situation from his vantage point. The emotions of another mean little because those are often unnoticed and undetected, as well as misunderstood. Joint attention (sharing in the viewing of an experience) and sharing in back and forth conversations are lacking.
- *Severe problems maintaining relationships.* The child misses the social cues that foster a relationship, such as seeking out another and engaging in behaviors that send signals that the relationship is valued. Conversely, the child may demonstrate an intensity in certain behaviors that push potential friends away. Individuals with

ASD may have difficulty initiating and sustaining conversation and often display a "stiff, plodding, one-sided conversation style" (Hull, 2017, p. 348).

- *Non-verbal communication problems.* The child often has difficulty voicing thoughts and feelings, or when she does voice them, others may find it abrasive and avoid her. Eye contact is often lacking, which may send the signal to a neurotypical individual that he is being ignored. The child often misses the subtle nonverbal cues that neurotypical children develop and rely upon to form and sustain relationships.

Regarding the area of repetitive and restrictive behaviors, two of the following behaviors must be displayed:

- Extreme attachment to routines and patterns and resistance to changes in routines
- Repetitive speech or movements
- Intense and restrictive interests
- Difficulty integrating sensory information or strong seeking or avoiding of sensory stimuli.

(American Psychiatric Association, 2013)

In addition to the diagnostic criteria, there are several co-occurring traits and behaviors that are often seen in individuals diagnosed with ASD. Due to the problems just described, individuals with ASD may appear to lack empathy. However, a truer way of seeing this is that the individual struggles to *show* empathy and communicate his feelings about a certain person or event. A contributing factor is that individuals with ASD sometimes struggle with the ability to grasp the perspective of another's viewpoint, or to identify and recognize another's emotional state. This characteristic is known as Theory of Mind (ToM) or mind-blindness, which Baron-Cohen (1995) states causes individuals with ASD to see other's behaviors as "confusing and unpredictable, even frightening" (p. 69). Children often are observed in social situations as though they are watching from the sidelines, frozen in place and not sure how to join in or what to do. Mind-blindness creates barriers in forming and sustaining relationships and can lead to the child feeling isolated, which can lead to feelings of self-rejection and despair (Hull, 2015).

Understanding one's own emotions and the emotions of others as well as interpreting the emotional state of another person is often a challenge for individuals diagnosed with ASD. Alexithymia, the "inability to recognize and give meaning to emotional signals in oneself and others" (Hull, 2012, p. 16), has many effects on the individual and especially children who are still in various stages of development. Alexithymia can result in chaos when the child with ASD experiences an emotion such as sadness, fear, or frustration, and creates problems in social functioning (Fitzgerald & Bellgrove, 2006). Badenoch and Bogdan (2012) discuss the rapid cycling of the sympathetic nervous system resulting in fight-flight-freeze behaviors when children with ASD are confronted with negative emotions. With little emotional control and coping skills, the child acts out behaviorally, which can become a repetitive cycle of responding when experiencing a negative emotion.

ASD and Co-Occurring Diagnoses

There are many co-occurring medical/physical diagnoses that can accompany ASD. Cognitive deficits and delays, which are more common in more severe forms of autism, cause difficulty in social development and awareness and language development, and create barriers in the educational process of the child (Durand, 2014). Epilepsy is another condition that often accompanies those diagnosed with ASD. Tuchman (2011) found that a person diagnosed with ASD is 10 to 30 times more likely to have epilepsy than those in the general population, and that the long-term outlook for a person with ASD and epilepsy is poor. Gastrointestinal (GI) problems and eating problems co-occur with ASD. Wang, Tancredi, and Thomas (2011) conducted a large study and found that 42% of children with ASD had GI issues, as opposed to only 12% of their neurotypical siblings. Eating problems such as refusing certain foods, craving other foods, and acting out during mealtimes are problems that many parents of ASD children report (Durand, 2014). Stress, which is a common part of the ASD child's world due to the triggering of the sympathetic nervous system (Badenoch & Bogdan, 2012), is believed to be a factor in GI problems, while sensory issues and hypersensitivity to texture are a factor in children with ASD having difficulty tolerating new and different foods.

Anxiety and mood disorders are among the most common 'psychiatric' conditions that co-occur with ASD at an alarming rate. Durand (2014) states that "roughly 50–80%" can be diagnosed with an anxiety related disorder (p. 58). The activation of the fight-flight-freeze response and release of neurotransmitters such as cortisol and adrenaline create a sense of disorder and danger, leaving the child feeling unsteady and unsafe. The behaviors that result in an anxiety-related diagnosis (obsessive-compulsive disorder, separation anxiety, phobias, etc.) are all connected to the child's attempt to restore a sense of safety and equilibrium. Depression occurs at rates of 25%–34% (Ghaziuddin, Ghaziuddin, & Greden, 2002) in individuals diagnosed with ASD. Problems from social situations, family stress, and trips to therapists, doctors, and special school classes leave children with ASD feeling overwhelmed, and many turn their negative feelings inward, resulting in overwhelming sadness and self-rejection (Hull, 2012).

Attention deficit hyperactivity disorder (ADHD) is yet another co-occurring diagnosis with ASD. When one considers the constant triggering of the sympathetic nervous system and the upheaval that results in high levels of anxiety, it seems logical that ADHD is part of the landscape for a child diagnosed with ASD. The demands of joining a confusing, fast-paced world often outweigh the child's psychological resources. A final problem that often plagues the child with ASD is issues with sleep (Durand, 2014). Trouble falling asleep, sleeping too much, and insomnia are all characteristics of those diagnosed with ASD. Sleep problems affect the mental and emotional functioning of the child, as well as academic performance and overall coping skills (Staples & Bates, 2011). From a family perspective, sleep problems of the child with ASD can create stress on the family system, and the bedtime routine is often a major problem area that is mentioned during the initial intake session.

The Power of Play and Relationship in Therapy With Children With ASD

Building relationships with children with ASD is challenging and very interesting to say the least. Some talk; some do not. Some talk so much that there is no room for your questions or comments. Many have no care for or awareness of boundaries, and time means absolutely nothing. Some are naturally kind and warm up to you quickly, while others refuse to come into your office because they do not like the color of the door. Some think and act on an adult level, dismissing your attempts at connecting with them with a seemingly smug indifference. Some will insult your taste in clothes, décor, and arrangement of your office. Others will comment on your 'yellow teeth' with a degree of honesty and sincerity that is almost endearing. They ask you all sorts of questions. "How can you be a good counselor if you're divorced?" "Do you masturbate?" "Why would a grown man have all these toys and want to play with kids. Are you weird or something?" Even great moments can bring unpredictable results. One boy was so impressed that I had in my possession an original Nintendo Game Boy with several games that he collapsed on the floor and sobbed. You may get a lecture on how disgusting it is that your end tables are dusty, while the very same kid picks a scab off the bottom of his foot and puts it in his mouth. In short, you don't know what may happen. Every child on the spectrum is different, and while the traits are similar, the manifestation of those traits and the personalities that accompany them can be displayed in a thousand different shades of color and intensity.

With the challenges come great rewards. The breakthroughs, while often slow in coming, do happen, and when they do, the joy is nearly indescribable to both caregivers and therapists alike. The boy who was unable to speak begins to share his thoughts and feelings through words. The girl who only could express herself through tantrums finds a voice and learns to control her impulses and outbursts. The young man who was so shy he barely left the house gets a part-time job and learns to drive. The young lady who self-harmed and pushed others away starts meeting with middle school kids to help them believe in themselves. The young man that was bullied and had constant conflicts with peers graduates high school, goes to college, and becomes a teacher and coach. The girl that openly told her parents and you that she hated coming to therapy brings her journal from home to show you what she put in it and tells you how you have helped her. The common denominator in all the cases, which are in either the challenging stage or the breakthrough stage, is relationship. The therapist is forming or has formed a therapeutic bond with the young person, which is the foundation on which all the work rests. Building the therapeutic relationship with children can be accomplished through play.

Play is the language of children. Play is how a child experiences the world around them and helps the child understand it. Play builds relationship and establishes trust between people. The therapeutic value of play with children is well-documented (Koocher & D'Angelo, 1992; Leblanc & Ritchie, 2001) and is effective with children with ASD (Hull, 2012). Because children with ASD often struggle to communicate verbally and have difficulty expressing themselves, play is a wonderful tool to help them communicate and work through frustration, fear, and sadness. Children with ASD and a co-occurring diagnosis face immense challenges because the non-ASD diagnosis creates disruption in the child's life that in many ways is already in chaos. As mentioned earlier, the brain of the ASD child is easily triggered into the fight-flight-freeze response due to sympathetic nervous system overload. However, play can provide the brain of the ASD child with a 'shock absorber' to cushion the effects of stress. Play also opens channels of learning in the brain to create opportunities for relationships to be established through a sense of safety and trust by pushing the brain from sympathetic nervous system activation into "ventral vagal activation" (Badenoch & Bogdan, 2012, p. 8), the place in the brain that gives us our sense of safety and where learning and relationship take place.

Play for the child with ASD may look very different from that of what most people consider play to be. However, as Rubin (2012) so eloquently describes, instead of determining whether the play of ASD children is either deficient or different, it "makes the most sense to conclude that it is both" (p. 31) because "to children who play in an autistic way, there are no distinctions between deficiency and difference—there is only the moment" (p. 31). I really cherish Rubin's sentiments, because as a therapist on the front lines of working with ASD children, I was discouraged a few years back as I combed the literature seeking techniques and strategies for play with these remarkable children, only to find heated debates about how children with ASD did not really play. Each day, I observed the play of children with ASD to be different, but it was play nonetheless, which inspired me to write about it. Eventually, I found other authors, such as Rubin, who offered play techniques that fit the 'different' style of play and allowed therapists like myself to help the child with ASD shift perspective, cope with negative emotions, and build self-worth while increasing social awareness and relationships. Children with ASD and co-occurring diagnoses will be experiencing significant amounts of stress. The regular pressure these children feel on a regular basis will be heightened by physical pain, and trips to doctors and specialists will be stressful to the caregivers as well as the child with ASD. Play therapy techniques employed by the therapist will lessen the effects of stress and give the child with ASD coping skills.

CASE STUDIES

The Case of Stephen

Stephen was diagnosed with ASD at age 5. He falls into the category of ASD known as 'higher functioning' (formerly Asperger's syndrome). Stephen's speech and ability to communicate are neurotypical in nature, but his social skill level, emotional maturity, and cognitive abilities are similar to those of children diagnosed with ASD. Stephen demonstrates the classic characteristics of ASD by his specified interests, inflexible thinking, and ToM deficiencies. When he was younger, Stephen struggled with gross and fine motor skill delays, and he required occupational and physical therapy to improve his abilities in these areas. Stephen has always struggled in school, which led to his parents having the testing done to determine the ASD diagnosis. Stephen has also been diagnosed with ADHD. Stephen has auditory and visual processing problems that impact his comprehension and severely hamper learning in nearly every academic situation. Stephen is currently 12 years of age. Academically and emotionally, he functions at around a third grade level. He struggles socially. While he is very friendly, his interests are not the same as those of his peers, although he tries hard to understand what they like and why they like that certain show or type of music. Because Stephen only talks about one or two interests repeatedly, his peers lose interest and tend to eventually ignore him. Stephen has difficulty remembering the details about a person, even family members, such as their age, birthday, or anniversary. He has difficulty telling time, marking the passage of time, or being aware of the monetary value of things. He struggles to remember how to do simple tasks, and his parents have remarked that each day feels like the same challenges are simply replayed, much like the movie *Groundhog Day*, starring Bill Murray.

Two years ago, Stephen was stricken with severe stomach pain and intense cramping that ultimately led to nearly nine months in and out of the hospital and multiple examinations, feeding tubes, and disruption of routine and family life. Eventually, Stephen was diagnosed with Crohn's disease. Already small for his age, Stephen's growth immediately stopped once the disease ravaged his gastrointestinal system. The Crohn's also impacted Stephen's ASD symptoms. Already fearful and triggered easily due to ASD, Stephen's fears escalated to the point where he refused to eat and drink, or even swallow saliva. Stephen's magical thinking, as evidenced by his denial of time or responsibilities ("If I sit here long enough, somehow I'll just be ready for school"), became worse as he became increasingly sick. Already a rigid thinker, the Crohn's disease that afflicted Stephen seemed to cement into one-way thinking common to ASD children and then pour molten steel over it to create an impenetrable structure in which no amount of logic and reasoning could penetrate. One example of this was when Stephen was in the hospital and his weight loss was nearing dangerous levels due to his refusal to eat. He told me that his thinking process was simple: if I don't eat or drink or swallow saliva, then I won't have any stomach problems because there won't be anything in my stomach to cause problems. The doctors, nurses, his parents, and family members all tried to show Stephen that his refusal to put anything in his stomach was making things worse, and that if he did not eat the hospital staff would have no choice but install a peripherally inserted central catheter (PICC line) so that his body could get vital nutrients. An excerpt of Stephen's conversation with his mother about the PICC line follows.

Mom: "You have to eat or they are going to put the PICC line in."
Stephen: "But I don't want the PICC line."
Mom: "Then go ahead and eat the pop-tart and drink the juice. It's your favorite."
Stephen: "But I don't want to eat or drink anything."
Mom: "Then they have to put the PICC line in you."
Stephen: "But I don't want the PICC line."

This conversation went on for about 20 more exchanges, but there was nothing anyone could do to make Stephen understand that he could prevent the PICC line by eating and drinking. To Stephen and his magical thinking, it made sense that he could refuse both and get what he wanted. After the PICC line was put in him, he was furious at his parents and the doctors. The challenges of a lack of ToM would not allow him to see that his refusal to swallow food or drink was what made the doctors put the PICC line in, nor could he see that the PICC line was saving his life. As I sat with him one day at the hospital, I realized that Stephen's will to resist eating or drinking was so strong that he was prepared to die rather than give in to something that he did not want to do. Despite having witnessed the challenges of ToM deficiencies in individuals with ASD for nearly 15 years, this was the most extreme form and it was difficult to watch, to say the least.

The Case of Angela

Angela was diagnosed with ASD at around 8 years of age. Her mother reported that she demonstrated the rigid thinking and obsessive tendencies common to ASD early in life. Social situations were difficult for Angela, and as she progressed in school she was bullied and lashed out at peers and teachers. Angela was plagued with sensory issues, which is common in children with ASD. She could only wear certain types of clothing and hated shoes and socks. When something irritated Angela, she would be upset for hours and often exhibited tantrums in public places such as malls and restaurants, prompting her parents to refuse to take her anywhere with them. Like many children with ASD, Angela also struggles with ADHD. Angela began to have gastrointestinal problems in third grade, which resulted in her missing a lot of school. Ultimately she was diagnosed with celiac disease, an autoimmune disorder in which the small intestine is damaged when foods with gluten are ingested. Many families with a child with ASD must limit or eliminate certain foods to help their child battle certain symptoms of ASD, which can cause a great deal of stress for the child and the family. Angela's family experienced a great deal of stress due to a complete shift in the foods that Angela needed to eliminate, and Angela and her two older siblings voiced their displeasure to Angela's mother. Mealtimes became difficult and became a trigger for Angela's anger and subsequent tantrums. When Angela was about ten, she was diagnosed with juvenile rheumatoid arthritis, also known as juvenile idiopathic arthritis (JIA). JIA caused inflammation of Angela's joints and caused waves of pain to shoot through her body when she performed even the simplest of tasks. Her brain, already prone to flying into fight-flight-freeze mode at the tiniest frustration, now was overwhelmed beyond belief by the JIA. Angela missed a great many days of school due to her battles with celiac disease, but when JIA entered her life, her school life became increasingly difficult. Holding a pencil or pen was often impossible, and Angela was unable to concentrate on her work due to the great pain she was forced to endure. Due to the constant pain and stress, Angela's mother decided to homeschool Angela. It was at this time that her mother decided to seek the help of a therapist for Angela.

Play Therapy Techniques With Stephen and Angela

Before I begin this section, I want to stress a very important factor that a therapist working with children with ASD and a co-occurring disorder must consider, and that is the element of attempting to see life through the eyes of the child. The therapist must spend time getting to know the child: his personality, how she processes information, his hobbies, her ways of coping with stress, and so forth. I have written in several places about the concept of the therapist to 'just be,' which is the concept of eliminating every distraction and agenda and simply joining the child in that beautiful space that Virginia Axline so poignantly expressed as the essence of child-centered play therapy (Hull, 2012). Children with ASD require a therapist that is willing to be brave enough to enter their chaotic and odd worlds; however, for children with ASD and a co-occurring disorder, the therapist must be prepared for heartbreaking amounts of sadness, fear, and frustration. For children with ASD like Angela and Stephen, whose co-occurring diagnoses bring intense physical pain, there is often the entering of a realm unknown by the therapist, who is usually neurotypical and removed from any ongoing and unrelenting physical suffering. By spending time getting to the child with whom we are working, we take the first step in establishing the therapeutic foundation and creating layers of trust and safety. It is well-known that a key element of play therapy's success lies in the relationship between child and therapist. When the child with ASD is joined in unconditional acceptance through play with a trusted adult, the child's brain shifts from sympathetic activation and chaos to a parasympathetic state and safety (Badenoch & Bogdan, 2012). The longer that a child stays in a state of play and relationship that produces the sense of safety, the more 'normal' this brain state becomes and the adult, whether parent or therapist, becomes a trusted ally.

Sand Tray With Angela

The sand tray has long been an effective tool for play therapists (Hull, 2017; Richardson, 2012). The sand tray provides the child with the opportunity to use exploratory and imaginative play in a private world that "goes beyond words while supporting children's endeavor to find the words that can describe that world and their experience in it" (Richardson, 2012, p. 210). The sand tray is useful for children with ASD in helping them articulate feelings and thoughts as well as increasing ToM and building social relationships. The sand tray was useful in my work with Angela to help her create a world through which she could express her innermost thoughts and emotions. Angela, despite her challenges, was very imaginative and loved to create. However, many days her JIA prevented her from holding writing utensils, so drawing or painting was not an option. She soon spotted the sand tray and smoothed out the sand and began to create designs in the sand with her finger. On her third visit to the playroom, Angela poured water in the sand tray to make it wet and moldable, and said that she wanted to sculpt figures using the sand. She made several sand 'snowballs' and placed them on one side of the sand tray. Next, Angela dug a deep trench and created an island. She surrounded the island with plastic barbed wire fencing from a military play set. She used some LEGO palm trees to decorate the island, and then carefully made one large sand snowball and placed it in the middle of the island. Then she placed the other sand snowballs across the trench in various positions. I noticed that the balls she placed outside of the trench were put in groups of two or three. Richardson (2012) recommends a phase of quiet contemplation so that the child stays with their creation, followed by a phase of joint attention where the "eye contact is with the sand tray" (p. 212) and the therapist uses questions and makes observations about the creation and the child's experience, "not facts about the world" (p. 212). This phase is important with children with ASD, as the eye contact with the sand tray and not the child can provide a sense of safety and creates the opportunity for dialogue between child and therapist. Also, the inquiry about the experience of the child during the creating phase can help a child with ASD explore deeper feelings and practice communicating those. After Angela was finished, she and I sat in silence and I kept my eyes on her creation, noting each detail in my mind. After a few minutes, I voiced observations such as "The big ball seems alone from the others," and "The other balls seem to be close together in groups."

Angela used a stick as a pointer and showed me what the creation in the sand tray meant to her. She said that the big sand ball represented herself and that the island represented how she felt isolated from other people. I assumed that by 'other people' she meant her peers from school that she no longer had contact with. However, the 'other people' she was referring to were her immediate family members. The groups of two or three balls were her mother and father, siblings, and grandparents. She said that she constantly felt like there was a connection between them, but that because of her disabilities, she felt shunned and forgotten. She said that because of her illness along with the ASD, it made her appear to her siblings as though she required special treatment. She said that she was very jealous of her siblings, particularly her older brother, who she said seemed to "have everything he wanted." I asked Angela about life on the island and what it was like. We used a feelings list to help her, because she struggled with putting feelings into words. *Despair, rejected, alone*, and *terrified* were some of the words that she circled. For positive feelings, she circled *satisfied*, and when I inquired about this, she said that at least living on the island was comfortable and familiar for her because "I have been there so long," she said. I asked her if she thought any of her family members knew how she felt and she said, "Probably not." "How do you think they might feel if they knew?" I asked. Angela did not respond. "I wonder what would happen if you found a way to let them know that you feel like you do?" I asked. "They might want to visit your island." At her next session, Angela again created the island of sand and placed a large sand ball in the middle to represent herself. I noticed that this time, however, she spent nearly the entire session decorating the island with a log cabin shelter and different colored rocks. When sharing her thoughts and feelings about the creation, she said that she decorated the island because she felt better about herself and her situation. She smiled and said that decorating the island was "fun" and she liked how it looked.

At her next session, Angela created her island and made the sand ball that represented herself, but I was surprised to see that she built a bridge and placed a few sand balls on her island. Angela explained that she had reached out to her younger sister and spent time with her. Also, she had reconnected with a few peers from school and her mother had arranged a time for them to spend time together. Over the next two sessions, more sand balls appeared on her island and Angela's sand ball crossed the bridge and joined other sand balls. "I'm off the island," she said as she placed the sand ball that represented herself on the mainland. The sand tray was a key tool in helping Angela express herself, understand her own emotions and thoughts, and raise her sense of value and worth. As her self-worth improved, Angela could connect with others, as evidenced in her representation of her thoughts and feelings in the sand tray.

LEGO Minifigures and Action Figures With Stephen

A common characteristic of children with ASD is "specified interests" (Hull, 2017, p. 3), which are interests to which the child's concentrated energy is drawn in a very focused and intense manner. One of Stephen's specified interests from a young age was the wrestlers from World Wrestling Entertainment (WWE), mainly John Cena, one of the most popular characters in the wrestling world. Stephen insisted upon bringing his collection of WWE figures to the playroom as well as a toy wrestling ring and stage, and I allowed him to do so. I immersed myself in the WWE world, letting Stephen teach me the characters and their special moves, as well as the songs that played during their introduction as they marched toward the ring. I wanted to see the world through Stephen's eyes, and one way of doing this was to understand his specified interest of wrestling and the WWE. The themes that emerged from Stephen's love of WWE were strength, power, and athleticism. He re-enacted matches that he had seen on YouTube move for move, and the excitement that Stephen felt was infectious.

Each day for Stephen was difficult and frightening because of the PICC line, forced feedings, and physical pain. His mother reported to me that Stephen's OCD tendencies and tic behavior had become so problematic because of his physical discomfort that he was put on anti-anxiety medication by his psychiatrist. The play sessions using the WWE figures gave Stephen a break from his pain and helped him focus on something other than his illness. During one session, Stephen said that his illness made him feel weak and powerless, and I asked him what he could think of that would describe how he felt. Stephen said it would be like being a wrestler who was pinned down and helpless. I asked him to play out a match and take on the role of the loser. He did, and I asked him what the experience was like for him. "Just like I feel every day," he responded. He then took several wrestlers and piled them on the figure that had just lost, which represented himself. "Actually, this is how it feels every day," he said. Then, he took the ball of figures in his hands and pretended to walk it around the floor. When I asked what was happening, he said that his figure had to carry all of the other figures as punishment for losing. When I asked him to explain, he said it felt like no matter what he did, it was always wrong and he stayed sick no matter what.

LEGO play can be a very effective play therapy tool (LeGoff & Sherman, 2006) to help children express thoughts and feelings and work through traumatic experiences (Hull, 2012). Stephen liked to play with LEGO and LEGO minifigures. He liked to play with the minifigures by changing them to look like his favorite wrestlers or characters from video games. Building with LEGO helped Stephen forget about his struggles and tapped into his creative abilities. I used LEGO to construct a hospital room, and we played out what it was like for him to stay for many weeks in the hospital. He chose a LEGO minifigure that represented himself, and he talked about his thoughts and feelings as he laid his minifigure in the LEGO bed. We constructed a replica of his living room and what it was like to be at home. I used various minifigures to represent his parents, doctors, and other family members so he could show me how he responded to them. Then, we switched roles and he commanded the minifigures that represented his parents or doctors while I played the role of Stephen. This produced a sense of delight in Stephen and also brought humor into the process. Hearing him laugh was thrilling after seeing him in so much pain.

Art Therapy With Angela

Art therapy is an effective tool with children with ASD to improve social, emotional, and cognitive functioning (Goucher, 2012; Hull, 2012). Children with ASD have been found to use "mental imagery" (Goucher, 2012, p. 299) most of the time to process information, whereas neurotypical children only use mental imagery when necessary, relying on other parts of the brain to process information. Goucher (2012) explains that this reliance on mental imagery explains why children with ASD struggle with acquiring language skills and struggle with putting thoughts and feelings into words. Angela loved to draw, color, and paint, although her JIA often prevented her from being able to hold drawing utensils. On the days when she could, she liked to draw something and color it in with markers and crayons. Angela's drawings were always of happy things such as her pets and spending time with her family and friends. She always used bright, vibrant colors. She told me that when she drew and colored, it made her forget that she was sick or had any problems. I used art and her love of it to help her process feelings of fear, anger, and frustration while she drew and painted. One picture she drew was of a dog with a very sad face and large frown. She then took bright colors and painted in the face of the dog and painted a big, happy smile over the sad frown. When I asked about it, she told me that is what she chose to do every morning. "I cover up my sadness so that it doesn't bother other people," she said. "That is why I love to draw and color, you can hide stuff and it is easier than in real life. But drawing and coloring help me deal with everything and I always feel better, so that's why I put the smile on."

Video and Tablet Games With Stephen

Technology provides play therapists with powerful tools to help children increase insight, improve impulse control, improve self-worth, overcome negative emotions, improve coping skills, and deal with the transitions of life such as loss, moving, or the divorce of parents (Hull, 2016). Games such as Minecraft are like a virtual sand tray, while games like LEGO Star Wars or Super Mario Bros. allow the therapist to join the child in game play, while metaphors like overcoming obstacles, developing new attributes, or leveling up can be drawn to help a child relate to real-world challenges and give them a way to express thoughts and feelings about those challenges. Stephen was a huge fan of Minecraft and was delighted to see a version installed on my iPad. Using Wi-Fi, Stephen and I joined and worked together to build, fight enemies, and gather resources. One main issue Stephen struggled with was creating a new 'normal' and grieving the loss of his previous abilities and activities. During the months he was in the hospital, he not only felt isolated, but also was upset at not being able to go to theme parks and water parks, which were things he loved to do. After his hospital stay, doctors continued to be puzzled at the irregularity in his digestive system and his lack of growth, and he was constantly being examined, tested, and going back and forth to doctors and specialists. During this stage, Stephen endured large amounts of acute pain and general overall discomfort, forcing him to stay inactive and isolated.

A main theme of my work with Stephen was helping him through this time of grief and adjusting to a new sense of normal. Using Minecraft, we set up a world in which we played each session. Stephen liked to switch back and forth between 'survival mode,' a mode in which the player begins with no resources and must defend against many enemies such as spiders and zombies, and 'creative mode,' a mode in which all resources are available and the player cannot be harmed by enemies and can also fly. Using the "prescriptive play therapy" approach (Schaefer, 2001, p. 58), which involves the play therapist presenting toys and materials designed to address a specific issue, I invited Stephen to play in survival mode. I used the enemies of survival mode and compared them to Stephen's current real-life enemies of pain, discomfort, fear, and sadness over the loss of his abilities and activities. This presented Stephen with a visual image that the enemies he faced in the real world could be dealt with, and while these enemies did not magically always go away, there were solutions and help that Stephen could rely on, such as eating and drinking what the doctors recommended, relying on his mother and father, and taking his medication. Minecraft play in survival mode helped Stephen see a new perspective that the Minecraft world was constantly changing, and each enemy and situation had a solution to either defeat it or escape it. Visual imagery in play is an important part of working with children with ASD, because it plays such a vital part in how children with ASD absorb information and relate to the world around them (Goucher, 2012).

The biggest obstacle and enemy that Stephen had to face was physical pain. Constant cramping and pain from bowel movements terrified him and made Stephen afraid to eat or drink. One of the most feared enemies in Minecraft is the skeleton, which shoots arrows from a bow and moves quickly to attack once the player is spotted. Stephen described his stomach pain like "darts and shots; like getting stabbed with something sharp." Because he associated pain with his body trying to digest food, he was resistant to eating. His parents and the doctors explained to him that the pain was from not having enough food in his stomach; he needed to eat to make the pain go away. I asked him if the pain he experienced might be like the arrows from a skeleton. He nodded with a frightened look on his face. We discussed how to face skeletons in Minecraft, such as being prepared with armor and weapons, and also being careful to avoid where they might be, such as dark caves or staying inside when it was night. I applied this to asking Stephen what he could do to minimize the pain, and he reluctantly told me that he knew that he needed to eat. "Okay, let's talk about some ways to help you make that happen," I responded. We made a list of the foods he liked and that the doctors told him he could eat, and he agreed to try. His mother told me that he did make an effort to eat, and eventually, his eating improved. It seemed to be helpful to create a picture with something that he loved, such as Minecraft, to help him overcome the issue of not eating.

Art and Technology With Angela

Angela's love of art was expressed through the technology of the tablet and coloring apps. There are several free apps available, and it was not hard for her to pick one. Angela liked to create her own designs using a thick, dark outline and then color in the various sections much like a mosaic or stained glass. Mistakes could be easily erased with the 'undo' button, and colors were easily changed with a mere tap of her finger. "I feel powerful," she said during one coloring session. The pictures she created were saved in the camera roll on the tablet. One picture Angela drew when she had a particularly challenging week had jagged edges and sharp lines. She used several dark colors of red, purple, and green. After she was finished, I asked her to name her creation and to explain it. "Chaos," she responded, nearly in a whisper. She explained that her week was hard. She had a lot of pain, found herself missing her friends from school, and had several arguments with her siblings and mother. "It just feels like everything is messed up."

Angela, like many children with ASD, struggled to see a situation from another's perspective. This was particularly difficult when she was feeling bad from her JIA. For example, if her mother helped her older brother with a school project, Angela's brain would tell her that her mother did not love her and might forget about her. This thinking would lead to behavior fueled by thoughts and feelings that ultimately got Angela into trouble. The coloring apps were helping in drawing out situations that Angela described at home using stick figures, because they could be easily erased and re-drawn in different poses or situations. The theme of her being jealous of her mother's time with her siblings continued to be a trigger for her anger and feelings of abandonment, which resulted in her acting out. Drawing out these situations using the drawing app were useful to help identify Angela's thoughts and feelings. I sketched out her mother and brother in one room, and she sketched a stick figure that represented herself. I then asked her to draw a thought bubble over her head. Then, I asked her to imagine what she was feeling and thinking as her mother was with her brother. Her main thoughts were "She doesn't love me" and "She will forget about me." I asked her to make a symbol in the thought bubble that represented those thoughts. She drew a small circle with a plus sign in the middle and an X. Next, I asked her to tell me the feelings that she experienced in this situation. "Anger and fear," she said. I told her to put a symbol for those as well, and she placed a large black dot and a pound sign. "Now," I said, "Make a face that shows how you look with those thoughts and feelings." Angela erased her original face and made a scowl complete with beady eyes and a frown. "What would have to happen to make you feel happy and safe?" I asked. "My mom would be with me," she replied. "Okay," I said, "Let's draw that." She erased her mother and put her next to her. I asked her to erase the symbols from the thought bubble and followed the same format of asking her to create symbols to represent her thoughts and feelings, which were positive because her mother was with her, and she made a happy face with a large smile. The symbols that she chose for her positive thoughts and feelings were hearts, stars, and tiny smiley faces.

Using this model, we drew several scenarios that included Angela's mother with Angela's siblings without Angela, and several with Angela present. Each drawing included me asking her to identify her thoughts and feelings using the symbols, as well as imagining what her mother might be thinking and feeling as well. Keeping in mind that children with ASD use visual imagery most of the time, and the effectiveness of thought bubble training (TBT) (Paynter & Peterson, 2013) to increase perspective-taking, I found that the use of the stick figures on the tablet created a flow that kept Angela engaged, and the easy erasing of drawings and adding new ones through the tools of the app helped her see pictures of thoughts and feelings. Over a few sessions, Angela's ability to see the situation with her mother and siblings from a different, more positive perspective improved. Her mother reported that while she still did not like situations in which her mother spent time with her siblings, Angela's negative behavior ceased. This technique was also useful in replacing negative thoughts with positive ones, and drawing out the different feelings that came from those thoughts. The use of symbols instead of words seemed to help keep the process simple and Angela engaged.

PERSONAL REFLECTIONS

I will briefly describe my personal reflections on both cases in this section. This section is intended to give the practitioner working with children like these a sense of preparedness, and help the practitioner to be at their cognitive and emotional best to deliver the very best care possible.

Emotional Reactions

It is impossible for a practitioner to be emotionally absent from the process of therapy with a child. We are, after all, human, and to be human is to experience emotions. Being present with a child in the playroom and seeing her world as she sees it brings an emotional component that not only creates connection but also is a large part of the therapeutic value of play therapy. I work with children with neurodevelopmental challenges on a regular basis, so I am used to slow progress and at times no progress or even regressions. I often feel a twinge of sadness at the child's frustration with a challenging situation and my own frustration that something that I am doing is not working. The result, however, is a renewed energy to further strategize with the family or teachers, present the child with a new play opportunity, or dive into research to learn more techniques and examine the process for some unknown factor that might be stalling forward progress.

The cases of Angela and Stephen, however, brought me to new levels of sadness and frustration, and these emotions were not so quickly transferred into positive therapeutic energy. I distinctly remember visiting Stephen in the hospital on a Saturday morning. He had already been there about five days, and I was confident that I could cheer him up and get him to eat. Inspired by Patch Adams, I went into clown mode, pretending to be a fumbling doctor with a silly accent and tripping over a gown that I pretended was my doctor coat. I blew up surgical gloves and we drew silly faces on them, and then I taped them up around the room with surgical tape.

We batted several around and Stephen laughed repeatedly as we played together. Then, we played Minecraft together, and during this time I asked Stephen to tell me about his fear of eating to gauge his level of resistance. As soon as I brought up eating, Stephen shut down. It was as if my cover was blown and he saw right through my song and dance. His eyes looked pained, as if sadness and fear joined forces and cut off any ability to communicate. He dropped his controller and fell silent. I felt helpless to do anything. I was reminded of the impenetrable walls of ASD and that in my neurotypical mindset everything was simple and made sense. In Stephen's world, the pain of physical suffering combined with the traits of ASD and made his world even more upside down. He regressed by years, not just a few months or by a few stages. I felt anger, both at myself and my limitations, and embarrassment. I felt like a failure at not being able to budge his will and shift his perspective. Working with children with ASD is often a clumsy waltz with feelings of failure because there are so many setbacks that occur with each developmental stage, but Stephen's case was like witnessing a total developmental landslide, and it was heartbreaking to witness and feel so helpless to stop it.

During the time I worked with Angela, I experienced the emotion of frustration, but I also found myself feeling immense sadness. I am usually very good at leaving the emotions that surface during sessions at the office, but with Angela's case I found myself thinking about it after the workday. I imagined her struggling at home with her siblings, trying so desperately to get attention. Part of her feeling safe depended on having people around her and paying attention to her, and I worked very hard to shift this perspective. Just when I thought we had turned a corner and reached a milestone, her JIA would flare up and she would regress. During family sessions with her siblings and mother, I worked hard to help them understand Angela's ways of thinking as we strategized solutions to help lessen family conflict and help Angela up the developmental ladder. Many people falsely believe that children with higher functioning ASD are somehow better off, but in many ways I think the elevated expectations of others due to the child appearing 'normal' creates emotional devastation for the child. Listening to Angela and how she felt often left me feeling sad, because while I could see that many of her thoughts were distorted, the emotions she experienced were to her very real and upsetting.

Cognitive Reactions and Countertransference Issues

I battled all sorts of negative thinking while working with Angela and Stephen. The main theme of these was interpreting the regression or lack of progress as something that I was doing wrong, or at very least not doing right. I am familiar with the lack of progress that comes with working with children with ASD, but the levels of regression due to the physical symptoms of the co-occurring diagnoses were new territory. I constantly had to re-route potential negative self-attributions through my therapist filter ("Is there something I'm missing?"), which drove me back to the literature regarding the nature of ASD and particularly what happens in the brain of a child with ASD who is in severe physical and emotional distress. This 'truth' helped me stay grounded and gave me a new appreciation for the emotional and physical strength of these children as they faced all kinds of relentless triggering because of the interplay between ASD and the co-occurring physical challenges.

The demands of investing extra energy into Angela and Stephen and their families created countertransference issues. Working with a specialized population like ASD and co-occurring diagnoses demands that the therapist do extra reading, be available for families to offer support, and communicate with physicians, psychiatrists, and other specialists to provide the best care possible. This extra investment may cause the therapist to feel personally connected to the client and the client's family, and create a dependence between the client and family members and the therapist or vice versa. I found myself thinking of Stephen and Angela and their family long after seeing them at the office or talking with them on the phone. Knowing that Stephen had an operation coming up the next day often kept me up at night, or reading an email about a particularly bad day for Angela due to a JIA flare-up created emotional reactions that I typically did not experience with other clients.

To battle the countertransference and negative cognitions, I had to do several things. One, consistently telling myself that I was doing the best I could was important to help me stay grounded. Second, journaling and consultation with a colleague was most helpful in having a place for my therapeutic brain to unload, release, and reframe thinking and subsequent emotional reactions. Third, boundary work was helpful by re-prioritizing my personal time with family and refusing to check email after certain hours. Fourth, channeling my negative emotions and thoughts into positive energy by taking time to research about Angela and Stephen's physical challenges and ASD helped me feel productive and warded off feelings of failure. Fifth, learning to accept my limitations was very important. I found that working with these cases brought me to the brink of realizing that while I love our field, play therapy has limitations, and I as a therapist have limitations. I realize that I do not like admitting it, but it is true. I was forced to accept this fact, and in doing so I found relief and reassurance that doing my best each day and with each case is all I can do.

SUMMARY

Working with children with ASD and co-occurring diagnoses, particularly physical health–related ones, is challenging. Children with ASD often experience co-occurring physical, neurological, and psychological diagnoses that further disrupt their development and cause chaos in the child's life and the life of their family. Play therapists who work with ASD must be prepared to address the numerous challenges facing these children. Children with ASD and co-occurring diagnoses are at risk for developmental delays due to the interplay of the co-occurring diagnoses causing disruption in the brain and body of the child. Play therapy is effective with children with ASD and co-occurring diagnoses to help the child develop a sense of self and learn coping skills to help the child reach important developmental goals.

REFERENCES

American Psychiatric Association. (2013). *Diagnostic and statistical manual of mental disorders: DSM-5* (5th ed.). Arlington, VA: American Psychiatric.

Badenoch, B., & Bogdan, N. (2012). Safety and connection: The neurobiology of play. In L. Gallo-Lopez & L. C. Rubin (Eds.), *Play-based interventions for children and adolescents with autism spectrum disorders* (pp. 3–18). New York: Routledge/Taylor & Francis Group.

Baron-Cohen, S. (1995). *Mindblindness: An essay on autism and theory of mind.* Cambridge, MA: MIT Press.

Centers for Disease Control and Prevention. (2014). *Autism.* Retrieved from: www.cdc.gov/ncbddd/autism/data.html

Durand, V. M. (2014). *Autism spectrum disorder: A clinical guide for general practitioners* (1st ed.). Washington, DC: American Psychological Association.

Fitzgerald, M., & Bellgrove, M. A. (2006). The overlap between alexithymia and Asperger's syndrome. *Journal of Autism and Developmental Disorders, 36*(4), 573–576.

Ghaziuddin, M., Ghaziuddin, N., & Greden, J. (2002). Depression in persons with autism: Implications for research and clinical care. *Journal of Autism and Developmental Disorders, 32*(4), 299–306. https://doi.org/10.1023/A:1016330802348

Goucher, C. (2012). Art therapy. In L. Gallo-Lopez & L. C. Rubin (Eds.), *Play-based interventions for children and adolescents with autism spectrum disorders* (pp. 295–315). New York: Routledge/Taylor & Francis Group.

Hull, K. (2012). *Play therapy and Asperger's Syndrome: Helping children and adolescents grow, connect, and heal through the art of play.* Lanham, MD: Jason Aronson.

Hull, K. (2015). Play therapy with children on the autism spectrum. In D. A. Crenshaw & A. L. Stewart (Eds.), *Play therapy: A comprehensive guide to theory and practice.* New York: Guilford.

Hull, K. (2016). Technology in the playroom. In K. J. O'Connor, C. E. Schaefer & L. D. Braverman (Eds.), *Handbook of play therapy* (2nd ed., pp. 613–627). Hoboken, NJ: John Wiley and Sons.

Hull, K. (2017). Children with autism spectrum disorders. In C. Haen & S. Aronson (Eds.), *Handbook of child and adolescent group therapy: A practitioner's reference* (pp. 347–356). New York: Routledge.

Koocher, G. P., & D'Angelo, E. J. (1992). Evolution of practice in child psychotherapy. In D. K. Freedheim, H. J. Freudenberger, J. W. Kessler, S. B. Messer & D. R. Peterson (Eds.), *History of psychotherapy: A century of change* (pp. 457–492). Washington, DC: American Psychological Association.

Leblanc, M., & Ritchie, M. (2001). A meta-analysis of play therapy outcomes. *Counselling Psychology Quarterly, 14*(2), 149–163.

LeGoff, D. B., & Sherman, M. (2006). Long-term outcome of social skills intervention based on interactive LEGO® play. *Autism, 10*(4), 317–329.

Levy, S. E., Giarelli, E., Lee, L. C., Schieve, L. A., Kirby, R. S., Cuniff, C., . . . Rice, C. E. (2010). Autism spectrum disorder and co-occurring developmental, psychiatric, and medical conditions among children in multiple populations of the United States. *Journal of Developmental and Behavioral Pediatrics, 31*(4), 267–275.

Paynter, J., & Peterson, C. C. (2013). Further evidence of benefits of thought-bubble training for theory of mind development in children with autism spectrum disorders. *Research in Autism Spectrum Disorders, 7*(2), 344–348.

Richardson, J. F. (2012). The world of the sand tray and the child on the autism spectrum. In L. Gallo-Lopez & L. Rubin (Eds.), *Play-based interventions for children and adolescents with autism spectrum disorders* (pp. 137–157). New York: Routledge/Taylor & Francis Group.

Rubin, L. C. (2012). Playing on the autism spectrum. In L. Gallo-Lopez & L. C. Rubin (Eds.), *Play-based interventions for children and adolescents with autism spectrum disorders* (pp. 3–18). New York: Routledge/Taylor & Francis Group.

Schaefer, C. E. (2001). Prescriptive play therapy. *International Journal of Play Therapy*, *10*(2), 57–73. https://doi.org/10.1037/h0089480

Staples, A. D., & Bates, J. E. (2011). Children's sleep deficits and cognitive and behavioral adjustment. In M. El-Sheikh (Ed.), *Sleep and development: Familial and socio-cultural considerations* (pp. 133–164). New York: Oxford University Press.

Tuchman, R. (2011). Epilepsy and encephalography in autism spectrum disorders. In D. G. Amaral, G. Dawson & D. Geschwind (Eds.), *Autism spectrum disorders* (pp. 381–394). New York: Oxford University Press. https://doi.org/10.1093/med/9780195371826.003.0026

Wang, L. W., Tancredi, D. J., & Thomas, D. W. (2011). The prevalence of gastrointestinal problems in children across the United States with autism spectrum disorders from families with multiple affected members. *Journal of Developmental and Behavioral Pediatrics*, *32*, 351–360. https://doi.org/10.1097/DBP.0b013e31821bd06a

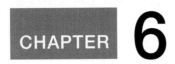

CHAPTER 6

Children, Cancer, and Child Life

Fostering Resiliency Through Empowerment

Meredith Cooper and Melissa Hicks

Truth is the torch that gleams through the fog without dispelling it.
—Claude Adrien Helvetius

The diagnosis of cancer can be devastating to a family. Providing thoughtful supportive intervention from initial diagnosis can help to mediate the potential negative psychological effects on children. Often these are typical families coping with an atypical situation. Given the appropriate information and tools, these families can emerge from the experience emotionally healthy and use the skills as a foundation for future life challenges.

This chapter will explore the developmental understanding and impact of cancer on children that will be used to inform interventions that are developmentally appropriate, supportive, and play oriented. A model of supportive intervention will be highlighted to address the typical psychosocial goals for children impacted by cancer. Special considerations will be addressed for situations in which the child himself has cancer or a sibling or parent is diagnosed with cancer. While it is essential to provide support to the entire family, this chapter will primarily focus on the direct interactions with children and adolescents.

CANCER IN THE FAMILY

One of the most devastating sentences a family can hear is "You have cancer." For most families, when those words are spoken by a medical team, nothing else is heard. All their fears, both real and perceived, come flooding to the surface. The actual family member diagnosed with cancer changes the implications and impact on the family, but regardless, the family is forever changed. Cancer is a family illness. Yes, one person is the patient and must undergo the treatment and subsequent side effects, but each individual in the family is impacted in unique ways. Many studies have highlighted the potential impact on all family members and the value of support for the entire family (Ellis, Wakefield, Antill, Burns, & Patterson, 2017; Hamama, Ronen, & Rahav, 2008; Howell et al., 2016; Meyler, Guerin, Kiernan, & Breatnach, 2010; Sieh, Visser-Meily, & Meijer, 2013).

Most families can come through with strength and resilience in the face of crisis. These authors fundamentally believe that families have the internal strength and resiliency to cope with almost anything given the needed tools and support. Those tools are often within them but need to be fostered to cope with this situation. Effective support for families coping with cancer is one that is based on a preventative model with opportunities for growth, and not on a deficit model. Current studies suggest that children impacted by cancer, whether they or their parents are the patient, were not only resilient but demonstrated psychological growth in relation to their cancer experience (Phillips & Prezio, 2017; Phipps et al., 2014; Wilson et al., 2016).

In their book, *Building Resilience in Children and Teens*, Ginsburg and Jablow (2011) identify the Seven Crucial Cs of Resilience. These are competence, confidence, connection, character, contribution, coping, and control. These can be especially helpful when focusing on intervention in a preventative model working with children impacted by cancer. Of relevance to this population and an area for intervention are competence, connection, coping, and control. For children with cancer, any opportunity to feel competent is important. Successfully coping with a procedure or advocating for themselves helps the child to feel competent in a challenging time. The child life specialist or play therapist can help the child achieve this through medical play. Utilizing a variety of medical supplies, the child can work through challenging procedures or situations. This medical play can also serve as an assessment tool to assess misperceptions or fears. Connection promotes resiliency in all family members. Family connectedness has been found to improve increased quality of life in childhood cancer survivors (Orbuch, Parry, Chesler, Fritz, & Repetto, 2005; Sharp et al., 2015). Additionally, Brown et al. (2007) reported that the perceived support from friends and family members helped to serve as protective factors for children adjusting to their mother's breast cancer. Effective intervention can help to enhance family communication and strengthen relationships (Phillips & Prezio, 2017). Support and intervention by a skilled helper can have a positive effect on coping and should be the priority when establishing therapeutic goals. Successfully navigating the cancer experience for children, regardless of who the patient is, can be especially empowering. Finally, providing as many realistic opportunities for control have value, especially during a time when families are confronting so much that is out of their control. Seeking out and offering even the smallest of choices promotes a sense of control. Non-directive play time is a perfect example of this opportunity for control. Other options for choice could be related to materials and what they choose to share with family members.

Of additional importance in this work with children impacted by cancer is family functioning as it relates to adjustment to illness. It has been documented that positive family functioning when coping with cancer has led to improved psychosocial outcomes (Brown, Daly, & Rickel, 2007; Ferro & Boyle, 2015; Hicks & Davitt, 2009, 2018 in press; Meyler et al., 2010; Orbuch et al., 2005; Phillips & Prezio, 2017; Sharp et al., 2015). In addition to connectedness and supportive relationships, a hallmark of this positive functioning is communication. These authors have found communication to be essential, and firmly believe one of the most important goals of the clinician should be to foster communication within the family. When working with children impacted by caner, the communication must be grounded with honest and accurate information. The quote at the start of this chapter speaks beautifully to this foundational precept. While often frightening and difficult, truthful communication can serve as a beacon in an uncertain time. When children are given truthful information, they understand they can rely on the adults around them. They will learn that they are given the best information parents have available to them and will inform them if or when situations change. This predictability can provide comfort in the unknown and decrease the anxiety that can be associated with filling in the gaps of information. It is the wise and skilled clinician that can gently guide parents to the use of truthful, non-threatening, and age-appropriate information and support.

WHEN THE CHILD HAS CANCER

It is estimated that 10,380 children in the United States under the age of 15 were diagnosed with cancer in 2016. Because of major treatment advances in recent decades, more than 80% of children with cancer now survive five years or more (American Cancer Society, 2016). This increase in survival makes it especially important to address psychosocial concerns from diagnosis to lay a foundation for coping with this and other potential challenges in the future. Child life specialists and play therapists possess the skills and tools to provide this supportive and proactive intervention. As ideally, there is a child life specialist in the hospital setting working with children diagnosed with cancer, this chapter will focus on practice outside the hospital walls.

As in all cases, a thorough intake and assessment is essential upon beginning work with a new client. The clinician will want to understand the child's developmental level and understanding, as well as past experiences, internal coping resources, illness-related factors, family functioning, and support structures to plan intervention accordingly. Each child's experience and perceptions are unique, but the following table (see Table 6.1) can serve as a framework for developmental understanding and impact of a cancer diagnosis on the child.

A set of psychosocial treatment goals should be established based on the assessment. Hicks and Davitt (2009, 2018 in press), suggest content areas for psychosocial adjustment evaluation. These general points include areas related to understanding of illness, role in treatment, integration into normal routines, and support systems in place. These goals should focus on adaptation and integration of the cancer diagnosis into the 'new normal' of the family. Goals of the clinician should relate back to these and promote adjustment in these areas.

TABLE 6.1 Developmental Understanding and Impact of Cancer

Developmental Age	Understanding of Cancer	Concerns Related to Cancer
Preschool Age (3–5)	One point of view Simple explanations of cancer Link events to one thing Illness caused by specific action or thought Will get better automatically if follow rules Relates cancer to familiar ideas	Many misperceptions related to causality Don't understand why you can feel worse to get better Fear of separation from parents and abandonment Fear of pain and procedures
School Age (6–12)	Understand more complex explanations Can see relationship between events Fewer misperceptions related to cause Views illness as a set of symptoms Getting better comes from compliance with treatments Can sense illness is serious Many think about dying	May receive misinformation from other sources Fear of pain and physical injury
Teens (13–18)	Complex relationship between things such as symptoms and role of treatment May ask more detailed questions Define illness by symptoms and limits on life but understand reason for symptoms Understand cancer can lead to death	Concerns related to impact on life such as school, peers, sports May also receive misinformation from other sources

Model of Support

Over the years, there has been conflicting data regarding the psychological impact of a cancer diagnosis on a child. The potential for anxiety, depression, and post-traumatic stress disorder has been cited (Ferro & Boyle, 2015; Brown et al., 2007). However, more recently, it has been shown that children display an emotional hardiness (Germann et al., 2015; Phipps et al., 2014; Sharp et al., 2015). A proactive approach that addresses strengths and protective factors may have an impact on this ability to exercise resilience in the face of crisis.

The following areas of intervention can help the child life specialist or play therapist to empower children, thus fostering this resiliency. With this population, both directive and non-directive play has value. When first diagnosed, there are many times when the child needs specific information to help support coping and lay a foundation for adjustment in the future. This is a time when the clinician may choose to do direct cancer teaching to ensure the child's understanding of their illness and treatment and assess misperceptions. The playroom should contain items for both types of intervention. As infection control is essential with this population, a review of restrictions should be completed with parents. When working with a 9-year-old boy with lymphoma, a well-stocked playroom and a non-directive intervention helped him process and cope with his restriction on eating food by mouth due to a complication of treatment. He was not permitted to eat food by mouth for over two weeks and was becoming increasingly frustrated. One day, he found the plastic food in the playroom and began throwing it around. One could see the frustration release through this activity, which he continued daily for almost two weeks. It evolved toward the end to throwing the food in buckets, as it made a good sound, and he would verbalize things like "got you in there" and "take that." Overall, this was an empowering experience for this child.

These intervention areas can be part of an effective plan for the child diagnosed with cancer. The child life specialist or play therapist can use many of the creative ideas in their toolbox to address these important areas to aid in the child with cancer's coping with their illness and mitigate any potential psychological sequelae. While identified when discussing the child with cancer, many of the interventions suggested in this chapter can be used for children in each of the three groups. The clinician needs to adjust the activity for the client's situation.

Understanding of Illness

It is important for the child to have an honest, developmentally appropriate explanation of cancer. Based on developmental level, the child may have misperceptions that can lead to even greater anxiety. When not given adequate information, children will fill in the gaps, often with misinformation. Common cognitive misconceptions are that cancer is contagious, it is caused by something someone did, or it is caused by a thought or wish. Additionally, some younger children believe that cancer causes hair loss, when hair loss is actually due to chemotherapy treatments.

It is likely this type of illness education will be done in the hospital; however, it is important to always reassess as the child is presented with a lot of information that will need to be reinforced. When discussing cancer with children, it is important to use appropriate language as to not inadvertently support a misperception or use a word that could have a double meaning. For example, many well-intentioned people will explain cancer using a good cell/bad cell scenario. In a younger child, who may feel they got cancer because they were bad, this language could reinforce that notion. Better word choices would be sick cell/healthy cell or normal cell/abnormal cell.

Additionally, it is important to note that children frequently process information related to the illness in small doses. This author has had situations where a discussion related to cancer and its treatments was started and the child would completely change the subject and want to move on to something else in the playroom. Children are skilled at 'self-dosing' themselves with the information that they can process at any given time. It doesn't mean they didn't hear you, just that they had taken in enough. In most cases, the child will revisit the information when they are ready, so maintaining opportunities for open communication is essential.

One possible way to support the psychosocial goal of understanding their illness would be through non-directive medical play, in which the child has medical supplies and equipment available to them to use to play out the scenarios they choose. Many children with cancer gravitate to medical play in the playroom. Having many materials available will allow for them to choose what they need. Many themes will emerge. Frequently, the theme of blood draws or central venous device access are played out. This is especially seen at diagnosis, because this is a frequent experience when arriving at a diagnosis and the initiation of treatment. Additionally, having a play hospital with figures in the playroom can be highly effective. When one is not available, children often turn play houses into hospitals to play through health care–related themes. This play will also allow assessment of the coping skills for such procedures, and when appropriate a more directive approach can be used to help define and employ coping skills for such procedures. Additionally, themes that have been described in children with illness are mastery play, providing support, fears, and withdrawal of blood (Nabors et al., 2013).

Another way to assess understanding would be through the "You Are the Expert" activity. This is empowering for the child and a wonderful assessment tool for the clinician. The child is told they are going to teach the clinician about their illness and asked what materials they may need. Allow the child to complete the exercise and make note of any misperceptions. Any misperceptions can be clarified by asking the child (as the expert) questions. Misperceptions related to causality and other concrete information should be addressed and personal perceptions processed with the child after the 'teaching' session is complete.

Expression of Feelings

Many feelings, and often conflicting ones, come with a cancer diagnosis. Children are thrown into a new and unpredictable world. Typical activities that allow for expression of feelings are appropriate. Expressive art activities have been especially useful with this population and serve as a vehicle for communication with their family, which has been highlighted as an important factor for positive adaptation (Orbuch et al., 2005). Giving children appropriate outlets for the expression of frustration and anger are important. Targets are an especially effective tool, as they have both the written/verbal expression and the physical release. A target can be drawn on poster board and the child lists what angers or frustrates them about cancer. When finished, they can throw wet toilet paper at the target and try to hit the words. As an alternative, if you have outside access, the targets can be drawn with chalk on the pavement and the child can use syringes with water to try and erase the words. Both activities can give a sense of control and empowerment to the child.

Some research suggests that there is a relationship between attitude toward illness and health-related quality of life. Focusing intervention on the modifiable factors such as illness-specific fears and attitude toward cancer can help to improve psychosocial outcomes (Canter et al., 2015). Identifying fears and confronting them can be an extremely powerful tool toward building resiliency and growth.

Communication

Open communication is essential to promote effective coping with illness. Honest, accurate, developmentally appropriate information should always be given. This communication must be within the family, but also with peers and others outside the immediate family. The child also benefits from learning to advocate for themselves, which gives back a sense of control that can often feel lost with diagnosis.

Activities to facilitate communication within the family are especially helpful. For example, some things may be difficult to say verbally, but a mailbox created for families to write and share notes could be a useful start. Working with the child and role-playing discussions with others will also be especially helpful. One specific activity to help the child with cancer and siblings would be an activity on perspective taking. Have each trace their two feet and cut them out, keeping one and giving one to the other person. On the shoes, have them write and identify what it may be like to 'walk in the other person's shoes.' This can be especially helpful when there may be some conflict regarding parental attention.

Psychoeducation

Data suggests a positive adjustment benefit when children with cancer are provided with psychoeducation regarding a variety of topics. This information should be highly interactive and individualized. Further, training-based education, where specific skills were taught and practiced, were shown to be more effective than simply information-based training (Bradlyn, Beale, & Kato, 2003). These areas can be related to coping skills training, problem solving, assertiveness training, and adherence to treatment regimes. Children with cancer are often confronted with painful procedures and treatments to eliminate the disease. Helping children to identify effective coping strategies and practicing them is an extremely important therapeutic goal. The establishment of coping plans for particular situations can be especially empowering. Both cognitive and behavioral approaches can be effective tools. These skills should be learned and practiced within the session so the child is then able to employ them as necessary.

Additionally, many children may experience anticipatory anxiety prior to procedures or hospital visits. Cognitive coping strategies, such as thought stopping and cognitive reframing, have been extremely useful for this author when addressing anticipatory anxiety. While it is not about the process, sometimes a concrete finished product can serve as a reminder for children of the skills learned. For example, creating a first aid kit for coping is one such concrete intervention. After discussing coping strategies that the child may find useful and practicing such skills, the child can 'add' them to their first aid kit. The opportunity for creativity is endless and at the discretion of the clinician and child. Bubbles, party blowers, a magic wand, timers, lists with positive reframe statements, and small aromatherapy containers are a few examples of what some children choose. The activity can be as simple as the child drawing a suitcase-type figure on paper and drawing or writing the skills inside it, or creating an actual first aid kit like the cardboard or metal ones purchased from a craft store. This author has even had different containers, such as boxes that are empty inside, each representing a different strategy the child can employ.

Children with cancer need to learn to function in the world with their diagnosis. Invariably they will be confronted with difficult situations. As noted earlier, problem-solving skills and assertiveness training can be useful tools for the child to access. These skills will help them with friends and family as they attempt to successfully reintegrate into normal routines. Role modeling and practicing with the clinician are important steps to empower the child to take action.

Germann et al. (2015) suggest that interventions that focus on the pursuit and attainment of goals can help to promote positive psychosocial adjustment. The clinician can help the child or teen to identify their goals, maintain their work toward the goal, and overcome the barriers to achieving the goal that cancer may place in their way. This author has seen how setting goals and having hope for the future can certainly give children and families encouragement in the moment and allow them to get through even the most difficult days.

Self-Concept and Redefinition of Self

The next area for psychosocial intervention is self-concept. The diagnosis of cancer can have an impact on self-concept, which needs to be assessed and addressed. One intervention done with older school-aged children and teens is mask making. On the outside, they paste things from magazines to indicate what they show the world about themselves, and on the inside, they paste things indicating their inner world. One adolescent with a brain tumor covered the whole front of the mask in brown paper. During processing, he indicated that he covered it because no one sees him at all. He had been having trouble with peers at school and feeling a lack of support especially in relation to his cognitive and physical changes. This activity done in group allowed others to share strategies for engagement and for the client to practice them in a safe environment.

A very important goal, particularly when working with long-term survivors, is helping them to integrate the cancer experience into who they are as a person without letting it define them. It is easy to fall into allowing the illness to identify them, particularly when they have had a lengthy treatment. Intervention to work on meaning-making can be helpful. Narrative therapy can be helpful tool to help them rewrite the script. Another helpful intervention has been asking clients to create a title of an autobiography and list the titles of different chapters. This can be a tool to assess and then process their sense of self. And finally, an expressive activity in which the client draws a road map through treatment, complete with speed bumps, road blocks, and rest areas, can be especially helpful for assessment and processing.

Normalcy and Support Systems

The next area for psychosocial intervention would be helping to promote a sense of normalcy and ensuring support systems are in place. Research by Rodriguez et al. (2011) has shown that most of the stressors a child with cancer experiences are associated with impact to normal functioning, such as attending school and interacting with family and peers. Canter et al. (2015) found that children who did not consider cancer to have a serious negative impact on their normal functioning reported higher quality of life. It is important that children can address the loss of normalcy after diagnosis, but they need to work to reframe it into a 'new normal,' as there will be changes that are out of their control. An activity that is particularly helpful for this would be a change tree. Have the child draw a tree trunk on a large piece of paper. Provide them with green, yellow, red, and orange leaves. Have the child identify things that have changed since diagnosis on all but the green leaves, and place them on the tree. Next, have the child identify things that have stayed the same on the green leaves and add those to the tree. The clinician can then process this, with the child highlighting that while some things have changed, many things have remained the same. The activity can be taken a step further in another session, but focusing on the trunk and roots and having the child identify what supports they have in place to help cope with their illness. This second part is an opening to the discussion of the reactions and support of those around them and how to interphase with others.

Fostering resiliency in the entire family should be a goal for intervention and support. A family intervention focusing on the strengths each member brings to the family in challenging times can help family members to focus on and tap into individual strengths in times of crisis. A family strength garden, an adaptation on the feelings garden described later in this chapter, can be one such intervention. A flower is created for each member in which the other members write a strength they bring to the family. Flowers are shared with each other and placed in the garden to revisit in the future.

Clinical Considerations Based on Phase of Illness

While working with children with cancer, there may be different therapeutic goals based on phase of treatment when the family seeks services. Next, various phases of illness will be briefly addressed to highlight potential specific stressors and impacts the child may be experiencing at that time. These potential concerns will also serve to inform therapeutic goals and intervention.

Initial Diagnosis

The diagnosis of cancer often comes as a complete shock to families. There are many unknowns. Children often experience a barrage of tests and procedures to arrive at the diagnosis, which can be extremely anxiety producing for them. Many families report that this is when they realize their lives will be split into two parts—before diagnosis and after diagnosis. They realize that life has forever changed. Children may have additional anxiety as they see the reaction of their typically in-control parents. The time between receiving the diagnosis and having a specific treatment plan is one of the most challenging times. The associated feelings of helplessness and lack of control are especially impactful at this time. Some adaptive responses during this time are understanding of illness, seeking information, expression of feelings, exercising appropriate control, and integrating treatment into lifestyle.

Treatment Phase

This time is highlighted by changing routines, many hospital visits, unpredictable side effects, and hospital admissions and finding ways to create a sense of normalcy. Intervention should focus on routines, promoting predictability whenever possible, and maintaining developmental milestones, as regressive behavior may be exhibited. Social and school intervention is especially important, as this is a time the child may return to school and have more interaction with peers. The child should be prepared for potential reactions from others and practice responses. Additionally, parents should be encouraged to maintain limits to send a message they are a child first, then a child with cancer. During this time, goals are the expression of needs, the family communicating openly, returning to normal activities and routines such as school and peer interaction, and normal limit setting.

Remission and Long-Term Survivorship

The end of treatment can bring some positive psychosocial outcomes such as high self-worth, good behavior, and improved mental health and social behavior (Wakefield et al., 2010). However, this can also be an especially anxiety-producing time for children and families, which some report is even more difficult than the treatment phase. During treatment, they are under the watchful eye of the medical team and have a set course of action. When treatment is over, although relieved to complete that phase, families can be especially anxious. Many express concerns about recurrence, as well as real and perceived concerns about late effects of treatment. Some older children and teens may experience survivor's guilt. It is very likely they formed a peer group of other children or teens being treated for cancer. Unfortunately, some will die from their disease, leaving others to question, why them and not me?

Many long-term survivors cope well and live psychologically well-adjusted lives (Germann et al., 2015). However, it is important to remember that with any time of significant growth or change there is the possibility for psychosocial upset. Some examples of these times are graduation, getting insurance for the first time, or having children of their own. Additionally, times when follow-up medical exams are scheduled can produce extreme anxiety. Sometimes the anxiety can be so significant that survivors elect to discontinue the recommended follow-up. This is an area where the additional support of the clinician could prove extremely helpful.

Relapse/Recurrence

This is an especially emotional time. Many feel that they did all they were supposed to and it still came back. Some, teens especially, question whether they can do treatment again. Fear can set in as they remember others that have relapsed and the outcome of their subsequent treatment. It is important to remember to reeducate the child on the diagnosis and treatments, particularly if it has been some time since the initial diagnosis and they are at a different developmental level or receiving a new type of treatment. One goal can be to support hope for the future, as this can be especially difficult at this time. Sometimes that hope for the future is all that can get them through each moment. One teen patient who had just received news of his second relapse wanted to focus solely on college applications. It was clear he understood he would not live to attend college, but it was an important developmental milestone for him and it gave him hope in the moments through his palliative treatment and allowed him to achieve some desired goals before his death.

WHEN A CHILD'S SIBLING HAS CANCER

As indicated, cancer affects the entire family. The siblings of a child with cancer are impacted in unique ways. Additional support for the siblings by a child life specialist or play therapist can be extremely beneficial. There are certain questions that may be raised by siblings that are universal, but the mode of expression depends on the child's developmental level. The understanding of cancer would be similar to that listed in Table 6.1, however, the impact on the siblings is unique. Other impacts on how siblings adjust are the length of hospitalization, the severity of the illness, the length of treatment, attention given to their feelings, the relationship with the child with cancer, and most importantly, the quality of the explanations given to them. It is equally important for siblings to have the same open, honest, and developmentally appropriate explanations regarding the diagnosis and treatment.

For preschool siblings, the focus may be on guilt or fantasy life. They still have misperceptions about cancer and what is going on when the family is separated. One 5-year-old brother reported that his sister got leukemia because she was jumping off the couch and they are not allowed to do that. In fact, the child was jumping off the couch and got significant bruising, which lead to the leukemia diagnosis. This is just one example that highlights the potential for misperceptions related to cause of illness that can be observed in both the child with cancer and other child family members.

In addition to feelings of sadness, guilt, and confusion, school-aged siblings often express feelings of inferiority or jealousy. Adolescent siblings can express resentment for being a surrogate parent for other children in the family, decreased time for social life, and being more dependent on family due to the situation instead of beginning to exert more independence from the family. Conflicting feelings and concerns can be experienced. This disconnect can be especially challenging for the child or teen to process. The following table illustrates common concerns and experiences for siblings of children with cancer.

When working with siblings, the psychosocial goals will be similar to those of the child with cancer; however, the lens will be adjusted to focus on their unique concerns as highlighted in Table 6.2. While there can be challenging emotions and reactions associated with a sibling's diagnosis of cancer, it can have some positive effects such as the development of empathy, closer relationships with the sibling, individual growth, and an enhanced self-concept. The objective for the helping professional is to help the child or teen turn the stressful situation into a growth-stimulating experience but focusing on strengths and resiliency.

TABLE 6.2 Impact of Cancer on Siblings

Possible Experiences of Siblings	Feelings, Concerns, or Questions of Siblings
Social isolation from family and friends	Fear of own health
Decreased parental attention and nurturance	Guilt and shame over causation
Lack of understanding of illness	Embarrassment over having ill sibling
Decreased opportunities due to financial implications of illness	Increased anxiety
Loss of familiar routines	Jealously
	Somatic complaints
Accept additional familial responsibility	Worry about brother or sister
Can affect school and peer relationships	Sad
Fighting and hostility	Angry
Withdrawal	Cognitive misperceptions related to cause
Attention-seeking behaviors	Resentment
Reject parents due to perceived abandonment	Protectiveness
Regression	

WHEN A PARENT HAS CANCER

The diagnosis of a parent with cancer is equally as devastating for the whole family as the diagnosis of a child within the family. It is believed about 18% of those adults diagnosed with cancer have a child under the age of 18 in their home (Weaver, Rowland, Alfano, & McNeel, 2010). The parent's first reaction is often twofold: what will happen to my child, and how can I protect my child? Their desire is for their child to continue their normal growth and development without the intrusion of cancer entering their lives.

Unique to this variation of a parent with the cancer is that it is theoretically possible for the child not to be told of the parent's diagnosis, because they will not directly experience the treatment. In addition, it is often not asked in the adult oncology setting if the patient with cancer has children in their home. No child life specialist is present to help guide parent and child in this variation of the cancer journey. This child life specialist has witnessed many parents who wish to 'protect' their child by not telling them of their cancer diagnosis and treatment. For one Hispanic family, it was not until the mother was dying in the intensive care unit that the teenage son was told his mother had cancer, despite her being in treatment for two years.

There is valid concern for a parent to worry about the impact of their cancer on their child. Research indicates that finding out that a parent has a serious illness, like cancer, elicits feelings of anxiety, confusion, sadness, anger, and uncertainty with respect to the illness (Semple & McCance, 2010; Visser, Huizinga, van der Graaf, Hoekstra, & Hoekstra-Weebers, 2004). Months after their diagnosis, parents note in their children emotional upset, problems with sleeping, concentration, and a drop in grades (Hilton & Elfert,1995; Zahlis, 2001). Recently a theoretical model has been presented to view a child's adjustment to a parent's cancer diagnosis, focusing on the

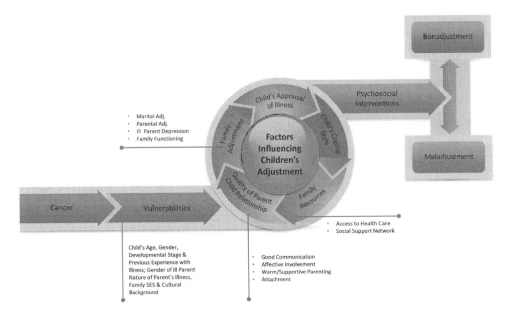

FIGURE 6.1 Model of Factors Influencing Children's Adjustment to Parental Cancer

Source: Adapted from the Resiliency Model of Family Stress, Adjustment and Adaptation (McCubbin & McCubbin, 1996)

whole family functioning rather than solely children's adjustment (Phillips & Prezio, 2017). This model, an adaptation of the resiliency model of family stress, adjustment, and adaptation, illustrates the interrelationship among child and family characteristics, family functioning and relationships, and child and adolescent well-being. While the vast majority of literature to date in this arena focuses on validating the impact of parental cancer on children, the model in Figure 6.1 moves on to recognize that with effective supportive interventions resiliency may be fostered, creating positive adjustment for children.

Children are incredibly perceptive and often speak of 'knowing something is wrong' before parents tell their child of the cancer diagnosis. Children have described to this child life specialist the phone ringing more than usual, hushed conversations behind closed bedroom doors, tears of parents, or additional visitors coming to the home unexpectedly. Even infants pick up on these nonverbal cues that something is amiss in their world, and can feel a sense of uncertainty at a time when their critical developmental task is establishing trust and predictability in their world. Parents do want to handle the crisis in a positive way, and the goal is always to help the family emerge from the crisis stronger than before the diagnosis. As noted earlier in the chapter, children have the capacity to cope and grow through the crisis when given appropriate support. Thus, helping parents to understand the need to tell their child of the cancer diagnosis in an age-appropriate manner is the first critical step of support when the parent has cancer.

As stated previously, an intake and assessment is the first step in this as well as all family cancer situations. Research is indicating that a parent's depressive mood and poor family functioning may be identifying factors for at-risk populations (Krattenmacher et al., 2012). Asking questions related to family communication and supports are important. In addition to assessing the child's developmental level, temperament, and any special needs, with this parental cancer variation there are additional critical questions to be asked. Operating outside the medical community, it is important to assess the parent's understanding of their diagnosis and treatment. It is not uncommon for this child life specialist to explain how cancer teaching is done for their child by showing a doll with central venous access to a parent, only to have the parent state that this is their first understanding/sight of their own central venous line. Many parents do not know the stage of their cancer. It is desirable to have a release of information to speak directly with the medical care team to share the support being given and gain appropriate, accurate medical information when necessary.

When possible, encourage parents to talk to their child soon after diagnosis, as this creates a sense of inclusion and trust. It is important for the clinician to assess the parent's own coping with this news and provide support for them or direct them to outside resources. The goal is for the parent to maintain control of their emotions to the point of focusing on the child and their needs during this important conversation. A helpful guide for parents and clinicians to reference in explaining a cancer diagnosis to a child may be found on the Wonders & Worries website (www.wondersandworries. org/for-parents/illness-discussion-tips/). In addition, referring to Table 6.1 on the developmental age of the child, their understanding of cancer, and likely concerns related to cancer is beneficial.

Working with the parent, it is important to help them focus on the questions that often come up with children. These questions include "Did I cause the cancer?" "Can I catch cancer?" and "What will happen to me?" The latter question is a good opportunity for the parent to tell the child what is happening now and to explain current symptoms and physical changes. This will lead to helping to explain what the next step is in treatment and the changes that the child will experience. This is also an appropriate time to tell the child that should something significant change with the treatment plan the parent will inform them. With this verbalized commitment, the child is more likely to move forward with their normal growth and development, enjoying activities with the certainty that they know 'the plan.' It also helps to emphasize open family communication, as children can easily overhear well-meaning friends or neighbors discussing their parent's illness. Creating the ground rule that the parent will come to the child with important information related to the illness and the child will come to the parent with questions or concerns is a critical component of family support.

It is important to reinforce to parents that children may need and want repetition. They may ask the same questions multiple times as they begin to process this new information and the feelings associated with it. Making open-ended statements to the child conveys willingness to talk about the cancer such as, "I told you I was going to the clinic yesterday. I wonder if you have any questions about that visit and how my cancer treatment is going."

Aspects of these difficult times play out in the changes that occur in family life. The physical symptoms of the illness and side effects of treatment are often upsetting for children to observe as they are a very tangible reminder of the illness. One child no longer wanted friends to come over to play, as she felt they would laugh at her now bald mother and she did not want her mother to be embarrassed. The physical changes and treatment protocols often create new routines. Days are filled with doctor appointments causing either reduced work or even stopping work. Mom can no longer drive car pool or may be too tired to help with homework. One child said when medical equipment was brought into his home, it "felt like our house shrank." The parent's room was no longer a viable option for both parents, and as the hospital bed took over the den, not only did this crowd out the other furniture, it created the need for the child to play more quietly than in the past. As these changes occur, new roles often occur for family members as well. Older siblings may be called upon to take on additional responsibilities both in terms of added household chores and assisting with younger siblings. A grandparent may come into the home to aid in support. It is advised that as consistent as possible caregivers are maintained to add predictability to the child's life and maintain as much normalcy with their care as possible. It must also be noted that almost all families are unsure of their financial status going forward as they anticipate medical care bills and expenses unknown to them.

With all these changes happening in the family, often in rapid succession once cancer enters the life of the family, it is easy to understand that one of the most difficult times for the child is when a parent is first diagnosed with the cancer. At the time of the diagnosis or later in treatment, separations often begin to occur for the child and their parent. This may be an actual separation with hospitalization, sometimes away from the city where the family lives, or it may be one or more symbolic separations. Examples of symbolic separations include no longer being able to help in the child's classroom for risk of infection. Fatigue or other treatment side effects may prevent the parent assisting with homework or watching the child's after-school sports. Also, particularly upsetting to the child is seeing the parent sick or upset. Sounds of vomiting of a parent after chemo may echo throughout the entire house. These reactions to treatment create bodily changes, most notably often loss of hair. This and other physical changes in the parent are a constant reminder to the child of the illness of their parent.

Model of Support

Similar to the child diagnosed with cancer, an effective treatment plan for the child with parental cancer includes providing the child with age-appropriate information about their parent's cancer, support communicating with their parents, family members and health professionals, and an environment where they can comfortably share their feelings about their parent's cancer and have their experiences normalized by peers (Ellis et al., 2017). Similar crucial components of age-appropriate understanding of illness, treatment and side effects, facilitated expression of feelings, and identified individual coping skills were also found to lead to improved parenting and amelioration of many children's issues (Phillips & Prezio, 2017) with the Wonders & Worries intervention.

Illness education as noted at the beginning of this chapter would be modified to recognize the child has not directly experienced the medical procedures or environment of the parent and has not had direct cancer teaching. The clinician or parent would begin the teaching of what cancer is with building blocks such as Duplos, body books with pictures of cells and white, round felt circles to represent healthy cells and larger, misshapen black felt circles to represent cancer cells. A sample dialogue could be:

> These blocks are put together to make towers and other things. Our body has a building block called a cell. All parts of our body are made up of cells. (Show pictures of various kinds of cells in body book.) These cells grow and make new cells. Sometimes cancer cells begin to grow and crowd out the healthy cells so they cannot do their job. (Lay black cells over the white cells demonstrating the crowding out of the healthy cells.) We do not know why cancer cells begin to grow in a person's body (usually).

It is possible for the clinician to model and rehearse with the parent cancer teaching for the parent to teach their child. It is also likely that the parent will wish for the clinician to be present to assist the parent with the cancer teaching or even conduct it with the parent present for validation and support.

Treatment for cancer may involve surgery before or after chemotherapy, as well as radiation. Chemotherapy, a strong medicine, may be the most detailed to explain, as it should involve providing the child with an understanding of the blood and other organs in the body affected by this strong medicine that seeks to eliminate fast-growing cells. Focusing on the three components of the blood, all fast-growing cells, and how each is impacted is important, as all have a direct relationship to the child's family life. When white blood cells are reduced, the parent may catch a cold or get another virus/infection more easily. This can be a confusing concept for children. While they cannot catch cancer, they and their friends must be mindful to wash their hands often, and at certain times the child may not have friends over to play or the parent may not venture out of the safety of their home to attend an activity or work. When red blood cells are affected, a reduced energy level for the parent often occurs. This can be misunderstood by the child and interpreted that they did something wrong that prevents the parent from wanting to be with them or do the things they used to do together. Finally, platelets may drop, causing bruising, nosebleeds, and other physical reminders for the child of the parent's illness.

An excellent activity to help children understand the various components of blood is "blood soup." If possible, a large pillow in the shape of a bone is used as a visual to explain the various parts of the blood. Inside the pillow are round felt shapes in the colors white, red, and yellow. As each is examined, state the purpose of each in the body. A flip chart can be made for the child to remember these components of blood and their role in the body. To make the blood soup, ask the child to add to a small Ziploc bag mini marshmallows (white blood cells), red hot candies (red blood cells), rice (platelets) and corn syrup (plasma). The child may add the amount they think is in their parent's blood.

Surgery to remove cancer often involves separation from the parent and additional caregivers coming into the home. Preparation for this is critical. Determining the timing of this depends on the child's age, with more advance notice given for older children than younger children. The explanation of the procedure may remain simple and should be based on what the child will experience, including who will be there to care for the child and what the routine will be during the absence of the parent and even the days of healing upon the parent's return. Explain how the child will be kept informed, and when and how the child may remain in contact with the parent or parents. Will there be a phone call, or can the child draw pictures to decorate the parent's room? Will the parent leave messages for the child to be read each day by the caregiver, or record a favorite story to listen to at bedtime? Part of this preparation, particularly if the child is to visit the parent in the hospital, is relaying to the child what will be experienced through their senses. What will the child see, hear, smell, and feel emotionally? Think this through from the child perspective and describing in child-friendly terms. Once the child has the information, the child has the choice of determining if they are comfortable with the visit. If the child does not wish to visit, validate this choice and help them find a way to convey their love to their parent in another way. It should be noted that this choice should only be offered to the child if the adults, including the medical team, feel it is appropriate and can avoid medical procedures unsettling to the child while the child is present.

Radiation involves a strong light focused on the area of the body where the cancer is to eliminate it. Often it is done repeatedly for several days or weeks. If possible, having the child visit the radiation center or taking pictures of the facility will help the child understand this treatment. In the Wonders & Worries playroom, a model radiation table is available that fits a Barbie-size doll for children to enact this process of cancer treatment.

With the preceding explanation of the impact of cancer on a child's life, both in terms of the changes in family life and the complexity of treatment, it is easy to see how important it is for the child to have opportunities to express their feelings. Supporting parents to ensure that these opportunities exist at home and in their child's world of school and outside activities is critical. Most readers will already understand what these opportunities may be to a large extent. What is perhaps new is helping parents to be aware that their child may be very sensitive to the stress of the parent at this time. Many children 'hold in' their feelings, not wanting to add stress to their parent's life. It is not uncommon for children to wait until treatments are over and it is 'safe' to show their own feelings. The importance of the clinician or other trusted adult that the child believes is safe and can facilitate the release of their feeling during the treatment phase is critical.

An excellent activity to help children express their feelings regarding the changes that are happening in their family and communicate these feelings to parents is the feelings garden. The comparison is made to a garden that contains many kinds of flowers, all beautiful. The child makes construction paper flowers and places on each flower a feeling they have experienced during their parent's cancer diagnosis and treatment. For younger children, these feelings can be selected from a prepared sheet of feelings and cut out, then glued to the individual flower. Older children may wish to use markers to label their flowers with their feelings. Each flower is then glued to a Popsicle stick and inserted into foam placed inside a flower pot. The pot can be decorated with paint markers and Easter basket grass laid over the foam. Taking this item home often elicits conversation in a gentler way between parent and child regarding the child's variation of feelings at this difficult time.

Closely tied to offering opportunities to express feelings is identifying and expanding the child's coping skills. Discern with the help of the parent the preferred coping techniques the child naturally gravitates to in their life. Do they prefer to be active, outside doing sports? Do they find comfort cuddling with their pet? Once these are identified, focus on explaining to the child what stress is and how there are ways to deal with it in a positive way. Discuss with them what they like to do, and begin to increase these to provide additional alternatives, especially for situations where their preferred means of stress reduction may not be available. In particular, work with the child, parent, and school to determine a plan for the child should he/she become anxious at school. One possibility is making a coping kit to be available as needed in the counselor's office composed of items utilized by the child, such as bubbles, drawing materials, a stress ball, or Play-Doh. Each item should be gone over with the child during a play session and identified as a preferred means of support by the child.

A last ideal component of support for children with a parent with cancer is the opportunity for them to be with peers also experiencing a parent with cancer. Research finds that this opportunity with peers normalizing their feelings and experience is beneficial. This carries the practical challenge of the child needing to be old enough to participate in group as well as other logistical obstacles such as schedules and traffic. Identifying age-appropriate children who have parents with similar disease stages is important. This child life specialist's experience is to group children of newly diagnosed cancer in a group. Stage four or final phase of life situations are not in the same group and often require individual support due to the likelihood of needing to offer anticipatory grief support. This therapist has also seen two middle schoolers at the same school realize they look familiar but did not know each other or that the other had a parent with cancer until in our group. With younger children, a fun game to connect children and help them realize things they have in common is called 'All My Friends and Neighbors'. In this game, a large circle is made of chairs with enough for each person to sit, except for one. Identify the person to be 'it.' Have this person stand in the middle of the circle with all others sitting in a chair. The person in the middle says "Welcome all my friends and neighbors who (name something about themselves)." Examples may be: like pizza, have a dog, or are afraid when they visit the hospital. All who can answer yes to the question run to join the person in the middle. The person in the middle then says "Goodbye all my friends and neighbors." Each person then scrambles to find a chair different from the chair they just sat in. The person left without a chair is the person who is then 'it' in the middle of the circle. The clinician should play and be in the middle from time to time, making statements related to illness that may be common for many of the children.

Ideally more will be done in the near future to extend this proactive component of support as awareness grows of the need for children who have a parent with cancer, both in the United States and internationally.

PERSONAL REFLECTIONS

Working as the first pediatric oncology child life specialist at Austin's children's hospital, two distinct experiences shaped my commitment to co-found Wonders & Worries, a non-profit providing professional support for children through their parent's illness. The first was working with an 8-year-old boy, John, who had leukemia. After three years of treatment, he was dying. Wise beyond his age, as so many children with cancer are, he knew he was dying. The medical team knew he was dying, his parents knew he was dying. I knew he was dying and knew he knew. But I and the medical team were not allowed to say anything to John by his parents. They felt that if this was verbalized, the miracle they desperately wanted and prayed for would not occur. I watched John stoically bear this burden alone until his death, not wanting to upset his parents, protecting his parents, by not saying the unspeakable. This very tragic example reinforced in such an extreme way how intuitive and perceptive children are in the midst of illness and the anguish of watching a child bear the emotional burden of illness alone.

The children's hospital at the time was located adjacent to our main adult hospital and affiliated. The ninth floor of the adult hospital was the adult oncology unit. Word that there was an oncology child life specialist at the children's hospital spread to the nurses on the ninth floor. While not officially having responsibilities there, I was called occasionally to that unit. Each time it was for a young mother in the final phase of her life, usually with less than a week to live. Realizing that there was a young child involved, a nurse would call and ask me to "do something." I was dismayed each time. What could this child have thought and felt for the months and maybe years of treatment their parent had endured? What could be done now—so little, so late? As a parent, I was heartbroken for the parent. How tragic, dying, leaving your child and not having the confidence that the psychosocial tools and support surrounding your illness had been put in place and that your child would survive your loss and even thrive with additional positive growth?

Over the last 15 years, I have seen the difference Wonders & Worries support makes as families navigate the difficult space of parental cancer. The incredible strength children muster in the face of great uncertainty when given honest, caring, professional support is especially impactful. I am so proud of each of the families we have served but I am especially pleased of the subject experts we have become and our plans to grow support for children who have a parent with cancer beyond Austin (Meredith Cooper).

It is an incredible privilege to walk beside families as they navigate the cancer experience. When families allow you to enter their world during one of their most vulnerable times, it is truly a gift that one should not take for granted. While it is rewarding work, it has the potential to be very difficult emotionally for the child life specialist or play therapist. Often, you are working with these families for the duration of treatment and, in many cases, this can be a very long time. There are so many children and families that come flooding to my mind when I think about my work. There was a school-aged boy I worked with for almost 2 years as a new child life specialist. He had little family support, and at times the nurses and I seemed like his closest and most consistent support. Working with him taught me about boundaries and the importance of maintaining them, as at times I may have been too close. It was a difficult but important lesson in self-preservation that I needed to learn early in my career, as the impact of his death was extremely devastating. Another teen, upon finding out that cure was no longer an option, sought me out to process all the things he would not achieve in his life, such as attending the prom or going to college. After moving through those losses, he immediately wanted to plan his funeral (complete with being dressed as a clown in the coffin—we could not convince his parents to fulfill that wish) and together share his wishes with his parents. Not easy work at all, but it certainly taught me lessons on the fragility of life, the things that are important when staring down your mortality, and the value of control even at the end of life. And finally, working with many children who have a parent with cancer, the importance of truthful information was reinforced. I particularly recall a very telling feelings garden done by a school-aged child. In this child's garden, there was one flower: 'suspicious.' She proceeded to talk about how she was suspicious because her parents always whispered when she was around. I had known the importance of honest and accurate information, but this encounter solidified it for me across populations impacted by cancer. I have seen firsthand that families can survive and even thrive through the cancer experience and emerge even stronger on the other side.

Throughout my career, I have worked closely with families from each of the situations we have highlighted in this chapter—the child with cancer, siblings of children with cancer, and families where the adult has cancer. What is clear to me is that each child and family I have worked with has left an imprint on me, and they have helped to shape who I am as a person and who I have become as a clinician. For this gift, I am truly grateful (Melissa Hicks).

REFERENCES

American Cancer Society. (2016). *Cancer facts & figures 2016*. Atlanta, GA: American Cancer Society.

Beale, I. L., Bradlyn, A. S., & Kato, P. M. (2003). Psychoeducational interventions with pediatric cancer patients: Part II. Effects of information and skills training on health-related outcomes. *Journal of Child and Family Studies, 12*(4), 385–397.

Bradlyn, A. S., Beale, I. L., & Kato, P. M. (2003). Psychoeducational interventions with pediatric cancer patients: Part I. Patient information and knowledge. *Journal of Child and Family Studies, 12*(3), 257–277.

Brown, R. T., Daly, B. P., & Rickel, A. U. (2007). *Chronic illness in children and adolescents (Advances in psychotherapy: Evidence-based practice)*. Boston, MA: Hogrefe Publishing.

Brown, R. T., Fuemmeler, B., Anderson, D., Jamieson, S., Simonian, S., Hall, R. K., & Brescia, F. (2007). Adjustment of children and their mothers with breast cancer. *Journal of Pediatric Psychology, 32*(3), 297–308.

Canter, K. S., Wu, Y. P., Stough, C. O., Parikshak, S., Roberts, M. C., & Amylon, M. D. (2015). The relationship between attitudes toward illness and quality of life for children with cancer and healthy siblings. *Journal of Child and Family Studies, 24*(9), 2693–2698.

Ellis, S. J., Wakefield, C. E., Antill, G., Burns, M., & Patterson, P. (2017). Supporting children facing a parent's cancer diagnosis: A systematic review of children's psychosocial needs and existing interventions. *European Journal of Cancer Care, 26*(1), 1–22.

Ferro, M.A., & Boyle, M.H. (2015). The impact of chronic physical illness, maternal depressive symptoms, family functioning, and self-esteem on symptoms of anxiety and depression in children. *Journal of Abnormal Child Psychology, 43*(1), 177–187.

Germann, J.N., Leonard, D., Stuenzi, T.J., Pop, R.B., Stewart, S.M., & Leavey, P.J. (2015). Hoping is coping: A guiding theoretical framework for promoting coping and adjustment following pediatric cancer diagnosis. *Journal of Pediatric Psychology.* https://doi.org/10.1093/jpepsy/jsv027

Ginsburg, K.R., & Jablow, M.M. (2011). *Building resilience in children and teens, 2nd Edition: Giving kids roots and wings.* Elk Grove Village, IL: American Academy of Pediatrics.

Hamama, L., Ronen, T., & Rahav, G. (2008). Self-control, self-efficacy, role overload, and stress responses among siblings of children with cancer. *Health & Social Work, 33*(2), 121–132.

Hicks, M., & Davitt, K. (2009). Chronic illness and rehabilitation. In R.H. Thompson (Ed.), *The handbook of child life: A guide for pediatric psychosocial care* (pp. 257–286). Springfield, IL: Charles C. Thomas.

Hicks, M., & Davitt, K. (2018). Chronic illness and rehabilitation. In R. H. Thompson (Ed.), *The handbook of child life: A guide for pediatric psychosocial care.* Springfield, IL: Charles C. Thomas.

Hilton, B.A., & Elfert, H. (1995). Children's experiences with mothers' early breast cancer. *Cancer Practice, 4*(2), 96–104.

Howell, K.H., Barrett-Becker, E.P., Burnside, A.N., Wamser-Nanney, R., Layne, C.M., & Kaplow, J.B. (2016). Children facing parental cancer versus parental death: The buffering effects of positive parenting and emotional expression. *Journal of Child and Family Studies, 25*(1), 152–164.

Krattenmacher, T., Kühne, F., Ernst, J., Bergelt, C., Romer, G., & Möller, B. (2012). Parental cancer: Factors associated with children's psychosocial adjustment—a systematic review. *Journal of Psychosomatic Research, 72*(5), 344–356.

Meyler, E., Guerin, S., Kiernan, G., & Breatnach, F. (2010). Review of family-based psychosocial interventions for childhood cancer. *Journal of Pediatric Psychology, 35*(10), 1116–1132.

Nabors, L., Bartz, J., Kichler, J., Sievers, R., Elkins, R., & Pangallo, J. (2013). Play as a mechanism of working through medical trauma for children with medical illnesses and their siblings. *Issues in Comprehensive Pediatric Nursing, 36*(3), 212–224.

Orbuch, T.L., Parry, C., Chesler, M., Fritz, J., & Repetto, P. (2005). Parent child relationships and quality of life: Resilience among childhood cancer survivors. *Family Relations, 54*(2), 171–183.

Phillips, F., & Prezio, E.A. (2017). Wonders & Worries: valuation of a child centered psychosocial intervention for families who have a parent/primary caregiver with cancer. *Psycho Oncology, 26*(7), 1006–1012.

Phipps, S., Klosky, J.L., Long, A., Hudson, M.M., Huang, Q., Zhang, H., & Noll, R.B. (2014). Posttraumatic stress and psychological growth in children with cancer: Has the traumatic impact of cancer been overestimated? *Journal of Clinical Oncology, 32*(7), 641–646.

Rodriguez, E.M., Dunn, M.J., Zuckerman, T., Vannatta, K., Gerhardt, C.A., & Compas, B.E. (2011). Cancer-related sources of stress for children with cancer and their parents. *Journal of Pediatric Psychology, 37*(2), 185–197. https://doi.org/10.1093/jpepsy/jsr054

Semple, C.J., & McCance, T. (2010). Parents' experience of cancer who have young children: A literature review. *Cancer Nursing, 33*(2), 110–118.

Sharp, K.M.H., Willard, V.W., Okado, Y., Tillery, R., Barnes, S., Long, A., & Phipps, S. (2015). Profiles of connectedness: Processes of resilience and growth in children with cancer. *Journal of Pediatric Psychology, 40*(9), 904–913.

Sieh, D.S., Visser-Meily, J.M.A., & Meijer, A.M. (2013). Differential outcomes of adolescents with chronically ill and healthy parents. *Journal of Child and Family Studies, 22*(2), 209–218.

Visser, A., Huizinga, G.A., van der Graaf, W.T., Hoekstra, H.J., & Hoekstra-Weebers, J.E. (2004). The impact of parental cancer on children and the family: A review of the literature. *Cancer Treatment Reviews, 30*(8), 683–694.

Wakefield, C. E., McLoone, J., Goodenough, B., Lenthen, K., Cairns, D. R., & Cohn, R. J. (2010). The psychosocial impact of completing childhood cancer treatment: A systematic review of the literature. *Journal of Pediatric Psychology, 35*(3), 262–274.

Weaver, K. E., Rowland, J. H., Alfano, C. M., & McNeel, T. S. (2010). Parental cancer and the family. *Cancer, 116*(18), 4395–4401.

Wilson, J. Z., Marin, D., Maxwell, K., Cumming, J., Berger, R., Saini, S., . . . Chibnall, J. T. (2016). Association of posttraumatic growth and illness related burden with psychosocial factors of patient, family, and provider in pediatric cancer survivors. *Journal of Traumatic Stress, 29*(5), 448–456.

Zahlis, E. H. (July 2001). The child's worries about the mother's breast cancer: Sources of distress in school-age children. *Oncology Nursing Forum, 28*(6), 1019–1025.

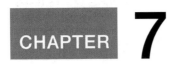

CHAPTER 7

Playing With Stigma

Medical Play for Adolescents With HIV

Kathryn A. Cantrell, Kerri Modry-Mandell, Jessica E. Pappagianopoulos, Sarah V. Grill, and W. George Scarlett

Meet despair with play, play that softens hard times and renews so as to thrive.
—Anonymous

Nikka was a 19-year-old female embarking on her college career when she was first diagnosed with HIV. The day of her diagnosis was also the day she had planned to go shopping with her best friend for her new dorm room. Instead, she spent the afternoon in the clinic, shocked by the results and fearful for her future. Suddenly, Nikka had to put aside her worries about college and instead focus on her health and the impact of an HIV diagnosis. She was scared. What would people, especially her family, think? She was overwhelmed. How could this even happen when she was being so careful? And she was daunted. How would it be possible to keep up with meds and classwork? What would her new social life look like?

I (KAC) met Nikka the second month into my position as a child life specialist at St. Jude Children's Research Hospital in Memphis, Tennessee. When I became the sole child life specialist for a clinic serving over 580 children, adolescents, and young adults with HIV throughout the greater Memphis area, I imagined I would be working with smiling school-aged children and babbling babies. In fact, many of the patients I worked with were as I had imagined. But most were adolescents suffering an illness experience wrought with violence, stigma, and shame. And while I had imagined I would be providing medical play interventions to preschoolers, ones designed to support adjustment to frequent needles and complicated medication regimes, the medical play in this setting, with adolescents experiencing discrimination due to their HIV status looked much different. Medical play for these adolescents was not just a mode for educating and for normalizing the hospital experience. It was also an expressive outlet for combating stigma and the despair associated with HIV.

Nikka benefited from the medical play designed to support her adjustment to an HIV diagnosis, one that carries stigma and discrimination. During our time together, she decorated a pill case to discreetly house her medications, wrote a play rehearsing how to disclose to new friends at college, and wrote a poem for other patients, educating them on what physical symptoms accompany her medications.

In this chapter, we elaborate from this opening example of Nikka and explain how medical play can be adapted for targeting adolescent patients with HIV. Before describing medical play interventions for this specific population, however, we will provide an updated account of the HIV experience for adolescents and the specific problems that medical play can help ameliorate. The chapter concludes with recommendations for implementing medical play while working with patients like Nikka.

HIV IN ADOLESCENCE: A DEVELOPMENTAL LENS

Young people ages 13–24 account for nearly 26% of all new HIV infections annually within the United States (Centers for Disease Control, 2012). Antiretroviral therapy, or regimens of daily HIV medication, allow adolescents to live healthy and productive lives. However, one of the leading barriers to taking antiretroviral medication for many is internalized stigma associated with HIV (Hazra, Siberry, & Mofenson, 2010). Stigma accounts for increased social isolation among adolescents (Battles & Wiener, 2002) and inhibits soliciting support for health management (Battles & Wiener, 2002; Hazra et al., 2010), which has a lasting health impact, as suboptimal medical adherence is the leading cause of AIDS progression and eventual death in adolescents with HIV (Zanoni & Mayer, 2014).

The human immunodeficiency virus, or HIV, is a virus that suppresses an adolescent's immune system, leading to more illness. Adolescents with HIV (AHIV) acquire the virus either perinatally, at birth, or behaviorally through sexual contact or intravenous drug use. Adolescents with perinatally acquired HIV must confront their mother's own diagnosis while adhering to lifelong treatment. For adolescents with behaviorally acquired HIV, issues of adjusting to treatment, medication adherence, and disclosure to sexual partners complicate an initial diagnosis.

A developmental lens aids in understanding how AHIV cope with their illness. Adolescents between the ages of 12–19 are constantly constructing and rehearsing their identities during social interactions. Normally they depend on peer relationships and intimacy to construct roles for themselves and to make deliberate decisions and choices, especially about vocation, sexual orientation, and life in general. When they are unable to rehearse roles socially due to social isolation, they can develop role confusion, a risk factor for mental health concerns in adolescence. For adolescents especially, it is the social stigma assigned to an HIV diagnosis that remains a central stressor accounting for social isolation, leading to role confusion and problems in identity development (Battles & Wiener, 2002).

Dan McAdams (2001), arguably today's leading theorist on identity development, explains that people create their identity through constructing stories about their lives and that narrative identity builds slowly over time as people share stories with others.

His work shows narrative identity emerging in late adolescence, as a function of societal expectations and maturation in formal operational thinking and as an ongoing means to answer the identity question, *Who am I?* However, when confronted with a stigmatizing illness, adolescents are less likely to talk openly about their diagnosis for fear of abuse and discrimination. This phenomenon impedes the storytelling process and identity development as a whole. In short, AHIV are silenced by their HIV and by the thought of their having to share their HIV story with their peers.

Stigma, which is associated with depressive symptoms, loneliness, and lower self-esteem, is an obstacle not just to identity development, but also to being physically healthy (Gadow et al., 2012). For example, AHIV often fear taking medication in front of peers due to the possibility of inadvertent disclosure (Martinez et al., 2012), and they often feel uncomfortable when asking questions of clinicians, questions whose answers are needed if they are to take proper care of themselves. Further, the negative connotation that is often attached to HIV, due to its association with taboo topics such as sex and death, instills fear in adolescents when attempting to disclose a diagnosis to family or friends. Adolescents are likely to refrain from disclosing diagnoses because they fear enduring emotional abuse, such as being blamed or judged, and because they fear being the topic of gossip (French, Greeff, Watson, & Doak, 2015). For example, one adolescent with HIV said this about what her peers might say if she disclosed: "Maybe she is having different partners. That is why she is HIV" (French et al., 2015, p. 1044).

Also, AHIV have expressed frustration due to peers' lack of education and sensitivity regarding HIV. They may fear rejection or discrimination by family and friends, or the possibility of being ostracized by individuals who incorrectly presume that HIV can be caught by simply talking or being in proximity (Hogwood, Campbell, & Butler, 2013).

This brief overview of how HIV and stage-related issues combine is meant to explain how a developmental perspective is crucial to understanding the experience of adolescents with HIV. What follows are details to foster further understanding of that experience.

Psychosocial Impact

Joseph was diagnosed with HIV at birth, shortly before his mother passed away due to AIDS. Raised by his grandparents, Joseph began working at his grandfather's hardware store when he was 16 years old. At 18, he began looking for other jobs to build his resume but quickly became paralyzed with anxiety. While working for his grandfather, Joseph never had to hide his pills or come up with excuses when he had medical appointments. But with new supervisors, Joseph is now worried about how to navigate a professional setting with an HIV diagnosis. He is faced with questions such as, "How much do I have to share?" "Will I be forced to lie?" "What if they find out? Could they fire me?"

The quality of HIV-infected patients' relationships is associated with how adaptively they manage the diagnosis (Macapagal, Ringer, Woller, & Lysaker, 2012). Stigma can prevent an AHIV from developing or maintaining those positive relationships needed in order to manage their illness. Disclosing intimate life events, including illness, loss, and family functioning, are necessary to establish close relationships. For AHIV, stigma may limit this ability, adding secrecy to new friendships or romantic relationships (Hogwood et al., 2013). In addition to limiting social support and open communication, stigma can impede educational efforts to enhance health literacy and, subsequently, to improve health behaviors. Without the ability to openly discuss their HIV diagnosis, adolescents are not able to share their knowledge about the disease with peers, thus preventing a progressive discourse on HIV prevention.

AHIV may also struggle with mental health conditions. The risk for depression or anxiety disorders is higher for AHIV compared to the general population (Gadow et al., 2012). For many AHIV, lower levels of social support, higher viral load, negative experiences disclosing to acquaintances, and identifying as LGBT significantly correlate with mental health conditions (Lam, Naar-King, & Wright, 2007). Adolescents who are perinatally infected with HIV face wide-ranging challenges, from developmental disabilities, stigma, and family death to toxic environmental factors, including poverty, racism, and violence (Mellins & Malee, 2013). Due to death or illness in the family, or family disruption, youth with perinatally acquired HIV may also experience multiple caretaker transitions (Mellins & Malee, 2013). These stressors combine with social stigmatization to increase the prevalence of mental health conditions, including clinical depression and anxiety (Gadow et al., 2012).

Mental health outcomes differ depending on the source of one's HIV. In a study of youth with perinatal HIV, 70% met the criteria for a DSM-IV diagnosis (Gadow et al., 2012). For youth perinatally infected with HIV, a higher viral load predicts depressive symptoms (Gadow et al., 2012). Likewise, youth with perinatally infected HIV are more likely to be on psychotropic medication than their peers without HIV (Gadow et al., 2012). Behaviorally infected youth are more likely to be concerned about stigma, putting them at an increased risk of depression. Furthermore, behaviorally infected youth are more likely to be male, be a member of a sexual minority, and have a history of substance abuse (MacDonell, Naar-King, Huszti, & Belzer, 2013). Regardless of these distinctions, it is clear that there is a need in AHIV care to address mental health, social stigmatization, and personal disclosure issues.

Relational Impact

Macy became diagnosed with HIV after she was sexually assaulted at age 13. Entering adolescence with a trauma history and a new stigmatizing illness made Macy question whether it was possible for her to feel loveable again. While working with her child life specialist, Macy described a boy at school who she had a crush on but shared, "He'll never date me because I am nasty now." When asked how she came up with the word "nasty," Macy explained, "Well, that's what my sisters say when they hear someone has HIV. That's why I'll never tell them. I'll never tell anyone—no one will like me if I say it out loud."

The HIV experience for youth impacts the entire family, and for youth living with HIV, having a supportive family is integral to their well-being and medication adherence (Vranda & Mothi, 2013). Many families live in fear of disclosure because of stigma. For parents of youth with perinatally acquired HIV, disclosure means confronting personal responsibility and acknowledging the behaviors that led the parent, as well as the child, to be infected (Vranda & Mothi, 2013). Furthermore, both parent and child can internalize shame, putting the family at an increased risk for mental health problems (Vranda & Mothi, 2013). Adding to the problems is the fact that the family having an AHIV often copes with discrimination, illness, lack of resources, and isolation. Thus, efforts to support each member of the household are necessary for augmenting adjustment and coping in the lives of youth with HIV.

Supportive communities also impact the quality of life for youth with HIV. Lack of support from communities can mean social isolation for AHIV, and social isolation, as mentioned, can lead to poor medication adherence for AHIV and depression (Kang, Delzell, Chhabra, & Oberdorfer, 2014). Therefore, in addition to supporting the family system, it is imperative to provide AHIV with a welcoming community to promote social support.

Physical Health Impact

Lance was diagnosed with HIV at birth and has been taking the same medication for as long as he can remember. Once he turned 19 and after a rough year transitioning to adult care, Lance began to have trouble remembering to take his medication. Because he had never forgotten in the past, he had been healthy and active in his life. With less adherence, however, he began feeling gastrointestinal symptoms associated with an increase in viral load. When talking with his former pediatric medical team, Lance described that his new clinic doesn't feel as supportive, and this may be confounding his adherence: "They are so rushed there. I never feel like I can talk openly about why it's hard to always remember. They just want me out the door. So I keep my head down and don't talk about it."

Near-perfect (> 95%) adherence to medication is necessary to achieve optimal viral suppression and to prevent antiretroviral drug resistance (Reisner et al., 2009). Unfortunately, for AHIV, lack of medication adherence is high and can result in poor health outcomes (Reisner et al., 2009). For youth with medical conditions, some degree of suboptimal adherence is common, especially for those with chronic conditions such as HIV (Zanoni & Mayer, 2014). For many AHIV, medication adherence can be supported by a number of interventions, including contingency management, MEMS caps, pillboxes, and caregiver supervision (Reisner et al., 2009). Despite these interventions, many youth cite social stigmatization, lack of community, and fear of disclosure as inhibiting the efforts of those intervening (Gunther, Foisy, Houston, Guirguis, & Hughes, 2014).

In short, while the psychosocial and relational impacts of an HIV diagnosis are extensive, the physical health implications of the diagnosis are also extensive, despite the fact that antiretroviral therapy has transformed HIV from a progressive, fatal infection to a manageable chronic illness (Hazra et al., 2010). Rather than focusing just on survival and avoidance of opportunistic illnesses, AHIV must now focus on long-term disease management, sexual partner disclosure, vocational aspirations, reproductive health, and transitioning to adult medical care. These and other challenges for AHIV make managing their illness difficult at best and impossible for many (Hazra et al., 2010).

After a lifetime of taking antiretroviral therapy, youth with perinatally infected HIV often experience treatment fatigue and apathy associated with medication burnout

(Hazra et al., 2010). Furthermore, transitioning to the adult medical care model takes time and advance planning, as the pediatric and adult chronic care models are vastly different. Such planning is often absent.

While youth with behaviorally infected HIV may not experience the same treatment fatigue as those with perinatally infected HIV, many experience a host of other complications. Youth with behaviorally infected HIV, particularly the Black LGBT population, are often unable to seek treatment in a timely manner, due to lack of access (Zanoni & Mayer, 2014). In particular, the incidence of new HIV infections in the Black LGBT population remains disproportionately high compared to the general population (Zanoni & Mayer, 2014), and it is not uncommon for youth from this population to experience a dual stigmatization of sexual minority status and HIV infection, resulting in increased internalized stigma, depressive symptoms, and subsequently increased disease progression (Kemeny, 2011).

In sum, an AHIV's ability to cope with the psychosocial, relational, and physical impact of HIV is significantly influenced by the stigma associated with the diagnosis. Medical play interventions for AHIV, play designed to address the problem of stigma (and resulting isolation), can help. In subsequent sections, we explain that medical play interventions that provide social and emotional support to combat the impact of stigma on AHIV lead to better management of the illness and better engagement in normal developmental tasks, particularly the tasks of forming positive, intimate peer relationships and a positive self-narrative for identity development.

MEDICAL PLAY FOR ADOLESCENTS WITH HIV

Within the field of pediatrics, many perceive play-based interventions as being appropriate only for children under 12 years, that is, before adolescence. But play-based interventions have been shown to also benefit adolescents, albeit ones specifically designed with adolescents in mind. In the coming sections, we consider the medical play interventions that support AHIV's coping and long-term development.

For this chapter, we conceptualize play broadly in order to capture the variety of experiences that may be described as playing or being playful—including moments of humor, games with rules, and flights of imagination that get embodied in storytelling, drawing, and other acts where imagination and expressing are highly valued. In play, the person playing usually feels in control, and usually it is the process of playing that is valued at least as much as reaching some goal.

Constructing Illness Narratives: Reflecting on the Past

As previously explained, constructing personal narratives about oneself is central to an adolescent's constructing a functional identity. For AHIV, this entails constructing and sharing illness narratives, narratives that incorporate HIV into an adolescent's overall life story, and hopefully, narratives that bring out positives, such as being resilient, being cared for, and having hope for the future. Although the creation of personal narratives is a natural activity, due to the stigma surrounding their diagnosis, it feels less so for many adolescents with HIV (Dean, 1995), hence the need for added supports that allow AHIV to tell their stories.

As a therapeutic outlet, constructing illness narratives presents the opportunity for AHIV to reflect on their experiences and discover more about themselves. AHIV may write and re-write their own story, transforming it from a negative experience into a positive one (Kleinman, 1988). Their stories can take various forms, including playful and artistic forms, such as can occur in creative writing, journaling, scrapbooking, and drawing (Rao et al., 2012; Pienaar & Visser, 2012).

One narrative intervention, the "Memory Box Initiative" (Vaandrager & Pieterse, 2008), can be especially relevant for adolescents who have acquired HIV perinatally and have lost a parent with HIV. These adolescents often are grieving while simultaneously adjusting to their own diagnosis. The memory box serves as a method of differentiating their parent's illness narrative from their own. The intervention, which is at once a narrative and a legacy project, begins with the adolescent placing a picture of a lost parent within a decorated box. Gradually, the adolescent may continue to add objects that represent and remind him or her of the lost parent.

Harnessing the Support of Peer Relationships

Adolescence is also a time for forming qualitatively different kinds of friendships than those established in childhood—friendships based less on activity and cooperation and more on dialogue, collaboration, and shared feelings that can foster intimacy and promote the development of positive identity (Sullivan, 1968). Furthermore, during adolescence, individuals are often focused on their own image and on how others may perceive them. As such, the challenges of engaging in social activities and forming one's identity are amplified when an individual receives a chronic diagnosis, especially one accompanied by a social stigma. Living with a stigmatizing diagnosis, whether acquired perinatally or behaviorally, may lead to actively avoiding taking up the developmental task of building friendships based on intimacy.

One strategy for cultivating friendships for AHIV is to have AHIV spend time with peers who share the same diagnosis, such as attending HIV-specific summer camps. Spending prolonged time engaging in playful activities and sharing experiences with other AHIV normalizes the daily challenges faced by AHIV, while simultaneously leading to their feeling socially connected and to their having the opportunity to learn and acquire information from peers. Indeed, there is research to bear this out. According to Gillard, Witt, and Watts (2011), an evaluation of an HIV/AIDS-specific summer camp showed that participants felt less socially isolated and formed friendships and also acquired more knowledge and information pertaining to their diagnosis, such as disclosure and medication adherence skills.

Online communities provide another medium for developing friendships with peers. For some AHIV, participating in confidential online communities may fulfill the desire for social connectedness while circumventing the challenges of face-to-face interaction. Online communities may manifest themselves in many formats, such as one-to-one chats, forums, or blogs. Rather than interacting in person, AHIV may take comfort in anonymously divulging a diagnosis or insecurities that may accompany their chronic experience (Bacigalupe, 2011). Further, AHIV may feel defined by their diagnosis, and thus the ability to autonomously create an avatar may promote playful exploration and discoveries about themselves that go beyond their illness.

In virtual worlds, AHIV can try on different identities. One such virtual world is known as "Second Life," a 3-D world created by one's imagination in which individuals with HIV can socialize and form connections (Boulos, Hetherington, & Wheeler, 2007). In examining virtual spaces, it becomes evident that such play environments can overcome both geographical (if there are no other AHIV living in proximity) and intangible barriers AHIV put up in an effort to shield themselves from social rejection.

Disclosing one's diagnosis to others is also a crucial part of AHIV's challenge to manage their illness and support their own development. Disclosure, a process that will manifest itself differently in each unique AHIV, may lead to increased parental support, improvement in peer relationships, and a reduction in the stigma attached to one's diagnosis (Hogwood et al., 2013). Further, there exists a positive association between one's antiretroviral medication adherence and the number of people to whom the adolescent has disclosed a diagnosis (Evangeli & Foster, 2014). AHIV may also utilize the disclosure process to promote education and raise awareness of HIV to others in the community (Mo & Coulson, 2008; Hogwood et al., 2013).

However, despite the positive outcomes stemming from disclosure, AHIV often are hesitant to disclose their diagnosis due to fear of rejection and ensuing loneliness. Therefore, it is crucial to foster a supportive, safe environment in which adolescents feel comfortable to disclose when ready. Supports such as providing opportunity to role-play the process of disclosure may be offered. Role-playing can assist adolescents in practicing how to tell friends why they sometimes may not attend social activities, may be absent from school, or may need to take medication during class. Adolescents may also practice how to respond to potential jokes or questions regarding HIV so that they are better prepared.

Personal narratives may also serve as a foundation for disclosure. When an adolescent feels prepared to disclose, there exist numerous mediums through which illness narratives can be expressed to others in creative and playful ways, such as creating songs, podcasts, films, and performing plays (Sliep, Weingarten, & Gilbert, 2004; Willis et al., 2014). These activities can initiate conversation between family members, peers, and the community about one's diagnosis. Narrative-based support groups have also been designed so that individuals can cope along with others (Garte-Wolf, 2011). Creating and sharing narratives may also provide insight regarding health literacy to clinicians. For example, if an adolescent forms an incoherent or contradicting illness narrative, it becomes clear that the HIV diagnosis is not properly understood and further diagnostic teaching is required (Ezzy, 2000).

Supporting HIV Management

Lyon et al. (2003) developed a pilot program aiming to increase medication adherence in adolescents. The intervention, designed for patients and family/friends, was composed of educational sessions with a 12-week curriculum that met biweekly in a group setting. The curriculum encompassed the following topics: the workings of HIV, importance of antiretroviral therapy, medication options, nutrition and exercise advice, communications with physicians, and methods of distinguishing between truth and fiction in how the media portrays HIV. Following each session, a summary of the educational material was presented in a game show format for participants. Results of the pilot study revealed an increase in adolescents' knowledge of HIV, confidence in the effectiveness of medication, trust in health care physicians, and improved adherence to medications.

In recent years, more innovative and playful interventions have been developed to increase health literacy in regard to HIV. One prominent example is LifeWindows, a computer-based intervention comprising 18 modules aimed at improving medication adherence among patients with HIV (Fisher et al., 2011). Examples of modules include "Journey Through the Bloodstream," which takes the participant on an animated journey while providing diagnostic education of HIV through explanations of important terms such a CD-4 count, T-cells, and viral load. In "Bill the Pill," an animated character demonstrates techniques for consuming pills that may be difficult to swallow due to large size, adverse taste, or side effects of nausea. "Skip Sisdose" employs humor as a

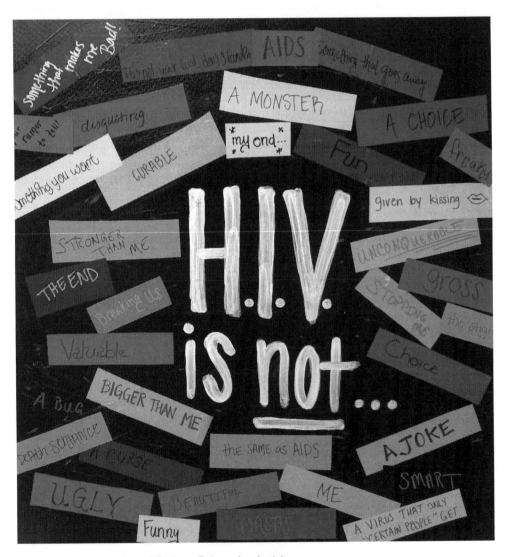

FIGURE 7.1 Examples of Patient-Driven Art Activity

method of describing the barriers of taking medication (e.g., challenges of remembering, or refraining from taking medication when peers are around due to a lack of privacy) and how to work around such obstacles. "Battle for Health" is an interactive video game where participants utilize strategies such as pillboxes and alarms to take medication at appropriate times in order to battle against infections. Players of the game can receive diagnostic education in a playful and humorous way. In evaluating the effectiveness of LifeWindows, Fisher et al. (2011) found that participants who had regularly engaged with the computer program had significantly higher antiretroviral medication adherence.

Although not precisely play, art therapy can be a means of expressing oneself in a playful manner, and has often been utilized to assist patients with medical complications in coping with psychosocial issues related to health (see Figures 7.1 and 7.2). Rao et al. (2009) conducted a randomized clinical trial to examine the impact of art therapy on physical health outcomes among patients with HIV. Individuals who had participated

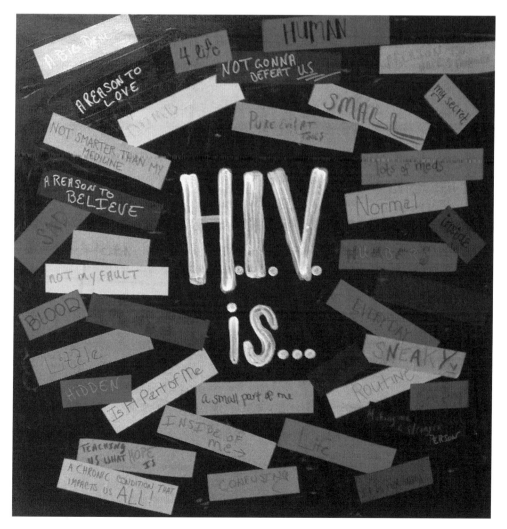

FIGURE 7.2 Examples of Patient-Driven Art Activity

in the art therapy session reported improved physical symptomatology in comparison to the control group, highlighting the benefits of art therapy. Given the potential obstacles that may arise when attempting to engage adolescents in art therapy, Malchiodi (2011) emphasized the importance for clinicians, keeping with a patient-centered perspective, to focus on work that is meaningful and that respects and supports the autonomy of the adolescents, and allows the adolescent to be the driver of each activity.

CHILD LIFE SUPPORT FOR AHIV: ATTENDING TO SPECIFICS

Due to preconceived notions that adolescents are not interested in medical play, Certified Child Life Specialists (CCLS) may refrain from integrating medical play into the care plans of adolescents. However, when play environments are designed with adolescents in mind, play can be used by CCLS as a crucial way to support AHIV and contribute to their positive health outcomes.

The Play Environment

With regard to creating a play environment for AHIV, their primary need is to have a space they can call their own (not shared with children or older patients), one that feels homey and helps create a sense of belonging and ownership. Unfortunately, the pediatric hospital has not always supported creating spaces for adolescents. The focus has been on children—with design and materials including wall animation/character prints, primary colors, plastic toys, juvenile media programming, and other child-friendly surroundings that are not particularly adolescent-friendly.

In contrast to child-friendly spaces, adolescent-friendly spaces include neutral colors, natural lighting, realistic images (e.g., of the natural world), comfortable age-appropriate modular furniture (couches, pillows, bean bags) arranged to promote socialization as well as alone activity. Similarly, in contrast to the games and construction materials for children, the loose parts and materials in spaces for adolescents should include up-to-date magazines, music, electronics (e.g., computer games), and whatever else it is that adolescents normally play with outside of a medical setting.

A designated adolescent-only space is optimal to show AHIV that they are valued and welcomed within the space. Such spaces can ultimately enable them to participate more openly and frequently in play that lightens their experience of being treated for HIV and that can lead them to better manage their problems dealing with stigma and developing positive identity.

CONSIDER THIS!

While parents and physicians often criticize the excessive amount of screen time that adolescents engage in, media use can be transformed into a positive tool to meet adolescents' developmentally appropriate needs! CCLS may facilitate adolescents in creating social connections online via appropriate chats, forums, blogs, and other online patient environments that can be tailored to the cultural interests of the AHIV. Play to their interests!

In addition to designing spaces for adolescents confined to a medical setting, CCLS can serve an important function by helping AHIV navigate the hospital or clinic. Hospitals and clinics are typically intimidating environments that AHIV will likely visit frequently. AHIV learning how to navigate these environments can instill a much-needed sense of being in control (Rollins, Bolig, & Mahan, 2005). To instill that sense, CCLS can conduct a "Clinic Scavenger Hunt," perhaps providing adolescents with clues leading to certain places in the hospital or clinic that may be important to know about, such as the cafeteria or playroom. Clues may also lead to certain pieces of medical equipment. The adolescents can be asked to take pictures with cell phones of the places and objects found. Upon return, they can compile the pictures into a meaningful collage via a mobile app.

Play Activities

Many adolescents with HIV do not feel comfortable asking questions of clinicians due to the stigmatizing nature of their diagnosis. In addition, they can be unsure of where to look and which resources to utilize when seeking information regarding HIV (Griffiths et al., 2012). Thus, they need supports to help them acquire a deeper understanding of the complexities confronting anyone having to manage HIV. In order to provide those supports, a CCLS may employ the following strategies.

Comic Strips

For how to communicate with doctors/clinicians and how to ask educated questions, comic strips provide the adolescent with an opportunity to draw in those they want to be portrayed in the strip, including themselves (see Figure 7.3). For adolescents who are new to their diagnosis and may not be ready for role-playing, comic strips can be a great way to scaffold up to dramatic play.

Film Screening With Conversation

To explore significant themes in relevant movies such as *Dallas Buyers Club* and *Me and Earl and the Dying Girl*, CCLS can host a movie night with a pre-/post-screening conversation. This interactive event creates a forum for open discussion and identification/examination of a variety of themes, including but not limited to humor, romantic relationships, stigma, illness, loss, and friendship. Films provide opportunities for discussion of salient topics without the need for self-disclosure.

Medical Games for Adolescent Groups

A CCLS can adapt almost any traditional card or board game to create medical play. For example, if an AHIV prefers to play chess, the game pieces can be replaced with medical equipment that can be woven into discussion during play. Further, a CCLS can ask adolescents to anonymously submit questions regarding a diagnosis, medications, sex, or daily challenges. The questions may then be compiled and displayed in a game show or trivia game format. This way, adolescents will have questions answered by clinicians and/or peers, gain knowledge of their diagnosis, and be presented with the opportunity to create connections with peers who have a shared diagnosis.

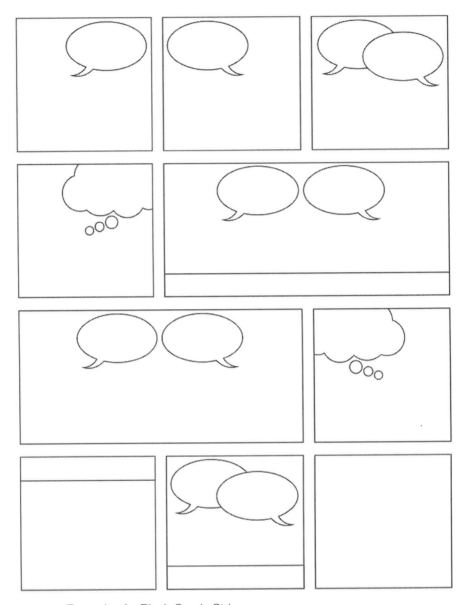

FIGURE 7.3 Example of a Blank Comic Strip

CONSIDER THIS!

Arrange furniture in spatial configurations that encourage social interaction and foster a sense of belonging (e.g., prep chairs/tables facing each other, particularly in a circled or squared arrangement to enhance communication and to support group work activities).

Learning From Peers

It may be more comforting for a newly diagnosed AHIV to learn about what has worked and what has not worked from a peer rather than from a medical professional. Thus, it is important to create environments that encourage communication between peers, fellow AHIV. These environments can be support groups, interest-based groups, and clinic mentorship programs. At St. Jude, AHIV create anonymous illness narratives to share their advice with peers, free from the fear of disclosure (Cantrell, Sutton, & Gaur, 2014). Themes of narratives include strategies for taking medication, starting a family, and disclosing to family (Cantrell et al., 2014).

Adherence to Medication

Many AHIV are wary of taking medication in public due to inadvertent disclosure to individuals in proximity and the potential judgments that may ensue. In order to combat this, CCLS can work with adolescents on meaningful art-making that serves a functional purpose. One example is "Pill Case Decorating," providing adolescents with art supplies and an empty pill case with the instruction to decorate it with any method of choice. The possibilities are endless, as adolescents can choose to adorn their pill case with an image of a favorite rock star or athlete, an inspiring quote, or even dress it up with some shiny 'bling.' The purpose is threefold. First, each time the AHIV needs to take their antiretroviral medication, the pill case will trigger a happy memory of this experience and may aid in reminding a patient to take one's pills. Second, an adolescent may disguise the case by decorating it so that it no longer resembles a pill case in order to avoid any stigma that may surround taking medication in a social situation. Third, this activity may also serve the purpose of rapport-building, especially if used as an introduction activity when an AHIV is newly admitted to the hospital/clinic.

CONSIDER THIS!

While the adolescent is designing the pill case, use this as an opportunity to get to know each other and to discuss any questions that may arise regarding use of medication or perceived stigma. Be sure to have a pill case handy that you can also decorate to help normalize the experience and balance the exchange of ideas and creative self-expression.

In addition to using the methods just explained, CCLS may assist AHIV in coming to terms with their diagnosis and building up confidence and ability to disclose their HIV status to peers, family, and/or romantic partners by implementing the following.

Embracing Mindfulness and Self-Reflection

There are water-based surface boards, sand gardens, soothing music, mandalas, and media available that provide the opportunity to gently create and re-create. These media can help adolescents to relax, reduce stress, and just 'let it all go!' Group mindfulness activities can provide AHIV an opportunity to model their relaxation skills for one another.

Expressing Oneself Via Dramatic Play

Dramatic play can provide adolescents with opportunities to use props/materials/music and designated safe performance space to explore their feelings, share experiences, and set personal/group goals around issues such stigma, intimacy, friendships, and disclosure. Dramatic play provides opportunity for AHIV to practice sharing (and working to come to terms with) their feelings in a non-judgmental and collaborative environment.

> **CONSIDER THIS!**
>
> For the LGBT population, drag is a form of self-expression that can help with identity development and self-esteem. At St. Jude, adolescents with HIV put on an annual drag show for their medical team and create performances specific to the HIV experience. They dress up in sequins, sing empowering lyrics, and dance all night long as the medical team cheers them on.

Creating Illness Narratives

CCLS can work with AHIV in creating illness narratives in fun and creative, yet also therapeutic, ways. Adolescents may choose to share their story through creative writing or drawing, or transform their narrative into a play, song, podcast, or film.

> **CONSIDER THIS!**
>
> A 15-year-old with HIV wanted to share his music with peers who also had the illness. As such, he composed and recorded an entire rap album for fellow patients. Song lyrics included instructions on how to take your medications, reassurance for decreased self-esteem, and hopeful messages about the future. It was a hit among the entire clinic and a great way to encourage helping others.

Practicing Role-Playing

Role-playing provides opportunity to help AHIV advocate for their own needs and play out their questions and/or insecurities. Role-playing can also provide opportunity for adolescents to get in touch with what is most important to them at the time (e.g., disclosure as it relates to dating/sexual experiences). Furthermore, role-playing can be a beneficial tool in practicing appropriate protocols, nuances, and ways of overcoming awkwardness while showing excitement, such as might be relevant for a first date or challenging peer encounter. Role-playing can also be important for working through feelings of worry and anxiety in a stress-free and supportive environment.

> **CONSIDER THIS!**
>
> While it is important that the CCLS provide one-on-one role-play with the AHIV to practice tailored/personal strategies, it is also beneficial and fun for the AHIV to role-play together. This promotes social connectedness and sense of belonging as the role-playing will be taking place in a safe space! Role-playing can be awkward; add humor and have some fun with it!

The Overall Play Relationship

One way to increase adolescent participation in play-based activities is to establish a sense of community. The benefits of play can be achieved most fully when adolescents are engaged and feel a sense of belonging in the space. To create a sense of community and belonging, rituals around play can help build trust and promote mindfulness, respect, and support. For example, each play session can begin with a circle-of-friends ritual, one that has each participant share with the group something they like about themselves and each other.

> **CONSIDER THIS!**
>
> You can also begin and/or end a play activity with a ritual that supports mindfulness/self-reflection (e.g., guided imagery, breathing exercises, meditation)—or better yet, a ritual that you and the AHIV/group tailor together!

CONCLUSION

Young people ages 13–24 years account for nearly 26% of all new HIV infections annually within the United States (Centers for Disease Control, 2012). The psychosocial impact of an HIV diagnosis in this population is exacerbated by societal stigma surrounding the diagnosis. As such, adolescents may refrain from disclosing their diagnosis due to fear of enduring emotional abuse. And when they don't disclose, they can be trapped in a permanent state of psychological isolation that seriously impedes their capacity to cope with their illness, make friends, and take on the developmental task of constructing a positive identity.

Medical play interventions can help by creating 'adolescent spaces' within hospital settings, by promoting age-appropriate play activities that empower adolescents to acquire a deeper understanding of their illness and its treatment, and by fostering connections among peers with AHIV, connections that foster self-confidence. For AHIV, there are myriad unique and complex challenges that can be addressed, understood, and expressed through play. Given that AHIV have been historically silenced, encouragement to play can work to overcome that silence and give them their voice that is needed for them to thrive.

REFERENCES

Bacigalupe, G. (2011). Is there a role for social technologies in collaborative healthcare? *Families, Systems, & Health, 29*(1), 1.

Battles, H. B., & Wiener, L. S. (2002). From adolescence through young adulthood: Psychosocial adjustment associated with long-term survival of HIV. *Journal of Adolescent Health, 30*(3), 161–168.

Boulos, M.N.K., Hetherington, L., & Wheeler, S. (2007). Second life: An overview of the potential of 3 D virtual worlds in medical and health education. *Health Information & Libraries Journal, 24*(4), 233–245.

Cantrell, K. A., Sutton, S., & Gaur, A. H. (2014). Pause, listen, share. *JAMA, 312*(4), 345–346.

Centers for Disease Control and Prevention (CDC). (2012). Vital signs: HIV infection, testing, and risk behaviors among youths-United States. *MMWR: Morbidity and Mortality Weekly Report, 61*(47), 971.

Dean, R. G. (1995). Stories of AIDS: The use of narrative as an approach to understanding in an AIDS support group. *Clinical Social Work Journal, 23*(3), 287–304.

Evangeli, M., & Foster, C. (2014). Who, then what? The need for interventions to help young people with perinatally acquired HIV disclose their HIV status to others. *Aids, 28*, S343–S346.

Ezzy, D. (2000). Illness narratives: Time, hope and HIV. *Social Science & Medicine, 50*(5), 605–617.

Fisher, J.D., Amico, K.R., Fisher, W.A., Cornman, D.H., Shuper, P.A., Trayling, C., . . . Dieckhaus, K. (2011). Computer-based intervention in HIV clinical care setting improves antiretroviral adherence: The LifeWindows project. *AIDS and Behavior, 15*(8), 1635–1646.

French, H., Greeff, M., Watson, M.J., & Doak, C.M. (2015). HIV stigma and disclosure experiences of people living with HIV in an urban and a rural setting. *AIDS Care, 27*(8), 1042–1046.

Gadow, K.D., Angelidou, K., Chernoff, M., Williams, P.L., Heston, J., Hodge, J., & Nachman, S. (2012). Longitudinal study of emerging mental health concerns in youth perinatally infected with HIV and peer comparisons. *Journal of Developmental and Behavioral Pediatrics: JDBP, 33*(6), 456.

Garte-Wolf, S.I. (2011). Narrative therapy group work for chemically dependent clients with HIV/AIDS. *Social Work With Groups, 34*(3–4), 330–338.

Gillard, A., Witt, P.A., & Watts, C.E. (2011). Outcomes and processes at a camp for youth with HIV/AIDS. *Qualitative Health Research, 21*(11), 1508–1526.

Griffiths, F., Cave, J., Boardman, F., Ren, J., Pawlikowska, T., Ball, R., . . . Cohen, A. (2012). Social networks—The future for health care delivery. *Social Science & Medicine, 75*(12), 2233–2241.

Gunther, M., Foisy, M., Houston, S., Guirguis, L., & Hughes, C. (2014). Treatment beliefs, illness perceptions, and non-adherence to antiretroviral therapy in an ethnically diverse patient population. *International Journal of Clinical Pharmacy, 36*(1), 105–111.

Hazra, R., Siberry, G.K., & Mofenson, L.M. (2010). Growing up with HIV: Children, adolescents, and young adults with perinatally acquired HIV infection. *Annual Review of Medicine, 61*, 169–185.

Hogwood, J., Campbell, T., & Butler, S. (2013). I wish I could tell you but I can't: Adolescents with perinatally acquired HIV and their dilemmas around self-disclosure. *Clinical Child Psychology and Psychiatry, 18*(1), 44–60.

Kang, E., Delzell, D.A., Chhabra, M., & Oberdorfer, P. (2014). Factors associated with high rates of antiretroviral medication adherence among youth living with perinatal HIV in Thailand. *International Journal of STD & AIDS, 26*(8), 534–541. https://doi.org/10.1177/0956462414545524

Kemeny, M.E. (2011). Psychoneuroimmunology. In H. Friedman (Ed.), *The Oxford handbook of health psychology* (pp. 138–161). Oxford: Oxford University Press.

Kleinman, A. (1988). *The illness narratives: Suffering, healing, and the human condition*. New York: Basic Books.

Lam, P. K., Naar-King, S., & Wright, K. (2007). Social support and disclosure as predictors of mental health in HIV-positive youth. *AIDS Patient Care and STDs, 21*(1), 20–29.

Lyon, M. E., Trexler, C., Akpan-Townsend, C., Pao, M., Selden, K., Fletcher, J., . . . D'Angelo, L. J. (2003). A family group approach to increasing adherence to therapy in HIV-infected youths: Results of a pilot project. *AIDS Patient Care and STDs, 17*(6), 299–308.

Macapagal, K. R., Ringer, J. M., Woller, S. E., & Lysaker, P. H. (2012). Personal narratives, coping, and quality of life in persons living with HIV. *Journal of the Association of Nurses in AIDS Care, 23*(4), 361.

MacDonell, K., Naar-King, S., Huszti, H., & Belzer, M. (2013). Barriers to medication adherence in behaviorally and perinatally infected youth living with HIV. *AIDS and Behavior, 17*(1), 86–93.

Malchiodi, C. A. (Ed.). (2011). *Handbook of art therapy*. New York: Guilford Press.

Martinez, J., Harper, G., Carleton, R. A., Hosek, S., Bojan, K., Clum, G., . . . The Adolescent Medicine Trials Network. (2012). The impact of stigma on medication adherence among HIV-positive adolescent and young adult females and the moderating effects of coping and satisfaction with health care. *AIDS Patient Care and STDs, 26*(2), 108–115.

McAdams, D. P. (2001). The psychology of life stories. *Review of General Psychology, 5*(2), 100.

Mellins, C. A., & Malee, K. M. (2013). Understanding the mental health of youth living with perinatal HIV infection: lessons learned and current challenges. *Journal of the International AIDS Society, 16*(1), 18593.

Mo, P. K., & Coulson, N. S. (2008). Exploring the communication of social support within virtual communities: A content analysis of messages posted to an online HIV/AIDS support group. *Cyberpsychology & Behavior, 11*(3), 371–374.

Pienaar, L., & Visser, M. J. (2012). An exploration of the experiences of adolescents living with HIV. *Vulnerable Children and Youth Studies, 7*(1), 66–74.

Rao, D., Desmond, M., Andrasik, M., Rasberry, T., Lambert, N., Cohn, S. E., & Simoni, J. (2012). Feasibility, acceptability, and preliminary efficacy of the unity workshop: An internalized stigma reduction intervention for African American women living with HIV. *AIDS Patient Care and STDs, 26*(10), 614–620.

Rao, D., Nainis, N., Williams, L., Langner, D., Eisin, A., & Paice, J. (2009). Art therapy for relief of symptoms associated with HIV/AIDS. *AIDS Care, 21*(1), 64–69.

Reisner, M. S. L., Mimiaga, M. J., Skeer, M. M., Perkovich, M. B., Johnson, M. C. V., & Safren, S. A. (2009). A review of HIV antiretroviral adherence and intervention studies among HIV—Infected youth. *Topics in HIV Medicine: A Publication of the International AIDS Society, USA, 17*(1), 14.

Rollins, J. A., Bolig, R., & Mahan, C. C. (2005). *Meeting children's psychosocial needs across the health-care continuum*. Austin, TX: Pro-Ed.

Sliep, Y., Weingarten, K., & Gilbert, A. (2004). Narrative theatre as an interactive community approach to mobilizing collective action in Northern Uganda. *Families, Systems, & Health, 22*(3), 306.

Sullivan, H. S. (1968). *The interpersonal theory of psychiatry*. New York: W. W. Norton.

Vaandrager, C., & Pieterse, H. J. (2008). The pen and the couch: Possibilities for creative writing and narrative therapy in South Africa. *The Social Work Practitioner-Researcher, 20*(3), 391–406.

Vranda, M. N., & Mothi, S. N. (2013). Psychosocial issues of children infected with HIV/AIDS. *Indian Journal of Psychological Medicine, 35*(1), 19.

Willis, N., Frewin, L., Miller, A., Dziwa, C., Mavhu, W., & Cowan, F. (2014). 'My story'—HIV positive adolescents tell their story through film. *Children and Youth Services Review, 45*, 129–136.

Zanoni, B. C., & Mayer, K. H. (2014). The adolescent and young adult HIV cascade of care in the United States: Exaggerated health disparities. *AIDS Patient Care and STDs, 28*(3), 128–135.

PART III

The Role of Medical Play in Childhood Medical Trauma

Integrative Attachment Informed Cognitive Behavioral Play Therapy (IAI-CBPT) for Children With Medical Trauma

Angela M. Cavett

Childhood traumatic events include experiences or negative contexts and experiences that result in acute and/or chronic physical, psychological, and relational distress, such as exposure to domestic violence, disaster, child abuse, and medical trauma (Cohen & Danielson, 2016). The rates of medical traumas are quite significant and include illnesses and injuries, particularly cancer, which is surprisingly common. For instance, 11,000 children are diagnosed each year with cancer (Kahana, Feeny, Youngstrom, & Drotar, 2006). Injuries are common, with about a quarter of youth per year involved in an unintentional injury, and this phenomenon is the leading cause of death in children, with males and children of lower socioeconomic status at even higher risk. The most common unintentional injuries are drowning and injuries sustained in motor vehicle accidents as an occupant of a vehicle or as a pedestrian; and is the second most common reason for hospitalization in children under 15 years of age (Grossman, 2000). Traumatic injuries sustained by others through war or abuse by parents or caretakers are intentional and frequently exacerbate the child's trauma reactions.

CHILDHOOD MEDICAL TRAUMA

Emotional Response to Medical Trauma

When a child faces medical concerns, he or she is confronted with a threat to safety from the illness and an anticipated or perceived threat to safety when considering or experiencing the therapeutic procedures. The child with medical issues may also be confronted with the adaptive stress placed upon a parent who is unable to protect him/her and at times are themselves involved in or experiencing medical procedures that are painful and threatening.

The physiology of trauma informs treatment. Neurological and bodily responses occur in response to threat of death, injury, or violence. These responses include changes in the hypothalamic-pituitary-adrenal (HPA) axis and noradrenergic and dopaminergic systems. The stress response is adaptive for a short period, but results in neurochemical and structural changes to the brain. Perception of threat impacts psychological functioning. When the threat is generalized to nonthreatening experiences and the child's reactions cause internal and external symptoms, the child may meet criteria for diagnoses such as post-traumatic stress disorder (PTSD), acute stress disorder, depression, anxiety, and oppositional defiant disorder.

Children who have experienced medical trauma from illness or injury are at risk of developing additional psychological problems. Chronic illness or injury can be traumatic for children (Graziano et al., 2016) . Children with cancer, for instance, in a study by Pelcovitz et al., (1998) had a 35% prevalence of PTSD. Between 19% and 32% of adolescents met criteria for post-traumatic stress disorder within 12 months of an injury (Zatzick et al., 2006). There are factors that put children more at risk. For instance, when injured children have depressive or anxious symptoms or when they dissociated at the time of injury, they are at higher risk of developing PTSD (Kahana et al., 2006). Among injured children, those who appraised themselves as being at a greater level of threat, and who experienced the trauma as more severe were more likely to develop PTSD (Kahana et al., 2006).

Marsac et al. (2016) developed a model specific to post-traumatic stress for injured children. Appraisals of the event related to the injury were important determinants of the child's risk. Children with medical trauma often exhibited problems related to anxiety, depression, and academic functioning. It was common for injured children to show post-traumatic stress symptoms. Additionally, these authors suggested that factors impacting post-medical trauma functioning included coping style, and that the initial appraisal of threat at the time of the injury impacted later functioning.

Although the focus of psychological treatment of traumatized children tends to be on the physical problems, emotional health is clearly at risk when a child has an illness or injury. Most children with post-traumatic stress from medical trauma are not initially diagnosed or treated (Rzucidlo & Campbell, 2009). Children with chronic illness (i.e., traumatic brain injury, asthma, diabetes, irritable bowel disease, cancer, pain disorders) benefit from cognitive behavioral therapy with parents involved in the treatment (Eccleston, Fisher, Law, Bartlett, & Palermo, 2015). Early assessment and intervention allows for identification and treatment of children and adolescents with medical trauma (Zatzick et al., 2008). Early symptoms of depression and post-traumatic stress predict later symptoms during the year following injury. According to Kahana, et al. (2006), social support of children with illnesses is protective against traumatic stress symptoms, and these authors also found that injured children with social impairments were more likely to develop PTSD.

Behavioral Response to Medical Trauma

Medical trauma affects all domains of the child's life. The child–parent relationship may be altered especially if the child does not have a parent present while hospitalized. If the parent is with the child at the hospital, the parent's reaction to the medical trauma may adversely impact the child. A child may need to travel for treatment outside of the area with which they are familiar, and different hospital environments and medical staff within them add another layer of adaptive demand on the child and his/her family.

The child's academic performance may reflect the impact of the medical trauma. Infrequent school attendance or stress responses such as lack of concentration may impede academic performance. School performance may be additionally impacted due to a focus on related concerns (e.g., pain, prognosis, the impact on parents). Participation in projects and group learning is impacted. School work may not be completed in a timely manner.

Social and extracurricular activities change with medical problems. The child may not be able to interact with friends and peers as often as in the past. Relationships, especially in childhood, require interaction. Injury or illness can impede time spent engaged in social activity. Extracurricular activities are often dependent upon consistency and practice, which can be a challenge for a healthy child but impossible when the child has chronic medical problems.

Childhood Medical Trauma's Impact on the Family

Medical trauma has an impact on the entire family. Post-traumatic stress symptoms are not only prevalent in children with medical trauma, as the family members of a child with chronic illness can also experience trauma, either primary or secondary (Graziano et al., 2016, Woolf, Muscara, Anderson, & McCarthy, 2016). Of the mothers of children with serious illness or injury, 12%–63% developed acute stress symptoms, and 8%–68% developed post-traumatic stress disorder (Woolf et al., 2016). Parents of children in automobile accidents were at increased risk of developing post-traumatic stress symptoms including PTSD. That risk increased dramatically if they relied upon thought suppression or engaged in maladaptive cognitions (Hiller et al., 2016).

The child and family would benefit if psychological care were integrated into treatment models (Graziano et al., 2016). Several areas are suggested for therapeutic focus including providing structure (i.e., routine), nurturing and social supporting (i.e., parent self-care, focused 1:1 time with each child), and strengthening of the marital relationship. The child's internalizing behaviors are reduced when caretakers are supportive of the child (Yasinski et al., 2016).

Social support for parents, siblings, and other family members is important. Often seeking out parents of other children who have had traumatic medical experiences can be one of the most healing supports. Not uncommonly, parents of children with medical trauma feel unheard or minimized in the medical arena. Although this dynamic seems to have decreased over the past few decades, it continues to be a real challenge that parents need to process.

Cognitive Behavioral Play Therapy for Medical Trauma

Cognitive Behavioral Therapy (CBT) developed from the integration of play therapy and cognitive behavioral therapies. Aaron Beck developed Cognitive Therapy (1963, 1964, 1972, 1976) based on the concept that cognition impacts emotion and by changing cognitions, emotions can be changed. Beck proposed that irrational thoughts were related to negative affect, and that helping patients develop more rational thought could lead to decreased pathology. Within Cognitive Therapy, it is not the situation one finds himself in but rather his cognitive assessment of the situation. Therapy can involve identifying and changing cognitions and actively replacing them with positive self-statements. Behavioral therapies are based on operant or classical conditioning and social learning theories. Operant conditioning explains how reinforcement and punishment can change the frequency of a behavior. Classical conditioning is based on associations between two stimuli, which results in a neutral stimulus developing the reaction of the stimuli with which it is linked. Modeling of behaviors and learning by the observer is described by Social Learning Theory. Susan Knell (1993, 2000a, 2000b, 2009) and Knell and Dasari (2009, 2010) developed Cognitive Behavioral Play Therapy (CBPT) to extend CBT to young children in a developmentally appropriate manner. CBPT is brief, instructional, and goal directed. As with other cognitive behavioral strategies, CBPT playfully and through the use of expressive/creative media allows the child to consider how thoughts impact feelings and behaviors.

Limitations of CBT and CBPT for Medical Trauma

CBPT is a modality of treatment that includes the power of play integrated with CBT techniques. However, CBT and CBPT have been criticized for respective limitations and weaknesses. First, relationship has been noted in several play therapies as the vehicle of change, and CBPT has been declared weaker in this area than other play therapies. The attachment relationship is typically neglected within CBT. The attachment relationship is especially important to functioning, and CBT and CBPT often do not adequately address attachment or relationship problems adequately. Second, although CBT and to a lesser extent CBPT are widely researched and empirically supported theories, their focus is on empirical validation of specific treatments and is limited in or fails to utilize science that does not 'fit' the CBT/CBPT basic premises. Third, although the strength of cognitive coping techniques can be utilized for conscious thoughts and are quite powerful, CBT and CBPT ignore or minimize the importance of unconscious thoughts. Memories of trauma are not always conscious. Fourth, verbal language in these treatment modalities is central. However, the language of children and especially those with trauma is expressed through nonverbal communication and play.

INTEGRATIVE ATTACHMENT-INFORMED COGNITIVE BEHAVIORAL PLAY THERAPY

I developed Integrative Attachment Informed Cognitive Behavioral Play Therapy (IAI-CBPT) to capture the strengths of CBT/CBPT while addressing their noted weaknesses, particularly their neglect of the importance of relationship in treatment. IAI-CBPT, a relation-based alternative to traditional CBT and CBPT, is a tiered, prescriptive, attachment-based treatment rooted in and dependent upon attachment and therapeutic relationship for its efficacy. Based upon the attachment between the child and his/her primary caregiver, the child's treatment is conceptualized through three tiers. Tier III addresses serious attachment and relationship issues in the parent–child relationship. It utilizes a primary focus on attachment-based interventions, preferably Theraplay (Booth & Jernberg, 2009). Theraplay is modeled after healthy parent–child relationships, and four dimensions of parent–child interaction are Structure, Engagement, Nurture, and Challenge, which reflect the relationship. Tier II reflects insecure attachment and relationship problems that are moderate. After the relationship is shifted to become healthier, cognitive behavioral concepts are applied. Finally, Tier I is similar to Cognitive Behavioral Play Therapy, as it can be applied effectively with children without primary or significant attachment concerns. Children who enter therapy with relatively secure attachment and relationship patterns with their primary caregivers begin therapy at Tier I.

IAI-CBPT is informed by Bruce Perry's research on the Neurosequential Model of Therapeutics (2009), which developed as a process that formally assesses and directs treatment sequentially through the deficits/symptoms (Perry, 1997, 2008a, 2008b, 2009). This is based on the triune brain and neural development. Treatment should reflect treatment based on the development at the time of the trauma. IAI-CBPT is consistent with the concept of Regulate, Relationship, Reason, which Perry suggests is optimal for treatment. For healing, the child must first be regulated, then in relationship, and finally reason can be used.

IAI-CBPT is (1) a prescriptive, integrative, component, and tier-based approach that is (2) rooted in attachment-style, parent–child relationship characteristics as well as the child's psychological symptoms/diagnosis, (3) is science-informed, (4) focused on the therapeutic relationship as the foundation for therapy, (5) developmentally appropriate, (6) play-based and as such, accepting of the child as she is and holds a vision/hope for positive change, and finally and most importantly, (7) individualized to the child. It comprises the following components, which will be fully articulated in the paragraphs to follow.

- Assessment
- Treatment planning
- Parenting
- Regulation/relationship/relaxation
- Executive functioning
- Affective awareness and modulation
- Cognitive understanding and strategies
- Behavioral awareness/modulation
- Narratives—Facilitating integration
- Termination.

Assessment and Treatment Planning

During the Assessment phase, the therapist considers the child within the system. The child's current functioning, prior mental health concerns, and current symptoms are noted. Assessment of parents' functioning must consider their stress and how available parents or guardians can be for the child. Parental mental or behavioral health concerns should be considered throughout treatment. The needs of siblings are also important. Assessment should also consider the family's ability to meet basic needs such as transportation, childcare, and food/shelter. The changes since the child's illness may be noted. Whenever possible, it is helpful to assess factors related to parents' and siblings' basic needs and level of family discord alone with the parents. This allows parents to give more details and does not risk the child feeling that their illness/injury 'caused' any problems that are noted. Spiritual beliefs and the importance of spirituality when dealing with medical illness/injury and stress may also be beneficial.

In terms of current functioning, the child's academic performance including attendance, grades, ability to complete required work, modifications to the work, and relationships with the teachers and school administration are important to assess. The child's social functioning including current friendships and time with peers, as well as how this relates to past social relationships, is noted. Social functioning would also include whether they are in activities such as music, sports, or clubs. The level of activity and changes from prior to medical trauma should be noted. Social supports outside of the family including extended family and community supports should be assessed. The support offered to the child and to each individual family member allows for comprehensive care.

A battery of testing may be given to assess symptoms, including but not limited to the Child Behavior Checklist (CBCL), Teacher Report Form (TRF), Youth Self Report (YSR), Children's Depression Inventory (CDI), Revised Children's Manifest Anxiety Scale (RCMAS), Trauma Symptom Checklist (TSCC), or Trauma Symptom Checklist for Young Children (TSCYC). To better understand the child's sleep and overall functioning, the clinician may utilize the Children's Sleep Habits Questionnaire (CSHQ), Adolescent Sleep Hygiene Scale (ASHS), or the Child Activity Limitations Interview (CALI). Assessing verbally for illness, pain, and treatment history are necessary. The Faces Pain Scale–Revised (FPS-R) can be useful. This includes onset, frequency, and patterns. For a thorough verbal assessment of pain, see Palermo (2012). To understand the child's thoughts about pain, the Pain Catastrophizing Scale for Children (PCS-C) may be used. The level of conscious awareness at the time of the injury/accident or during different periods of treatment as well as during the interview should be assessed. Understanding whether the child has dissociated and in what situations and for how long is useful information. The assessment of children with medical concerns includes how their medical experiences have impacted them. This includes the disease process and the procedures used for treatment. The attachment style of children with medical trauma is also assessed. Medical trauma impacts attachment and parent-child relationship. The MIM can be utilized to better understand the dyad and address concerns utilizing Theraplay.

Treatment Planning

Treatment planning is dependent first upon the attachment style. For Tiers III and II, the first goal is to improve the attachment style and relationship with the primary caregiver. As the relationship becomes healthier, other concerns become the focus. Tiers III and II are not the focus of this chapter. Tier I treatment is similar to CBT for children and adolescents. Psychological concerns, both internalizing and externalizing, are addressed with the focus directed by the assessment results. The child or adolescent is included in the treatment process.

Treatment planning is done collaboratively and individualized for the child and family. Play-based interventions such as "Stepping Up to Success" (Cavett, 2009, 2010a) and "Finding Fairies" (Cavett, in press) are utilized. These playful approaches allow the child's voice to be heard in a process that with standard CBT is often adult-driven. The interventions may also provide a visual that can be brought back out during the course of treatment to provide a visual of the treatment process.

Parenting

Parenting skills are utilized in IAI-CBPT throughout the treatment. The first level of parenting skills relates to attachment and helping the parent become more attuned to the child. The goals are to increase compassion, connection, acceptance, and safety for the child from the parent. This is heavily based upon the work of Bowlby (1951), Ainsworth, Blehar, Waters, and Wall (1978), Main and Solomon (1990), and Perry (1999). Parenting skills are taught and processed in therapy related to each of the treatment components. For instance, the parents learn relaxation, cognitive coping, and affect modulation strategies as their children do. The parenting component focuses on psychoeducation, skills, and support for the parent in applying the strategies. For young children, having a parent learn and display the strategy is necessary in order for the child to learn and apply it. For instance, cognitive strategies can be seen in very young children, but it seems based on parents demonstrating it and talking through the process with the child.

Parents of children with medical trauma and medical problems are essential in their children's recovery and resilience. Children are attentive to their parents. The parent is better able to help the child if they appear calm and confident. Coakley (2016) suggests that parents 'fake it' to help their children to be more calm. This can be helpful. Learning to become calmer even in times of anxiety and stress through coping skills is helpful for the parent and the child. Children are extremely perceptive, especially to their parents. Although it is true that putting on a game face can seem helpful, and in some instances may be best, it is unlikely that children will not see through that. Therefore, it is essential that the parent work through the process related to the child's medical trauma and learn coping skills themselves.

The presentation of the parent is an essential aspect of how the parent can comfort and respond to the child. The early relationship between parent and child is important, as the template for their interactions is already set. This is reflected in what the research indicates are 'problem' children in pediatric settings. Those children who are unable to call on their secure internal working models or consider adults and caregivers as safe and comforting are not calm in a setting that has cues of danger (i.e., needles, machines, and people racing about). To enhance the relationship between the parent and child is helpful for children with insecure attachments and who have medical trauma. In the here and now, the presentation of the parent is crucial, perhaps one of the most crucial and unappreciated aspects of the environment while in the hospital or following medical trauma. The importance of a calm presentation by the parent is communicated to the child, and the child, regardless of the words/cognitive reframes a parent or professional encourages, will react to the parent's presentation including their voice intonation and facial expressions. To help the parent express their thoughts and feelings can be helpful, but it is also important to work on what they portray. The anxiety, fear, mistrust, or anger felt by the parent is reflected into the child.

Regulation/Relationship/Relaxation

The foundation for all other components is regulation/relationship/relaxation. The child who feels dysregulated and unsafe has difficulty learning any higher level skills. Ideally children can rely on the parent–child relationship to establish regulation and relationship. Tier III and II work within IAI-CBPT is based on establishing the internal regulation and dyadic regulation. Regulation and relationship are aspects of this component that are woven throughout the treatment. Relationship is about attunement and understanding, empathy, and responsiveness. Through relationship, a child learns of safety. Without relationship, the child feels a sense of mistrust and fear. A primary goal for Tiers III and II is to improve the relationship between child and parent, increase the child's sense of safety within that relationship, and help the parent to attune to the deep needs of the child beyond his/her presenting behaviors. For Tiers III and II, interventions such as Theraplay may be utilized in order to create a change in the child's attachment style. Tiers III and II are primarily focused on attachment/relationship.

Polyvagal theory describes the co-regulation of others, especially a parent and child dyad. Safety is a critical part of secure attachment. Cues are read interpersonally and these cues result in a perception of safety or danger. Polyvagal theory suggests that we read "cues of safety" and "cues of danger" (Porges, 2015). Neuroception is a neural process, distinct from perception and sensation, capable of distinguishing environmental (and visceral) features that are safe, dangerous, or life-threatening. Porges describes social connectedness as what enables proximity and co-regulation of physiological state. Voice, face, and touch can help with downregulation when feeling fear.

Within the concept of safety is the paradox of feeling pain and fear for bodily integrity when faced with a medical procedure. For children, the concept of medical procedures such as an injection or surgery, which both hurt and at times make the body look different, can induce fear. The older the child, the more cognitive concepts can be utilized to provide psychoeducation about the procedure and how it is effective in helping the child. It must be considered, however, that the evidence that the child has such as a sensation of pain, not 'stopping' when he or she asks to have the procedure stop, is that what is being done to them is hurting them. The triune brain and the natural reaction of the nervous system to fear and threat, pain, and attachment disruption are all considered within the treatment. The attachment disruption can result as the parent is not able to provide safety and may even be seen as taking part in what feels like pain to the child. IAI-CBPT allows for psychoeducation about the brain's response for the parent and as much as is developmentally possible for the child.

Relaxation and Mindfulness

The tiers of IAI-CBPT indicate different strategies for children at different tiers. For very young children and for those with medical trauma that impact their attachment style, Theraplay (Booth & Jernberg, 2009) is likely the treatment of choice to help the child calm and relax. Interventions may include bubble-blowing in the mother-child dyad and using lotion while looking for a child's special spots. For young children and those with attachment concerns, coaching the parent to respond to the unconscious cues of safety or threat, as informed by polyvagal theory (Porges, 2015) is important. This can be done by addressing specific nurturing behaviors and how the parent does them. Rocking, singing lullabies, and providing physical contact are helpful at Tiers III and II. Singing lullabies is a crucial aspect of parenting infants and young children and has been noted across centuries. Winnicott (1971) suggested that lullabies can be auditory transitional objects. When lullabies are culturally based, parent-selected, and personalized, they are considered a song of kin, which has been found to be especially beneficial for both improved neonatal functioning and parental emotional well-being (Loewy, Stewart, Dassler, Telsey, & Homel, 2013). Anxiety was reduced in parents when they sang songs of kin after working with a music therapist.

The components of relaxation when done with a child at Tier II or I, including relaxation scripts, imagery, and progressive muscle relaxation, is a higher level skill that can be taught with the parent–child dyad as well as independently to children. These are common CBT skills, but when applied to children who need a more regulatory/relationship, intervention may not be sufficient. Often in therapy, parents, teachers, or medical professionals may say that the child knows coping skills but does not use them. Often this may be because we expect children to be able to utilize skills independently. When a child has unmet attachment needs, or as their energy ebbs and flows, the clinician, and more importantly, the parent must assess whether the child really needs to have a parent do the coping skills with them. For children at Tier II or I, these skills can be effective.

For children with medical trauma, medical problems, and pain, relaxation techniques are helpful. Pain can be reduced with relaxation techniques. Relaxation also helps the child relax physiologically, which reduces stress and, indirectly, pain. Psychoeducation about sensory experience and affect/memory/thoughts can be helpful. The parasympathetic nervous system responds to relaxation with decreased breathing rate, heart rate, body temperature, and blood pressure. Cortisol levels change related to relaxation exercises. Immune response is facilitated with relaxation. Psychoeducation may include the therapist, parent, and child discussing associations and how experiencing the sensation or even thinking about them can improve mood. Examples that may be given are feeling happy when smelling cookies or pumpkin pie, or feeling scared when smelling 'hospital smell,' calm when petting the child's dog, or soothed from a specific type of touch (i.e., scratching or firm rubbing but not soft or tickly touch). Practicing evoking the sensory memory can be helpful.

Two general types of breathing can be beneficial: relaxation breathing and mindful breathing. Relaxation breathing is aimed at relaxing the child. Mindful breathing is aimed at helping the child learn to focus his or her attention on the breath. Although both can be helpful, focusing on one or the other until they are well-learned is likely best. Yoga can also be beneficial with poses selected for sessions. The use of yoga should be done after consulting the physician about whether a pose or type of yoga would be acceptable for the specific patient.

When teaching breathing skills, puppets enhance the experience for young children. Toys such as *Sootheze* are stuffed animals that can be heated in a microwave or cooled in the freezer (by an adult) for relief of pain or discomfort or to increase the relaxation effect. *Sootheze* have flaxseed and herbs including lavender, rose petals, eucalyptus, and hyssop. They can be found online at www.sootheze.com. *Meditation for Teens* by Bodhipaksa is a CD that adolescents seem especially drawn to. Eline Snel's *First Aid for Unpleasant Feelings* helps older children and adolescents focus on their breath during unpleasant feelings. This involves not pushing away the negative feelings but instead giving the feelings loving attention. This can be helpful with an adult, who can discuss how pain cannot be pushed away, but by refocusing on the breath, the child may be able to learn tolerance.

Guided imagery is a technique that draws the child away from the medical concerns including pain. Guided imagery teaches the child to use the mind to concentrate on pleasant experiences and memories and to create new and imaginary ones. *Healing Images for Children* by Nancy Klein (2001) provides relaxation and guided imagery scripts for children with medical illnesses. Her scripts are specific to medical procedures or experiences, including waiting for appointments, taking medicine, help with painful sensations, surgery, and radiation.

Progressive muscle relaxation (PMR) is the tightening and relaxing of muscle groups. This is often done from head to toe and can be made into a game even for young children. For instance, Eric Carle's "Head to Toe" game can be used as a prompt, as described in Cavett (2010b), to focus on muscle groups from head to toe. Pretending to be raw and then cooked spaghetti can also be a playful PMR (Cohen, Mannarino, & Deblinger, 2006).

Executive Functioning

Learning to control concentration on or away from aversive stimuli is a skill often used by and with children with medical trauma. At the extreme, dissociation can be perceived as an adaptive coping response to situations of extreme trauma. It allows for survival when life is threatened. To allow for this response at times when it can be helpful may be considered. When children are no longer experiencing an extremely painful procedure, it can be adaptive to help them learn to alter their response and move to an engaged and fully present awareness. Even when it is not adaptive, it is important that children's experiences are validated as normal and 'what our bodies do to survive' at that time but do not need later. When altering focus, it is helpful to utilize grounding techniques. These can be done to allow the child to focus on sensory stimuli in the present moment. Within IAI-CBPT, children at Tiers II and III are more likely to have experienced dissociation or altered attention due to the trauma. The joint attention of parent–child play-based interventions can assist in drawing the child into the present and into relationship. For children at Tier I, who are less likely to historically or currently dissociate, executive functioning may have been less impacted by the trauma.

John Bowlby supervised James Robertson in a project of observing children in institutions including hospitals. He produced the film *A Two-Year-Old Goes to Hospital* (Robertson & Bowlby, 1952). The project involved video sampling of the child's behavior. The film brought to the public the experience of a young child separated from his mother while he was hospitalized. It provides a historical view of the perception of abandonment that informs our work today. Understanding the relational and regulatory aspects of attachment informs the use of executive function within therapeutic interventions across the regulation/relationship/relaxation experiential continuum.

Psychoeducation

Psychoeducation for children with medical trauma is done for each of the components (e.g., affect modulation) as well as for the child's specific illness or injury, pain, and the effects of trauma and loss. Doctor kits have been a long-time staple of most play therapy rooms. Dress-up toys may include a white coat, toy hospital, and ambulance, as well as doll figures representing adult and child figures that can be utilized as the child, parent, doctor, and other medical professionals. Band-Aids have significant utility in play therapy with children with medical trauma. In recent years, the toys available to use in psychoeducation during play therapy have increased dramatically. Organs, cells, and several bacteria are available as stuffed toys. *Smartlab Squishy Body* is a toy that allows children to see muscles, bones, and organs. The child can play with each of the organs and use an organizer to identify them independently. Young children may use the *Body Puzzle* by Belenduc as an introduction to the body. Each layer of the puzzle allows a deeper look into the body from the normal clothed presentation to the skin to muscles and bones and organs. The process of taking apart/putting together may allow for a feeling of control and mastery while providing the cognitive processing of general medical information about body basics. Psychoeducation may also rely on toys that are models of body organs or systems such as the *Miniland Circulatory System Model* or the *Miniland Anatomy Torso*. Games such as *Snacks and Bladders* and the *Anatomix Game* allow for a playful way of learning how the body works.

Affective Awareness and Modulation

Affective understanding within IAI-CBPT is critical, as the relational experience of affective connection is foundational. The child must feel heard and understood. Focus on attunement between therapist and child is also of great importance. The therapist listens deeply, attends to, and validates the child's experience. Assisting parents to learn to more responsively read their children's cues and respond to them is a focus of therapy. Parents learn to validate the child by accepting their emotional experience.

Children learn what emotions are and the common facial features displayed when experiencing them. Even very young children with medical trauma identify common feelings such as being overwhelmed, sadness, defeat, hopelessness, anger, frustration, and irritability. Emotions can be quantified and classified to various degrees depending upon the child's developmental level. Psychoeducation related to the physiological experience of feelings allows children to better and more quickly identify their internal experience. Children with medical trauma often include feelings related to fatigue and exhaustion as well as pain. Learning to 'measure' feelings can be done simply such as "small, medium, or large anger" or a Likert scale of faces or numbers. Strategies such as *Feelings Abacus* (Cavett, 2010a) can be helpful in quantification. Emotional expression is addressed in therapy, including helping parents and children understand possible behavioral expressions of emotions. Often, helping parents and children learn to come to agreement about how unpleasant emotions such as anger can be expressed in the family can be critical. Emotional understanding also includes understanding the emotional expressions of others and other's emotions and thoughts (theory of mind). Children learn affective modulation.

Affective modulation within IAI-CBPT is research-based (Gross, 2007). This work suggests that emotions can be modulated and this can be conscious or unconscious. Emotion regulation is done using five families of strategies (Gross, 1998). These include Situation Selection, Situation Modification, Attentional Deployment, Cognitive Change, and Response Modulation. Situation Selection refers to choices made by the person (or parent) that expose the child to certain situations. Parents can assist with situation selection with verbal prompts or problem solving. The relationship between the parent and child is influential. For instance, toddlers under stress are assisted not only by the mother's direct intervention but also by their attachment when the parent and child have a secure attachment (Nachmias, Gunnar, Mangelsdorf, Parritz, & Buss, 1996). The second point of affect modulation is Situation Modulation, which refers to making positive changes in the child's immediate environment to assist in helping the child to regulate emotions such as anxiety. The third step is Attentional Deployment, which is the directing of their attention to alter mood. The use of distraction and concentration facilitate this. The specific ways that distraction or concentration are utilized can result in it being beneficial or a hindrance. The fourth point of affect modulation is Cognitive Change, which relates to how situations are perceived. The cognitive appraisal can change affect response. Gross's research has shown that how a child perceives situations and utilizes Cognitive Change as an affect modulation skill is critical in the child's regulation. This parental regulation can be in the form of information shared with the child or specifically giving guidance on how to express emotions. This process, repeated throughout development, results in general perceptions held by the child. The final point of affect modulation is Response Modulation, which alters the response. This can include altering physiological reactions, such as changing the breath or using an alternative reaction such as exercise when angry. It also relates to expressing emotion differently than it is experienced internally. This is often done to coincide with social norms.

Cognition/Cognitive Understanding and Strategies

Beck (1972, 1976) proposed that thinking impacts feelings. Cognitive restructuring consists of identifying thoughts that are unhelpful and changing them to thoughts that may be more adaptive/helpful. Cognitive techniques are taught in IAI-CBPT, especially with children at Tier I. Cognitive coping begins with awareness of thoughts and how they impact mood and behavior. The therapist discusses how thoughts, feelings, and behaviors relate to one another using the cognitive triangle. Using the *Magnetic Cognitive Triangle* (Cavett, 2010b), the older child or adolescent can use magnets of feelings, thoughts, and behaviors to process their experiences and the changing process including alternative thoughts. Thought stopping and distraction are often used in medical settings to help children cope with pain and other distress.

To learn alternative thoughts, therapists begin by listening to the child and identifying thoughts that may contribute to their distress. Maladaptive language used such as catastrophizing or all-or-none thinking can be noted. It is important to acknowledge the child's reality and that their thoughts are common among children with medical trauma. Suggesting slight alternatives that allow for more hope and less rigidity can be beneficial.

Very young children may feel that the illness or medical procedures were/are their fault. Young children may also fear that they will make others sick. It can be helpful to use externalization, which allows the disease to be seen as the enemy and the cause of the pain or discomfort. This dialogue allows the parent and doctor, whom the child may have seen as sources of pain from procedures, as partners in fighting the disease. Using plush toys to show the organs, cells, and microbes can be helpful at this point in treatment.

Paris Goodyear Brown (personal communication, 2016) developed an intervention that is helpful for thought stopping and changing to alternative thoughts. A TV is created out of a box or other art material. The child is asked to draw pictures, including a picture of the distressing thought. For a child with medical trauma, this may be a representation of pain. For a child with a medical trauma such as drowning followed by intrusive thoughts of the drowning, the incident can be represented in the drawing. Several alternative thoughts can be drawn. It seems that the focus on the alternative pictures including using crayons, markers, paint, glitter, and stickers can allow the child to be drawn into the positive/calming pictures. After the pictures are drawn, the therapist stands behind the TV and places a picture in the 'screen' so the child can see the picture. The distressing picture is placed in the screen. The child can 'change the channel' and the therapist replaces the distressing thought (picture) with a calming thought (picture). A remote control is used for the child to pretend to 'change the channel' on the TV.

Children may comment that "nothing helps" or "I cannot manage the pain." As an alternative, the clinician may note that "there are some things that can help" and "there are things we can do to help you manage the pain." Often children with medical trauma, especially those with chronic pain, may feel like professionals do not understand them. It is vital that the child and parent realize that as the clinician, you believe that the symptoms are present and that you trust that the team is doing what is necessary. This may be done directly by gently confronting the perception "nobody believes me" and suggesting that the professionals do believe but realize the body and mind are connected. This allows the therapist to discuss how behavioral health is part of the system that allows for care that is as important as medical care. Our role is to use the research to allow the child to use behavioral, emotional, and cognitive strategies to cope.

Often children with medical trauma feel that "this is ruining my life." This may be discussed (using play strategies such as the *Magnetic Cognitive Triangle*, for instance) by noting that the medical concerns are real but the child has a choice (depending upon what the realistic choices are) as to how much the symptoms such as pain interfere with life. The child may state, "I can't handle pain," but be encouraged to use strategies that help such as breathing techniques or imagery. Older children may be encouraged to change how they react to discomfort. Across the cognitive coping skills, having parents help during the learning and initial implementation stages is essential. Parents can help the child to become more independent over time and depending upon age, attachment/relationship with parents, and current reactions to medical concerns.

My language with parents of children with medical issues is collaborative and acknowledges the desire to be able to protect the child and how this feels threatened when a child has a medical trauma or chronic pain.

> Our expectations of ourselves as parents can get in the way some times. This is true across many situations including when your child has chronic pain or medical problems. You expect to take away pain and your child expects it too. I remember the first time my daughter fell and got a bump. She expectantly looked to me and was calm and available. I went to her with outstretched arms. I was calm, concerned, and fully present. I kissed her bump and all was well. This is possibly the most challenging concern for parents when they have a child with serious medical issues. You are no longer able to kiss the owie and make it go away. Unfortunately, even the most educated and skilled doctor may not be able to take away the pain. When you come to see me, as a psychologist, I can help you think about where you are at now with your child's pain or medical problem and work with your perspective so that you and your child can learn to function within your new reality.

A difficult reality is that the child has medical concerns that the parent cannot control and may continue to feel pain. The therapist can help the child and the family to learn to live within this new normal. Learning to accept the pain and try to cope with it is a goal for CBT.

Behavioral Awareness and Modulation

For children with medical traumas, the areas of their lives impacted by the trauma may require direct behavioral intervention. These may include school attendance/avoidance, homework performance, activity planning, and sleep behaviors. Often, pain and illness behaviors that were adaptive in the short term become areas to focus on for behavioral change. Behaviors such as sleeping during the day can be considered pain behaviors that are often not adaptive after the acute medical concern is resolved. Routine is necessary for children after trauma and is often challenging for parents to reestablish (Rokholt, Schultz, & Langballe, 2016).

CBT is helpful to decrease avoidance. Altering thoughts can be part of behavioral change. For instance, a child who has stayed home from school may think, "I may feel pain at school and I do not want anyone to notice this." The therapist and parent may need to help the child understand that although some behaviors post–medical trauma may seem intolerable, with practice and gradual exposure the behaviors will become more possible and the child will feel better being able to function more normally. The child and parent may work with the therapist to develop a gradual exposure to the feared/anxiety-provoking stimuli (i.e., school attendance). Behavioral interventions may include operant conditioning, such as giving a reward for meeting a behavioral goal or giving a consequence for not meeting a goal.

Expectations for children after medical trauma, even those with ongoing pain, should begin to return to normal if possible. This may begin by having the child get their own snacks and drinks. Often when a child has medical trauma, parents and even siblings may rally to the child and do tasks such as this. However, to function more fully, the child should gradually return to age-appropriate chores. Chores such as cleaning the bedroom can be considered. School, both academically and socially, can be a significant adjustment for children with medical trauma and those who continue to require medical treatment. Returning to a normal schedule is helpful for children who have experienced medical trauma, including many who continue to receive medical care but are no longer hospitalized. A medical doctor decides when to medically clear a child for school. Often a therapist can be instrumental in helping this happen. This may include developing a behavioral plan that eventually increases the number of hours and/or days the child is at school and in the classroom. Rewards may be helpful in assisting with a behavioral plan. Consequences such as losing screen time if not in school for a given amount of time may be of additional utility. Helping the school provide accommodations so that expectations are consistent with each child's needs is crucial.

Sleep is often a problem for children during medical care or following medical trauma. Children may have difficulty falling or staying asleep and their sleep quality may be poor. Furthermore, behaviors developed during the initial medical trauma may negatively impact sleep. The lack of sleep may result in more significant problems. For instance, children with chronic pain often have developed poor sleep habits such as sleeping during the day. The sleep of children with type I diabetes impacts the onset and progression of the disease (Perfect et al., 2016). A first line of treatment is to help the parents assess current sleep-related behaviors and begin to utilize healthy sleep hygiene skills. Sleep hygiene includes understanding that sleep is important and that it impacts one's health. The bedtime routine is necessary to address clinically for many children. The child should have the same routine each evening, which may include bath, snack, book, prayers/gratitude for people, back rub by parent, and sleep. Some parents feel that using lotion with lavender is helpful. Helping parents set limits, including not allowing electronics or caffeine or limiting activity before bedtime, are related to getting adequate sleep.

It is important to help families understand that there are strategies for managing pain and medical procedures. These strategies may or may not reduce the child's perceived pain. The strategies will likely help the child, and the rest of the family, learn to function and regain some control over aspects of their lives that have been impacted by their medical issues.

During acute episodes of medical need, behaviors develop that are adaptive. These may not serve the child well as the medical concerns are resolved. This is especially true if the child continues to experience pain. Coakley (2016) describes the process as *redefining comfort*. The child may have behaved in ways that promoted early medical care, such as sleeping in or having parents, siblings, or others assist with tasks. However, as the child returns to normal functioning, those same behaviors may impede progress. Therefore, it is helpful to work with the child and parent to define what behaviors will be expected and setting up means to reach those behavioral goals. Coakley suggests that the child is encouraged to move from passive to active means of comfort. For instance, having children return to school or be expected to complete chores may be the goal.

Researchers have categorized coping skills in different ways, including two types described by Cheng and Chan (2003): *Control Coping* and *Avoidance Coping*. Control Coping includes "distraction, social withdrawal, self-criticism, blaming others, wishful thinking, resignation and emotional outburst" (p. 47). Therapists can encourage children and parents to develop strategies that allow for coping in the moment and for long-term benefit. These strategies may vary depending upon the child's current medical concerns and how functioning is impacted. Avoidance Coping, which may rely on similar mechanisms, is far less adaptive.

Narrative

Therapeutic goals (to process the trauma narrative by a specific session) must never impede the sense of safety. As safety increases, the ability to step up to a higher tier is created and the treatment can become more like standard CBT for children. Within IAI-CBPT, narrative is used in several ways. First, bibliotherapy is used for psycho-education and to address clinical issues that are like the presenting problems of the child. For medical trauma, this may include personalization of their understanding of the illness or injury. Second is Problem/Solution Narrative, which includes the issues brought to the session that relate to concerns since the last appointment that are articulated with speech or through play. Initially the child's version of the story may only include the problem. With or without therapist intervention, the child may use therapy to consider solutions for the problem. Third, Trauma Narrative is a specific story presented by the child, typically with the assistance of the therapist, to express traumatic events. For instance, a child who was in a car accident may have a trauma narrative that includes both the accident, the emergency care, and ongoing medical care. Having healing and resiliency narratives that are within the trauma narrative or that follow are helpful for the child.

Narrative allows for integration of the child's experiences. This includes the strengths and struggles of the child as well as the trauma and resiliency. The integration of the narrative, built on the earlier components, allows the child to connect the dots of their experience. The attachment literature supports the integrated narrative, even when a person has had trauma, as the indicator of secure attachment and psychological health. From a CBT perspective, the trauma narrative allows for exposure at titrated doses that allow for learning to look at and process the traumatic event. The elements of the trauma that were not directly traumatic but that were interpreted as such are addressed. This may include smells, sounds, or people who were involved in the medical care. For one child in my practice, seeing flowers was a trigger of medical trauma because he and his mother had been sent several bouquets of flowers while he was hospitalized. His parents could realize that his responding to flowers at his parents' anniversary seemed to trigger behaviors from him. As they processed this both as parents and with him, they could have him process his internal reactions to them and verbalize it. Without recognizing his experience and how it impacted his current functioning, this may not have been resolved. For children with extensive medical trauma, a *Life Narrative* like those written by children who are adopted can be helpful. The trauma narrative provides a framework for processing the experiences. Part of the working through of the narrative for children with medical trauma is to process experiences of invalidation by medical professionals. Often this includes a narrative of the parent understanding the child but not feeling heard by the medical professional. The future is also important to consider with children's narratives. This must be informed by the child's current medical condition and their prognosis. How the child will move forward as well as any grief or loss issues must be addressed. Resiliency narratives are important to all traumatized children. These are stories about when the child has been able to show and experience resiliency. Resiliency narratives tell of successes when the child was faced with a challenge or difficult situation and could problem solve, emotionally persevere, and overcome the situation. It is also helpful to have family narratives of resiliency. By helping the child identify with the family narrative of resiliency, she can see examples of times when a family member, such as grandma, was able to bounce back from a stressor. When family members have had similar challenges, the child can be told of how others could make it through. Specific methods for narrative telling have been designed for children with medical trauma. For instance, the *Beads of Life* approach allows adolescents diagnosed with cancer to discuss aspects of their selves including but not limited to their disease (Portnoy, Girling, & Fredman, 2016).

Termination

Termination allows for the processing of the therapy. Discussing the course of treatment and the progress made within the relationship is essential. This includes acknowledging that the child needed assistance at times but now can have others provide support or use strategies independently at times. Loss and grief is often experienced by children with medical trauma and termination of therapy brings with it another loss. Therefore, tying the child to community during the time of termination and jointly noting resiliency factors are essential. Termination can allow for discussion of future episodes of care by stating when the child or parents may want to seek out therapy again.

When a child or adolescent is seen in therapy for psychological responses to the physical illness or pain, the family is an integral part of therapy. The parents and often siblings are included in components of treatment to support the child. This also helps each other member of the family. A parent of a child with medical trauma summed up therapy with her child like this: "You have really helped Olivia. But you have helped us too. This has been three in one therapy."

CASE STUDY

Tyron

Three-year-old Tyron came to the office for his first therapy visit following a one-week hospitalization and surgery for a bowel obstruction six months earlier. In recounting his time in the hospital, his mother noted that his sister became ill during that time and she had to return to her home several hours away and was not able to find childcare for his siblings for two days. During that time, he was not accompanied by a family member. His mother noted that when she returned to the hospital, he seemed inconsolable at first, not seeming to respond to her presence and later showing anger toward her. At the intake, he appeared anxious, tugging on his mother and wanting to be held often throughout the session. His mother reported that he cried often and appeared anxious when he was not in the same room with her. His presentation was consistent with separation anxiety and a specific phobia to medical procedures including being examined. Post-traumatic stress disorder was ruled out.

At 3 years of age, Tyron was seen for family therapy with his mother and often his father when his schedule allowed. The Marschak Interaction Method (MIM) was administered to provide guidance related to the parent–child relationship. Eight sessions of Theraplay were implemented as the Tier II phase of IAI-CBPT followed by Tier I. Tyron's parent–child relationship was strengthened with a focus on Nurturing, Engagement, Structure, and Challenge. He and his parents improved their connection through nurturing activities. His parents learned about parenting, including setting limits and providing structure.

For children like Tyron with histories of trauma, parents often have difficulty setting limits. Tyron learned about regulation and relaxation techniques through play, including a progressive muscle relaxation technique using a 3-foot Batman made of hard plastic and a small soft stuffed dog. He and his parents learned to tighten like the Batman and loosen and flop like the dog, which he named "Maggie" after his own dog. Dancing, moving, and lying on the floor while tightening and relaxing allowed for better understanding of physiology of the continuum of being tight to relaxed and his ability to actively make changes in this process. His parents could observe his limitations around self-regulation in calm and stressful situations and were coached on how to provide adequate support as needed. Emotions were included in play with directive techniques including using emotions puzzles and puppet play with skits about various emotions and coping skills. He utilized a large plush toy, *Meebie*, which has Velcro facial features reflecting various emotions/expressions. He often used the Velcro Band-Aids on *Meebie* to reflect "his hurts" and "places where he was poked." His parents were coached to integrate emotional language into their lives with both pleasant and unpleasant emotions. Even at 3, he was able to learn some ideas about the relationships between feelings, thoughts, and behaviors. The therapist read the book *The Three Little Pigs* while using a three-headed dragon to point out the character's feelings, thoughts, and behaviors. The puppet was later used while Tyron's mother or Tyron told short stories about things that had happened since their last session. The *Mirrored Cognitive Triangle* was utilized. Tyron's parents were also asked to write their feelings, thoughts, and behaviors on a worksheet of the cognitive triangle. They were given a second cognitive triangle worksheet to discuss how their own perceptions, thoughts (both spoken and unspoken), and behaviors impacted and were reflected in Tyron. Tryon and his parents co-narrated his time spent in the hospital. Narration included his mother bringing pictures each session. This narration included an understanding of Tyron and who he and his family were before, during, and after the hospitalization. The hospital experience was touched on in the first narration session, with gradual exposure to more in-depth discussion of experience, including eventually talking about his being alone in the hospital as well as some of the painful procedures that occurred, sandwiched with narration of family and individual strengths that provided support in his recovery physically and emotionally. He also played with the medical kit and utilized the toy hospital and figures (e.g., child, doctor, nurse, mother figures) as he and his mother co-constructed his narrative. The early work on affective understanding and cognitive coping allowed for processing of his narrative. He was seen for six months, at which time his symptoms reduced.

At 7 years of age, Tyrone returned to the office. This time he was experiencing difficulty at school and to a lesser extent at home. His parents said, "He doesn't remember the surgery much. It doesn't seem related to the current acting out. It seems like just a school thing." His parents reported that the teacher complained that he seemed to 'space out' and expressed concern that he may have ADHD. It was noted that he had been asked to leave the classroom and stand in the hall on several occasions, as his teacher felt his behavior was disruptive. His sessions included a parent check-in, directive intervention, and nondirective play. The parent check-in typically was 5–10 minutes and included dyadic work including Theraplay interventions, some new and some that had been used in his earlier work. Directive techniques focused on affective understanding, modulation, and cognitive coping and typically made up the majority of the session (30–40 minutes). Strategies related to anger management and executive functioning skills (e.g., picture schedule of school tasks) were provided. He and his mother reviewed and elaborated on his narrative of medical trauma. While discussing his short time away from his mother at 3 years of age, his therapist noted that he had felt abandoned and wondered if he felt abandoned when he had to go to the hall at this time in his life when his teacher felt he was not paying attention in class. Consultation with the teacher allowed her to understand his medical trauma history and possible dissociation, as well as triggers such as abandonment. She seemed to consider that his behavior may have been a trauma reaction instead of ADHD. The teacher was encouraged to use short engaging rituals as points of connection with Tyron in lieu of sending him to the hall. This was reported to be beneficial, reducing his 'zoning' and also improving his teacher–student relationship. During his nondirective play, he utilized the *Meebie* (large purple stuffed animal with Velcro parts). He constructed a *Meebie* with Band-Aids in many sessions and commented that "He had an owie. He hurts a lot." At times he used first person, stating "I hurt a lot" as he played with *Meebie*. He would then construct an obstacle course in the office using balance boards, balance beam, plastic 'stepping stones,' stilts, and sacks (to hop in). He would move through the obstacle course and the therapist would track his movement, stating "You are moving your body. You are strong and safe." For several sessions, he constructed a 'hurt' *Meebie* during the nondirective period followed by the obstacle course play. He would show movement and what seemed like 'escaping' behaviors while being verbally tracked by the therapist. He then would seem to find comfort and safety, plopping onto the beanbags. He asked to have his mother come back to the office to show her the obstacle course, and she became his point of safety and comfort after completing the course. He referred to her as "safety." After several sessions, this play decreased and it seemed that there was an integration of his physical and emotional need for safety and connection. This integration allowed for affective, cognitive, and bodily experience during each component.

SUMMARY

Integrative Attachment Informed Cognitive Behavioral Play Therapy (IAI-CBPT) for children with medical trauma is a promising adaptation of the traditional Cognitive Behavioral Therapy, and Cognitive Behavioral Play Therapy and Trauma-Focused Cognitive Behavioral models of treatment that are widely used and researched today. With its additional grounding in and focus on attachment and the therapeutic relationship, this model brings a more holistic approach into the arena of child trauma treatment and to the challenging realm of medical trauma.

REFERENCES

Ainsworth, M.D.S., Blehar, M., Waters, E., & Wall, S. (1978). *Patterns of attachment.* Hillsdale, NJ: Erlbaum.

Beck, A.T. (1963). Thinking and depression part: Idiosyncratic content and cognitive distortions. *Arch Gen Psychiatry, 9*(4), 324–333.

Beck, A.T. (1964). Thinking and depression: Theory and therapy. *Archives of General Psychiatry, 10*, 561–571.

Beck, A.T. (1972). *Depression: Causes and treatment.* Philadelphia: University of Pennsylvania Press.

Beck, A.T. (1976). *Cognitive therapy and the emotional disorders.* New York: International Universities Press.

Booth, P., & Jernberg, A. (2009). *Theraplay: Helping parents and children build better relationships through attachment-based play.* San Francisco: Jossey-Bass.

Bowlby, J. (1951). *Maternal care and mental health.* World Health Organization Monograph (Serial No. 2).

Cavett, A.M. (2009). Playful trauma focused-cognitive behavioral therapy with maltreated children and adolescents. *Play Therapy, 4*(3), 20–22.

Cavett, A.M. (2010a). Putting the puzzle pieces of resiliency together. In L. Lowenstein (Ed.), *Assessment and treatment activities for children, adolescents, and families. Volume 2: Practitioners share their most effective techniques.* Toronto: Champion Press.

Cavett, A.M. (2010b). *Structured play-based interventions for engaging children and adolescents in therapy.* West Conshohocken, PA: Infinity Press.

Cavett, A.M. (in press). *Integrative attachment informed cognitive behavioral play therapy.* West Conshohocken, PA: Infinity Press.

Cheng, S. T., & Chan, A. C. (2003). Factorial structure of the Kidscope in Hong Kong adolescents. *Journal of Genetic Psychology: Research and Theory on Human Development, 164,* 261–266.

Coakley, R. (2016). *When your child hurts: Effective strategies to increase comfort, reduce stress, and break the cycle of chronic pain.* New Haven, CT: Yale University Press.

Cohen, J. R., & Danielson, C. K. (2016). Effects of childhood traumatic event experiences. In M. K. Holt & A. Grills (Eds.), *Critical issues in school-based mental health: Evidence-based research, practice, and interventions* (pp. 164–176). New York: Routledge.

Cohen, J. R., Mannarino, A., & Deblinger, E. (2006). *Treating trauma and traumatic grief in children and adolescents.* New York: The Guilford Press.

Eccleston, C., Fisher, E., Law, E., Bartlett, J., & Palermo, T. M. (2015). Psychological interventions for parents of children and adolescents with chronic illness. *Cochrane Database System Review, 15*(4), Art. No.: CD009660.

Goodyear-Brown, P. (2002). *Digging for buried treasure: 52 Prop-based play therapy interventions for treating the problems of childhood.* Nashville: Paris Goodyear-Brown.

Graziano, S. Rossi, A., Spano, B., Petrocchi, M., Biondi, G., & Ammaniti, M. (2016). Comparison of psychological functioning in children and their mothers living through a life-threatening and non-life-threatening chronic disease: A pilot study. *Journal of Child Health Care, 20*(2), 174–184.

Gross, J. J. (1998). The emerging field of emotion regulation: Divergent consequences for experience, expression, and physiology. *Journal of Personality and Social Psychology, 74,* 224–237.

Gross, J. J. (2007). Emotion regulation. In M. Lewis, J. M. Haviland-Jones & L. Feldman Barrett (Eds.), *Handbook of emotions* (pp. 497–512). New York: The Guildford Press.

Grossman, D. C. (2000). The history of injury control and the epidemiology of child and adolescent injuries. *The Future of Children, 10,* 23–52.

Hiller, R. M., Halligan, S. L., Ariyanayagam, R., Dalgleish, T., Smith, P., Yule, W., . . . Meiser Stedsman, R. (2016). Predictors of posttraumatic stress symptom trajectories in parents of children exposed to motor vehicle collisions. *Journal of Pediatric Psychology, 41*(1), 108–116.

Kahana, S., Feeny, N., Youngstrom, F., & Drotar, D. (2006). Posttraumatic stress in youth experiencing illnesses and injury: An exploratory meta-analysis. *Traumatology, 12,* 148–161. https://doi.org/10.1177/1534765606294562

Klein, N. (2001). *Healing images for children: Teaching relaxation and guided imagery to children facing cancer and other serious illnesses.* Watertown, WI: Inner Coaching.

Knell, S. M. (1993). *Cognitive-behavioral play therapy.* Northvale, NJ: Jason Aronson.

Knell, S. M. (2000a). Cognitive-behavioral play therapy. In K. J. O'Connor & C. E. Schaefer (Eds.), *Handbook of play therapy: Volume 2 Advances and innovations* (pp. 111–142). New York: John Wiley & Sons.

Knell, S. M. (2000b). Cognitive-behavioral play therapy with children with fears and phobias. In H. G. Kaduson & C. E. Schaefer (Eds.), *Short-term therapies with children* (pp. 3–27). New York: Guilford.

Knell, S. M. (2009). Cognitive behavioral play therapy: Theory and applications. In A. Drewes (Ed.), *Effectively blending play therapy and cognitive behavioral therapy: A convergent approach* (pp. 117–133). New York: Wiley.

Knell, S. M., & Dasari, M. (2009). CBPT: Implementing and integrating CBPT into clinical practice. In A. Drewes (Ed.), *Effectively blending play therapy and cognitive behavioral therapy: A convergent approach* (pp. 321–352). New York: Wiley.

Knell, S. M., & Dasari, M. (2010). Cognitive-behavioral play therapy for preschoolers: Integrating play and cognitive-behavioral interventions. In Charles E. Schaefer (Ed.), *Play therapy for preschool children* (pp. 157–178). Chicago: University of Chicago Press.

Loewy, J., Stewart, K., Dassler, A., Telsey, A., & Homel, P. (2013). The effects of music therapy on vital signs, feeding and sleep in premature infants. *Pediatrics, 131*(5), 902–918.

Main, M., & Solomon, J. (1990). Procedures for identifying infants as disorganized/disoriented during the Ainsworth strange situation. In M. Greenberg, D. Cicchetti & E.M. Cummings (Eds.), *Attaching in the preschool years: Theory, research, and intervention* (pp. 121–160). Chicago: University of Chicago Press.

Marsac, M.L., Ciesla, J., Barakat, L.P., Hildenbrand, A.K., Delahanty, D.L., Widaman, K., . . . Kassam-Adams, N. (2016). The role of appraisals and coping in predicting posttraumatic stress following pediatric injury. *Psychological Trauma: Theory, Research, Practice and Policy, 8*(4), 495–503.

Nachmias, M., Gunnar, M., Mangelsdorf, S., Parritz, R.H., & Buss, K. (1996). Behavioral Inhibition and stress reactivity: The moderating role of attachment security. *Child Development, 67*(2), 508–522.

Palermo, T.M. (2012). *Cognitive-behavioral therapy for chronic pain in children and adolescents*. New York: Oxford.

Pelcovitz, D., Libov, B.G., Mandel, F., Kaplan, S., Winblatt, M., & Septimus, A. (1998). Posttraumatic stress disorder and family functioning in adolescent cancer. *Journal of Traumatic Stress, 11*, 205–221.

Perfect, M.M., Beebe, D.W., Levine-Donnersetin, D., Frye, S.S., Bluez, G.P., & Quan, S.F. (2016). The development of a clinically relevant sleep modification protocol for youth with Type 1 Diabetes. *Clinical Practice in Pediatric Psychology, 4*(2), 227–240.

Perry, B.D. (1997). Incubated in terror: Neurodevelopmental factors in the 'cycle of violence'. In J. Osofsky (Ed.), *Children in a violent society* (pp. 124–148). New York: Guilford Press.

Perry, B.D. (1999). *Bonding and attachment in maltreated children: Consequences of emotional neglect in childhood* (CTA Parent and Caregiver Education Series-Volume 1, Issue 3). Child Trauma Academy Press: US.

Perry, B.D. (2008a). Child maltreatment: A neurodevelopmental perspective on the role of trauma and neglect in psychopathology. In T. Beaucharine & S.P. Henshaw (Eds.), *Child and adolescent psychopathology* (pp. 93–129). Hoboken, NJ: Wiley.

Perry, B.D. (2008b). *The neurosequential model of therapeutics: Practical applications for traumatized and maltreated children at home, in the school and in the clinical settings*. DVD: Child Trauma Academy.

Perry, B.D. (2009). Examining child maltreatment through a neurodevelopmental lens: Clinical application of the Neurosequential Model of Therapeutics. *Journal of Loss and Trauma, 14*, 240–255.

Porges, S. (2015). Making the world safe for our children: Down-regulating defence and up-regulating Social Engagement to 'optimize' the human experience. *Children Australia, 40*, 114–123.

Portnoy, S., Girling, I., & Fredman, G. (2016). Supporting young people living with cancer to tell their stories in ways that make them stronger: The beads of life approach. *Clinical Child Psychology and Psychiatry, 21*(2), 255–267.

Robertson, J., & Bowlby, J. (1952). *A 2 year-old goes to the hospital*. DVD. Retrieved from: www.robertsonfilms.info

Rokholt, E.G., Schultz, J.-H., & Langballe, A. (2016). Negotiating a new day: Parents' contributions to supporting students' school functioning after exposure to trauma. *Psychology Research and Behavior Management, 9*, 81–93.

Rzucidlo, S.E., & Campbell, M. (2009). Beyond the physical injuries: Child and parent coping with medical traumatic stress after pediatric trauma. *Journal of Trauma Nursing, 16*(3), 130–135.

Winnicott, D. (1971). *Play and reality*. London: Routledge.

Woolf, C., Muscara, F.L., Anderson, V., & McCarthy, M. (2016). Early traumatic stress responses in parents following a serious illness in their child: A systemic review. *Journal of Clinical Psychology in Medical Settings, 23*(1), 53–66.

Yasinski, C., Hayes, A. M., Ready, C. B., Cummings, J. A., Berman, I. S., McCauley, T., . . . Deblinger, E. (2016). In-session caregiver behavior predicts symptom change in youth receiving trauma-focused cognitive behavioral therapy (TF-CBT). *Journal of Consulting and Clinical Psychology*, *84*(12), 1066–1077.

Zatzick, D. F., Grossman, D. C., Russo, J., Pynoos, R., Berliner, L., Jurkovich, G., . . . Rivara, F. P. (2006). Predicting posttraumatic stress symptoms longitudinally in a representative sample of hospitalized injured adolescents. *Child and Adolescent Psychiatry*, *45*(1), 1188–1195.

Zatzick, D. F., Jurkovich, G. J., Fan, M. Y., Grossman, D., Russo, J., Katon, W., & Rivara, F. P. (2008). Association between posttraumatic stress and depressive symptoms and functional outcomes in adolescents followed up longitudinally after injury hospitalization. *Archives of Pediatric Adolescent Medicine*, *162*(7), 642–648.

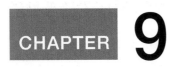

CHAPTER 9

Trauma-Focused Medical Play

Jenaya Gordon and Suzanna Paisley

> I learn my best from and am impacted most by my personal struggles. Therefore, I will join with children in their struggles. I sometimes need a refuge. Therefore, I will provide a refuge for children . . . I cannot make children's hurts and fears and frustrations and disappointments go away. Therefore, I will soften the blow. I experience fear when I am vulnerable. Therefore, I will with kindness, gentleness, and tenderness touch the inner world of the vulnerable child. Therefore, I will provide a refuge for children.
> —Gary Landreth

When working with children, there is nothing more gratifying than knowing you have made a difference. During a time of darkness, fear, pain, and confusion, there is light, clarification, control, and relief that can be provided to a child by being present and supporting play. Echterling and Stewart (2008) recognize that "because you intervene at a crucial point in a child's life and a family's history, a seemingly small intervention can make a profound difference for years to come" (p. 193).

This chapter will explore how trauma-focused medical play can transform the story of illness and trauma into one of understanding, hope, and empowerment. Children face various frightening and overwhelming challenges in health care environments. Referrals for medically traumatized patients can be challenging for clinicians who question if they possess the tools to help. Certified Child Life Specialists' (CCLS) experiences confirm that the acknowledgment and support of a child's trauma with medical play promotes resiliency for future medical experiences, encourage control, and provide opportunities for growth. Individual case studies will detail the struggles faced by pediatric patients and exemplify the resolve found through the power of play. This is all accomplished utilizing children's natural form of communication—play, a safe modality for children to explore and master their experiences while finding resolutions.

THE TRAUMATIC PROCESS

Forgey and Bursch (2013) assert:

> Illness- or treatment-related trauma (iatrogenic trauma) in children can be caused by frightening experiences they have in a health care setting, such as receiving a serious

diagnosis, experiencing painful or distressing procedures, coping with unfamiliar and complex medical technologies, being in the hospital without the support of a parent, and suffering repeated losses related to one's underlying illness or disability.

(p. 1)

According to Hosier (2014), 'traumatic play' is a typical behavior exhibited by young children after experiencing a trauma. The play can be concrete or symbolic and is often repetitive. The opportunity to process medical trauma through play with a supportive clinician or caregiver allows a child to communicate their story, express feelings, gain control, and rewrite the ending of the trauma. Utilizing play as the modality alleviates the limitations of developmental level, the need to verbally communicate events and emotions, or the hindrance of being confined to a hospital bed. Through trauma-focused medical play, the child can find a place of safety, create a plan, and find meaning, while their emotions are normalized. The child finds resolve and creates a narrative through nonverbal expression.

Many trauma-focused therapies are initiated weeks, months, or years after the traumatizing event and are often structured to take place over a dozen or more sessions. In contrast, CCLS are uniquely positioned to facilitate trauma-focused medical play soon after the event, during medical treatment, and often in as few as one or two meaningful interventions. According to Jones and Peterson (2012), "Studies have shown that the optimal time for intervention is during the first few weeks following trauma" (p. 15). When children and adolescents receive timely and crucial interventions, the play aids in their understanding of the diagnosis, treatment, and trauma responses while shifting cognitive distortions and creating new narratives.

Medical Trauma

Steele and Malchiodi (2008) describe trauma as "a terrifying experience that weakens or destroys our sense of safety and power" (p. 268). That experience may be the direct result of a medical team diagnosing and treating a child. Medical trauma, also called illness or treatment-related trauma, "results when a medical experience is perceived by the child as mentally or emotionally overwhelming" (Kisiel et al., 2010, p. 8). A child's emotional response in the health care setting can be impacted by constant contact with the medical team, often confusing and frightening medical interventions, and physical pain during and after procedures or treatments (Marsac et al., 2014). Parson (2014) asserts, "Invasive medical procedures are potential sources of trauma that inevitably become stored as emotional memories for children" (p. 126). Damaging the emotional being can be an unintended consequence of healing the physical being. Children and adolescents can suffer for years as a result of this paradox.

Medical trauma can be caused by something as simple as an IV catheter placement or as complicated as receiving a new cancer diagnosis. That pain and lack of control during an IV placement may cause a lifelong fear of needles. Assumptions can never be made as to what may alter a child's emotional state.

Levine and Kline (2006) describe this form of trauma as:

The initial 'pain experience' leaves a deep (traumatic) imprint on the nervous system which is then re-activated during later procedures. Medical/surgical procedures are by their very nature the most potentially traumatizing to people of all ages due to the feelings of helplessness that come from being held down, at the mercy of strangers, and in a sterile room when you are in unprecedented pain! Having to remain still while you are hurting and being hurt is the epitome of the terror of immobility! It is the prescription for trauma!

(pp. 198–199)

Longitudinal studies show the long-term effects of childhood adversity when a child's social and physical environments are negatively impacted. Adversity in the child's delicate and besieged ecology "can have measurable effects on his or her developmental trajectory, with lifelong consequences for educational achievement, economic productivity, health status and longevity" (Shonkoff et al., 2012, p. 234).

In the past few decades, the field of developmental neurobiology has yielded crucial information that continues to impact several pediatric and child-focused professions. It is now understood that when a child experiences prolonged and repetitive stress, the neural networks can physically change and become maladaptive (Perry, 2009, p. 244). Such changes can result in the child's inability to discriminate between actual and perceived dangers, leading to a prolonged state of stress response and anxiousness (Marsac et al., 2014, p. 4). "The development of executive functions such as decision-making, working memory, behavioral self-regulation, and mood and impulse control" may also be negatively impacted (Shonkoff et al., 2012, p. 237). A child has a far better chance of healing from the medically traumatic experience when they receive processing support following each event. Their understanding of what took place improves while they integrate the story, find power over the trauma, and create plans for coping with trauma reminders and future medical experiences.

Perry (2009) states:

The presence of familiar people projecting the social-emotional cues of acceptance, compassion, caring, and safety, calms the stress response of the individual . . . This powerful positive effect of healthy relational interactions on the individual—mediated by the relational and stress-response neural systems—is at the core of relationally based protective mechanisms that help us survive and thrive following trauma and loss.

(p. 246)

Multiple examples will be explored regarding play's impact on medically traumatized children. Case studies include Jane, whose bowel suddenly perforated; Max, who was alert while receiving chest compressions; Sam, who experienced multiple intubations and extubations while awake; and Zoe, who had an emergency amputation.

THE INS AND OUTS OF PROCESSING

Assessing the Appropriateness of the Intervention

A solid knowledge base of the child's history is crucial for assessing the appropriateness of processing. Factors to consider before moving forward with the intervention include prior trauma history, abuse, neglect, and psychological disorders. Prior to processing, complete a chart review, speak with medical and psychological teams (if applicable), and meet with the family to gather relevant information. Processing should never be done if there is an open investigation with law enforcement or family services. While the focus of the play may be on the medical experiences of the patient, other powerful experiences can be played out and revealed by the child. That is a role for a trained therapist, psychologist, or psychiatrist and out of the scope of practice for CCLS.

For the play to have therapeutic benefits, the individual needs to feel safe, calm, and regulated. Processing should not be initiated if the child is in a hyperaroused state or cannot self-regulate. Signs of hyperarousal include increased heart rate, increased blood pressure, and shallow breathing. Children in the emergency department (ED) or the intensive care unit (ICU) are often not emotionally or physically ready to process. Additionally, the clinician might consider medications received by the child, upcoming difficult experiences or procedures, and availability of caregivers to continue to support the child after the intervention.

Presenting the Intervention to Parents/Caregivers

When a clinician presents the idea of processing, it is often met with relief and gratitude from caregivers. They empathetically feel their children's pain and fear but struggle in knowing how to help. It can be comforting to explain that guiding children through sharing their narratives, revising their interpretations, and finding empowerment and safety can transform traumatic experiences. A clinician can introduce the intervention to caregivers in the following way:

> Part of my role is to help children process what has happened to them in the hospital. It can be helpful to give children the space to talk about it. If he isn't ready, that's perfectly fine. It's up to him and he is in control. If he wants to, I will slowly walk with your child through what happened. I will always follow his cues, so if it becomes too much, we can stop. The most important piece is called 'returning him to a place of safety'. This helps him move through the worst part of the story (instead of stopping there) so we focus on what was helpful (or would have been helpful) in the moment, what is being done to help now, and how he can be empowered moving forward.

What certain adults interpret as the most traumatizing part of a child's story may not be what the child needs to process. "Describing trauma as an experience of feeling totally unsafe and powerless to do anything about a situation gives parents a much more meaningful understanding of their child's struggles" (Steele & Malchiodi, 2008, p. 268). When introducing the idea to parents/caregivers, emphasize that this is the child's time to tell their story and there may be differences between what traumatized the child and what was most difficult for the caregiver. Recognize that children may choose to process with someone other than a caregiver. Caregivers can become emotional when the child is telling their story. This can distract from the intervention and cause their story to end prematurely. Some children may avoid sharing details of their story to protect people around them. Encourage the caregiver to step out of the room while the child processes when the caregiver has experienced their own trauma or cannot cope with hearing their child's experience (Forgey & Bursch, 2013).

Acknowledge the caregivers' reaction while advocating for what is best for the child during processing.

Explain to caregivers that because processing trauma through play can be a stressful experience for a child they should allow a break after the intervention. Children often will want to hold onto the figurines they have chosen to represent themselves and others in order to continue to play out their experiences. For example, when the CCLS began to gather the toys after processing with 5-year-old Sam, he held tightly onto the figurines representing himself and his parents. Sam played with those figures throughout the day. When the clinician can normalize play and educate caregivers on how to bring the child to a safe ending, the child's emotional safety is supported and caregivers' feelings of helplessness are decreased.

Processing With Jane

This case study highlights the importance of preparing caregivers prior to processing. Eleven-year-old Jane was admitted to the hospital with a history of Crohn's disease with a septic bowel that suddenly perforated. She was rushed into surgery and given an emergency ostomy. Jane had been on a ventilator (intubated), underwent drain placements, and experienced many painful dressing changes. After transferring to an inpatient unit, she was referred for processing due to her struggles coping with the hospitalization and medical procedures.

After utilizing figurines to play out getting sick at home and having the father figurine carry Jane to the car, Jane played out the ride to the hospital. The specialist stated, "Your Dad knew exactly what to do to keep you safe and get you help." This narration caused Jane's father to cry. The specialist normalized the father's tears to Jane and asked if he would like a moment outside while the play continued. Jane's father chose to stay, and the specialist reiterated that this was Jane's time to tell her story. Jane's story will be revisited throughout the description of processing steps.

Introducing Processing to Children

Prior to introducing processing to a child, check with medical professionals and caregivers to ensure that that there will be few or no interruptions. Place a sign on the door and ask the medical team not to interrupt. Processing can take a lot of energy, so ideally the intervention should occur when the child has rested and is comfortable.

A clinician can explain the intervention to children and adolescents in this way:

Part of my job is to help kids talk about what has happened while they've been in the hospital. Some kids say it really helps to talk about the scary/upsetting thing that happened and to share their thoughts and feelings. Other kids say they don't want to talk about it just yet; either way you are in control and it is your choice. Would you like to share with me what happened?

While the intervention is aimed at healing, the idea of processing a traumatic experience may be too much for some children. Teens seem to be more adept at verbally declining the intervention, while children may resort to giving non-verbal cues. A child might cover their head with the blanket, turn away, change the subject, or try to minimize the event to indicate they do not need support. Steele and Malchiodi (2012) stress, "In trauma-informed care, children must always have the choice to say 'no' to any intervention we propose or 'stop' to any intervention in progress that is activating. For safety to exist, children must experience some level of control" (p. 91). Before proceeding with the intervention, review the various feelings that may arise during the play and explain that they can choose to stop at any time. Emphasize that they are in control and your role is to support them in telling their story while keeping them safe.

It is the responsibility of the professional to read cues, normalize a child's feelings, and help create a plan to share their story with a trusted adult when ready. If the cues from the child indicate that they are not ready to proceed with the intervention, explain to the child, "It helps to not let the scary thoughts stay stuck inside your head. When you are ready to share your story, what adults can you talk to?" If the caregiver is comfortable supporting the child through the process and bringing the child to a place of safety when the story has concluded, a mixture of trauma and non-trauma toys can be left to allow for processing on their own. Discuss the steps of processing with parents and caregivers and provide written information and resources.

When given the choice to process, the child is often ready to share their story without hesitation. For example, 11-year-old Jane was tearful from pain and anxiety when the child life specialist entered the room, but her breathing slowed and her body started to relax when the specialist offered the intervention. Jane exclaimed, "Yea!" and clapped when the CCLS provided the chance to process.

PROCESSING STEPS

Gathering Materials

When a play session begins, a trusting relationship between practitioner and child is initiated with a child making choices. The child can feel a sense of control when given the opportunity to choose toys that represent the various individuals in the story, including themselves, therefore, having a variety of toys is optimal. The representative figurines selected by the child tell their own stories. A toy choice can show the patient as powerful or meek and the medical staff as heroic or terrifying. For example, Sam chose the largest superhero figure (see Figure 9.1) to represent himself and a protective dinosaur as his father, while Jane chose soldiers to act as the surgical team in the operating room (OR), where she felt the most vulnerable.

When a private office or play space is available, supply a play hospital with medical items, a playhouse, medical equipment, emergency vehicles, cars, figurines including action figures and soldiers of different genders, figurines of various ethnicities, genders, and ages, as well as animal and dinosaur figurines. Often in the hospital setting, children are not able to leave their beds so there is not enough room for all the suggested toys, however certain select items can support a successful processing session. Keep a

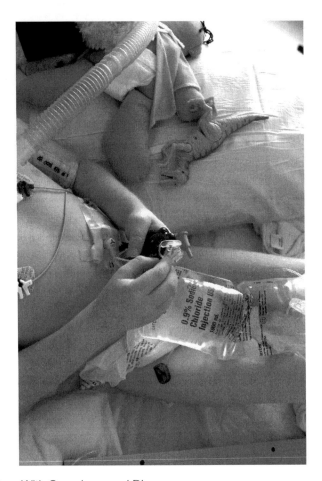

FIGURE 9.1 Sam With Superhero and Dinosaur

bedside processing kit available to allow for a readiness in the professional and a variety of choices for the child. Items for bedside kits include a mobile play hospital, medical play equipment, various action figures and animals, emergency and non-emergency vehicles, and a blank cloth doll with markers. It is not possible to bring every toy into the room that the child may need. When a specific item is not available, a child's imagination becomes a powerful tool. In Sam's case, he utilized his own suctioning tube as the intubation tube while playing out being extubated.

The Story Begins

"Through play, children and families take control of the story by expressing their feelings, enhancing their self-esteem, gaining self-control, acting out possible resolutions, and reinvigorating themselves. Play is one of your most powerful crisis intervention tools" (Echterling & Stewart, 2008, p. 201). After items are chosen and the child is ready to participate, the professional can invite the child to begin to share their story through play. "What were you doing right before this happened/you heard what happened?" "Using these toys, can you show what happened?" Jane described playing at home when she began to feel sick. Her father found Jane vomiting, and took her to the hospital. Jane moved the figurine representing herself into a corner, moved the father figure over to that area who then carried the Jane figure to the toy car.

To continue moving the story forward, ask open-ended questions. When asked, "What happened next?," Jane moved both figurines into the car and moved them to the doctor's office followed by the hospital. Jane's figurine was bent over in pain. Before moving on to another part of the story, make sure the child has finished that step: "Is there anything else you want to tell me about this part?" and continue to prompt, "Then what happened?" Jane resumed the play by placing her figurine on a hospital bed surrounded by doctors and stated, "I'm scared, they're not telling me what's going on." While helping move the story forward, keep in mind that the child must be the one to set the pace. During Zoe's play session, the CCLS held the moment, pausing in silence, after Zoe created a necrotic foot on her doll. Zoe set the pace, and the played moved forward when she was ready.

Levine and Kline (2012) emphasize:

> Children should never be forced to move through an episode too fast or forced to do more than they are willing and able to do. It is important to slow down the process if you notice signs of fear, constricted breathing, stiffening, or a dazed (disassociated) demeanor. These reactions will dissipate if you simply wait, quietly and patiently, while reassuring the child you are still by his side and on his side.
>
> (p. 202)

At each point of the session, include the child's feelings and sensory experiences. Questions to ask throughout the session include "What were you thinking and feeling?" and "What did you see/hear/smell/feel?" While Jane described the OR experience, she moved her figurine to the OR and surrounded herself with army figurines that represented the surgical team (see Figure 9.2). "I wanted my daddy! Why wouldn't

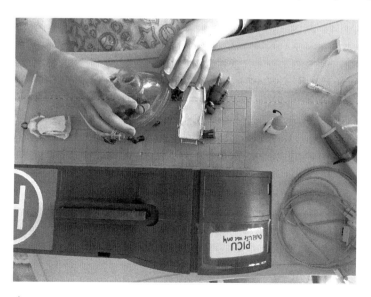

FIGURE 9.2 Jane

they let my daddy come with me?" she exclaimed. Jane then placed the mask over her figurine's face. After prompting from the CCLS, Jane stated, "I felt alone and cold."

As the child leads the medical play intervention, they will often communicate in their own way when the session is over. Jane pushed the toys aside and took deep breaths. Sam began demonstrating hyperarousal behaviors and became agitated. The CCLS saw his heart rate increase on the monitor and initiated bringing the play to a safe ending with regulating breaths. Max, who was 3 years old, physically turned away from the processing toys when he was finished.

Self-Regulation

The clinician can encourage self-regulation to help ease the unavoidable stress caused by playing out traumatic experiences. Throughout the session, model deep breathing for the child and encourage caregivers to do the same. For example, Jane was taking short, quick breaths, and the monitor showed her heartbeat increasing. The specialist put her hand close to the play to get Jane's attention and loudly began to take slow breaths in and out. Children also have their own ways of self-regulating. Max began playing with his own toys when he needed a break, then returned to the medical play when he was ready. Open-ended questions also prompt self-regulation. Steele and Malchiodi (2012) explain,

> From a safety self-regulation standpoint, providing children with consistent and frequent opportunities to describe the range of reactions, sensations, feelings, and thoughts they are having about what they are doing, what we are doing, or what we might be talking about, gives them a voice.
>
> (p. 93)

Concluding at a Point of Safety

When the child concludes their story, the clinician will return the child to a point of safety. "As with any encounter with someone in a crisis situation, you will want to leave the child on a positive note, feeling a greater sense of hope and resolve" (Echterling & Stewart, 2008, p. 201). Ask questions to encourage a feeling of safety. "When did you know you were going to be ok?" "Who is helping you now?" Children often identify family members as support systems. If appropriate, include the medical team in your safety statements; for example, "The doctors and nurses are here to help your body get better" and "We are all here to keep you safe."

There are times during a hospitalization that the child may be unsure if they are safe. In Sam's case, he did not yet feel like he was going to be OK. The uncertainty gave the specialist the opportunity to talk to Sam about who was helping him to feel safe and to get better. For Jane, the continuation of daily dressing changes made it difficult for her to recover and create coping plans in between each procedure. The CCLS used the play session as an opportunity to play out what had happened and scenarios in which Jane would feel safe during future dressing changes. During the session, Jane put the father figurine by the side of the Jane figurine and had the figurine take deep breaths.

This provided Jane with a sense of control and mastery. The specialist emphasized, "You know exactly what you need to do to feel safe during your dressing change."

Recreating the Story

One of the goals of processing is to empower the child to recreate their own ending. After the retelling of the story is complete, support the child in playing out a different ending: "Can you play out what you wish would have happened?" "What would you like to say to (the doctor, nurse, etc.)?" Sam used this opportunity to physically fight off the medical team while they were extubating. In the recreated OR, Jane, with her dad by her side, had the doctors tell her what was going to happen during and after surgery.

Playing Out the Future

Children can feel a sense of control and empowerment when they role-play a hospital discharge or a future procedure, examinations, and doctor's visits. Guide the child in creating a coping plan and a plan for communicating how the medical team can help. "What can the medical team/you/your family do to help you feel safe?" "What will it be like if/when you have another (insert medical procedure)?" Offer education on how to effectively cope with emotions. "What are some things you think you could do to help your body calm down if that happens?"

Jane was having multiple daily dressing changes for her ostomy. During the play session, Jane had the figurine representing Jane look away while holding the father figurine. Jane's figurine stated "be gentle" to the medical team. The CCLS modeled deep breathing and encouraged Jane's figurine to breathe and think of a happy place during the procedure. Jane stated, "I'm thinking of playing with my dog." The CCLS guided Jane through the different senses experienced when playing with her dog, including how her dog felt against her skin, the smell of her dog, and the different colors of the dog's fur. This plan was shared with Jane's nurse to give her another layer of control over her dressing changes.

CASE STUDIES

The following case studies demonstrate the power of play when words do not come easily.

Zoe

Zoe was a cheerful 14-year-old girl with developmental delays. It was thought that she functioned cognitively around a 7-year-old level while her verbal skills were approximately the level of a toddler. One day her foot felt like it was asleep, and she lost her balance and fell. As her foot began to turn black, her family brought her to the hospital. Zoe had developed a blood clot in her foot that quickly caused her foot and lower leg to necrotize. After much effort, it was decided that her leg could not be saved. Zoe would undergo an amputation to save her life.

The CCLS was called with the news that Zoe was being rushed into surgery within the hour. Everyone was appropriately worried about explaining to this child that she would return from surgery with her lower leg gone. Zoe's current ventilator use/status and mild sedation added concern. These factors, combined with Zoe's developmental delay, made for a complicated surgery preparation. The CCLS met with the caregivers privately, assessed Zoe's developmental level and created a plan. The preparation for surgery and amputation was brief and concrete. The specialist told Zoe,

> Your foot is very sick, that is why it is black and hurts. Your sick foot is causing your leg to be sick too, which is why it is turning black. The doctors have done everything they can to stop the sickness from spreading, but it is making the rest of your body sick. The only way to keep your body safe and healthy is for the doctors to carefully remove your foot and the bottom part of your leg.

The CCLS then explained surgery and that Zoe would be given a special "hospital sleep medicine" to ensure that she would be safely asleep during the surgery and that she would not see anything, feel anything, or be scared while the doctors helped her. Due to the breathing tube, Zoe was unable to speak but could nod to yes and no questions. The CCLS stated common fears and misconceptions, one by one, and allowed Zoe to nod if she related to those concerns. Zoe indicated that she was not scared or worried and that she understood what was happening.

A few days after the surgery, once Zoe was off the ventilator and able to speak, the CCLS offered to help Zoe process what had happened. The specialist provided a doll that looked similar to Zoe and asked Zoe if she wanted to amputate the doll's leg to match her own. Zoe clapped and exclaimed "Yea!" The specialist brought a medical play kit, scissors, markers, and a sewing kit. Zoe was asked to use the doll to share her story. Zoe pretended the doll was walking then showed the doll falling down. With her limited verbal skills, Zoe told her story by saying "Me asleep and fell. Hurt foot. Foot black." Zoe understood that she was at home, her foot felt like it was asleep, and the numbness caused her to fall. She observed that her foot and leg were turning black from the necrotic tissue. The CCLS agreed with Zoe's telling of the story and asked her to "show me with your doll how your foot looked." Zoe smiled as she reached for the markers. She proceeded to color the doll's foot and leg black, brown, and purple. Zoe held up the doll, pointed to the foot and made an exaggerated "owie" sound. The specialist echoed the sound Zoe made and added, "Wow, that foot is really hurt. I wonder if it was scary to see it black and brown and purple." Zoe answered with a low, quiet "Yea." The specialist matched Zoe's tone and added, "Yea, it was really scary." The specialist held silence in that moment until Zoe was ready to move on. She looked up and pointed to the scissors. The CCLS matched Zoe's excited expression and asked, "Oh, do you think she should have surgery?" Zoe smiled and exclaimed "Yea!" The specialist agreed and added, "That foot is just too sick. It's no one's fault that it got sick or that it just can't get better. It's time to have surgery to protect the rest of her body from getting sick." Zoe agreed and grabbed the scissors, but the specialist paused and asked, "Do you think she should get sleep medicine so that she's not scared and not hurting?" Zoe laughed, answered "Yea" and engaged with the medical play items. She used the stethoscope to listen to the doll, a syringe to put medicine in the IV tubing, and then placed the induction mask carefully over the doll's face.

The CCLS then helped Zoe carefully cut the discolored foot and leg. Once it was removed, Zoe definitively stated, "Foot sick. Foot gone. Doctor has foot." The specialist asked what Zoe would like to do with the foot, and if Zoe would like to say goodbye to it. Zoe reacted without emotion, swiftly threw the foot in the trash, and returned her focus to tending to the doll. The specialist sewed the opening closed as Zoe carefully held the anesthesia mask on the face. When finished, the doll was handed back to Zoe and she carefully wrapped the leg first with gauze, then in a bandage that matched her own (see Figure 9.3).

Once the "surgery" was completed, Zoe removed the mask from the doll and held her up to the sky, announcing "Like me!" Zoe giggled, clapped, and hugged the doll for several minutes, admiring her leg. To conclude the intervention, the specialist reiterated that it was not Zoe's fault that her foot got sick and addressed a common

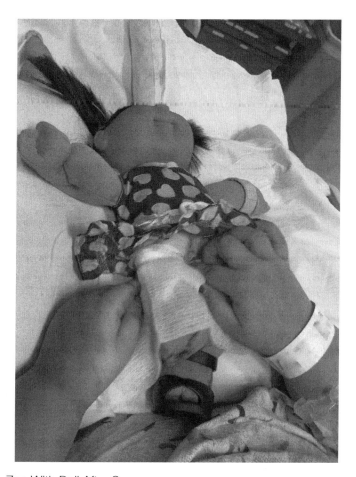

FIGURE 9.3 Zoe With Doll After Surgery

misconception that the foot may be returned to Zoe later. Zoe nodded in understanding. It was also explained that Zoe's other foot is not sick and will not be amputated. Zoe appeared relieved with this news as she sighed, smiled, pointed to her healthy foot and said "foot not sick."

Following the trauma-focused medical play, Zoe showed great pride in her doll. She showed everyone who walked in the room, explaining "Like me!" as she held the doll up. She even named the doll "Mini Zoe." Throughout the rest of Zoe's hospitalization, she received support from the child life team. Zoe continued medical play to process the traumatic medical event, address her fears of being hospitalized, and practice being independent. A CCLS and child life intern helped Zoe to create a "prosthetic" leg out of clay and provided a wheelchair for the doll. Zoe's mother admitted that the idea to medically play out a doll's leg amputation with Zoe initially sounded a bit morbid. However, she quickly saw the therapeutic value and how the intervention returned control to Zoe over an otherwise terrifying situation. Zoe responded well to emotional support, education, and medical play. It was suggested that she might benefit from such services in the community following her discharge.

Max

Max was a 3-year-old with a complicated medical history, including a tracheostomy. Max and his family were accustomed to hospital admissions, and his mother thought no different of this particular hospitalization. That was until Max announced, "I am going to die." Max's mom, Sheila, was taken aback and assured her son that he was not going to die. For days, he continued with his proclamation and would not let Sheila leave his side. Then one day in the ICU, Max looked at his mother, stated, "I'm going to die" and then immediately became unresponsive.

Sheila watched, stunned, as Max's heart rate dropped to zero and the medical staff rushed into action. She collapsed outside of the glass door of her son's ICU room and helplessly sobbed. After receiving chest compressions, Max's heart began beating. Following this event, Max became terrified of doctors, blue scrubs, and the medical environment in general. Max seemed to remember the code and referred to the doctors as monsters who were hurting him. He described receiving compressions as the doctors "pushing on my stomach" and stated, "God was holding my hand."

Child life had been involved in Max's care all his life and now was faced with supporting him through a terrifying medical event. The CCLS met with Sheila to introduce the idea of helping Max process the medical trauma through play. Sheila was open to the intervention and appreciative. When asked if he would like to share his story, Max agreed.

Max actively engaged in play with the medical helicopter and toy hospital. He focused his play on the helicopter but would occasionally set up the "hospital room" with "oxygen," "machines," and "doctors." The CCLS utilized tracking responses as Max quietly played with the hospital. Through his play and verbalizations, Max expressed that he did not feel safe in the hospital "because they poke" him, but he did feel safe in the helicopter. Max then shifted his focus away from the medical play toys toward his toys from home, possibly as a way of self-regulating. The CCLS acknowledged this by saying, "You want to take a break from playing about the scary thing that happened and just play with that toy right there."

After a few minutes, Max returned to the hospital set. Sheila prompted him to share his experience around coding. Max set up all the adult figures around the hospital bed of the little boy. He moved the tiny IV pole and other equipment around the bed as well. Max verbalized the experience being "scary" and that it "hurt." Max emphatically repeated a word, which seemed to be related to the code but which was indecipherable. He became frustrated when no one correctly guessed what he was saying. The CCLS instead focused on the tone and franticness Max was communicating by repeating the language Sheila had reported Max using earlier. "It was so scary and really hurt when the doctors were pushing on your tummy," expressed the CCLS. This statement resonated with Max, as he calmed and continued arranging the hospital figures.

The CCLS repeatedly validated that the code experience was painful and frightening. The CCLS and Sheila explained that even though it hurt, the doctors were helping Max's body by pushing on his tummy. This CCLS asked if he worried "They (staff) will push on your tummy (compressions) again," to which Max answered, "Yes." CCLS stated, "No one is worried that will happen again. If we are worried they need to push on your tummy again, we will tell you," to which Max nodded. Max then began to focus on his own toys and turned away from the medical play. In order to fully end at a point of safety, the CCLS asked Max who helped him during the code. He was able to identify that Sheila was present and protecting him. The CCLS and Sheila agreed and reminded Max that he was safe. The CCLS validated that Max was done playing about what happened for now and was ready to play with his own toys. The CCLS stayed to engage Max in non-directive play to ensure he had returned to a state of calm.

Following the intervention, Sheila and the CCLS spoke outside of Max's room. The specialist explained some of the therapeutic techniques, including validating reactions, naming feelings, clearing misconceptions, tracking play, and returning Max to a point of safety. During the conversation, the specialist suggested it might be beneficial for Max to see a play therapist to continue processing the medical trauma and to return control to Max. Sheila agreed with the CCLS, and Max engaged in play therapy after discharge from the hospital. Sheila later explained how Max's memory shifted from terror to pride through the opportunity to share his story and receive therapeutic support. Max openly tells people, "I told my Mommy I was going to die and then all the machines went off. God pushed on my stomach and the doctors saved me. I almost didn't make it but my hospital saved me." Max has great pride in "his" hospital and his ability to survive.

Sam

When 5-year-old Sam came to the hospital, he had yet to have a clear diagnosis. What the medical team knew was that Sam was previously healthy, but had gone into respiratory failure with left facial nerve palsy, muscle weakness, and seizures. Sam transferred from a different hospital after two failed extubations and re-intubations. Significant to the child life team was that Sam remembered both failed attempts and had been intubated and awake for 11 days since transferring hospitals. Sam was now in the pediatric intensive care unit (PICU) and recently received a tracheostomy.

The CCLS introduced the idea of processing his medical experiences through play two weeks into Sam's admission and both parents agreed. They shared Sam's experiences with various medical procedures and how each seemed to negatively impact him. According to Sam's parents, Sam had become more "physically aggressive" and frustrated with everyday cares. At that time, Sam was not yet verbally communicating after the extended intubation and newly placed tracheostomy.

Prior to processing, the CCLS built rapport with Sam by talking about the various toys and stuffed animals on his bed. Sam engaged with the CCLS and agreed to have her come back to visit again after he rested and received medications. When the CCLS introduced the idea of talking about what has happened to him in the hospital, Sam immediately looked at the CCLS, smiled, and gave her a hug. Sam had a story he needed to tell, and he appeared grateful for the opportunity. A variety of toys and figurines were provided by the CCLS, and Sam chose carefully. His choices told their own story: a large superhero figurine became Sam, a large green dinosaur became Sam's father, a princess became Sam's mother, medical figurines became nurses, and one scary looking monster figurine became the doctor.

Sam chose to start his medical journey by strapping his "Superhero Sam" to a hospital bed, while "Princess Mom" moved in and out of the ambulance. The CCLS narrated along the way: "Sam can't move in that bed," "Mom is right next to Sam," and "Sam does not know what's going to happen." After repeatedly playing out his ambulance experience, Sam moved to the play hospital. Methodically, Sam played through medical procedures, utilizing play items and real medical equipment. While playing out the lumbar puncture (LP), Sam placed his action figure in a kneeling position and began thrashing his action figure back and forth. Sam was dramatically exhibiting how his action figure was in pain and feeling out of control as the medical figures tried to hold him down. The CCLS included emotions Sam may have been feeling throughout the play: "Sam does not feel safe," "Sam's scared," and "Sam wants to go home." Later, his parents told the CCLS they previously thought Sam was not aware of the LP because of the medications he was given.

Sam continued with other medical experiences as the CCLS narrated the scene. Sam made the play medical team place the nasogastric (NG) tube on Superhero Sam to represent the EEG testing. Incorrectly, the CCLS narrated Superhero Sam getting an NG tube instead of an EEG. Sam immediately stopped his play, looked at the CCLS and shook his head no. When the CCLS stated, "Sam is not getting an NG tube, he's getting an EEG," the play continued. The IV tubing was used along with the play medical team to play out IV placements and shots. Throughout the various scenarios, Sam placed the mother or father figurine by Superhero Sam's side.

The last experience Sam played out was his extubations and re-intubations, while using his own suctioning tube as the breathing tube. This was the first time he introduced the "monster doctor" into the play. Sam had Superhero Sam thrashing around while the monster doctor attempted to take out the breathing tube and put it back in. The CCLS narrated for Sam, "I'm scared," "You're hurting me," and "No, leave me alone!" When the play finished, "Dinosaur Dad" hugged Superhero Sam. "Sam feels safe with Dad," stated the CCLS. The CCLS asked if there were any other parts of the story Sam would like to tell. Sam shook his head no and appeared tired.

The CCLS then asked Sam what he wished would have happened. He took Superhero Sam and began to kick and hit the monster doctor. The CCLS narrated along the way, "Leave me alone," "You can't hurt me," "I'm in control!" As Sam finished, the CCLS began to take loud calm breaths to calm the energy in the room and model self-regulation. When Sam appeared more relaxed, the CCLS stated, "When we play, you can do almost anything you want as long as everyone is safe, but when you are not in your play sessions, the medical team and doctors are not for hitting and kicking." Sam calmly nodded in agreement.

The CCLS returned Sam to a point of safety by asking, "How did you know you were going to be OK and safe?" Sam shook his head no. The CCLS immediately followed with "You don't know if you are going to be OK and you don't feel safe here." Sam nodded his head yes. CCLS normalized this feeling and focused on the procedures Sam played out, asking "How did you know you were going to be OK after those procedures?" Sam pointed at his mother and father. The CCLS expanded that idea, stating "Mom and Dad knew where to take Sam to help him get better" and "Mom and Dad are there to protect Sam and make sure he is safe." The CCLS also emphasized that the medical team is there to help Sam's body get better. The CCLS concluded the intervention with a grounding imagery activity, explaining that Sam can use it anytime he feels unsafe, in pain, or during a procedure. The CCLS recognized Sam as visibly tired after the intervention and encouraged Sam's parents to continue practicing deep breathing and the grounding activity to promote coping and calm. Sam was steadfast in his need to hold on to certain figurines. The CCLS confirmed the parents' understanding of how to support Sam's play while bringing him to a point of safety. The CCLS saw the need for additional medical play sessions, along with opportunities for expression of feelings. Throughout his hospital stay, the child life team carried out those interventions for increased coping and mastery.

CLINICAL AND COPING CONSIDERATIONS

Trauma Reminders

Children may re-experience a traumatic event or have trauma reminders in various ways. Nightmares, hyper-arousal symptoms, avoidance behaviors, and recurring memories of the trauma are common. Trauma reminders may be triggered through various stimuli and senses. The taste of saline, the sterile smell of an operating room, or a beeping alarm can all bring up memories of the traumatic experience. "Exposure to emotionally traumatic events is common among children who are treated in pediatric medical care settings, and it is important to recognize the emotional reactions that children might develop as a response to the trauma" (Shemesh et al., 2005, p. 582). During the initial intervention, educate families and children about trauma reminders and help create a coping plan for when they happen.

Siblings

Such emotional pain is not limited to the patient but extends to siblings as well. "Trauma can occur when someone is exposed to intense, distressing events either directly, by observing others' experience trauma, or vicariously, by learning of other's trauma events" (Ward-Begnoche, 2007, p. 84). Siblings often are present when providers share terrifying and confusing information and/or diagnoses. Frequently, siblings are observers to the medical event that brought their sibling to the hospital, as well as the painful medical procedures that happen bedside. Siblings witness parents and family members exude fear and sadness as they tell and re-tell the medical details. They stand in the background, often feeling overwhelmed and helpless, while watching loved ones struggle. Although specialists support these children by providing activities and education about diagnoses and procedures, their unique medical trauma often gets forgotten. Processing through medical play allows the telling of their own stories and possibly decreases the likelihood of medical procedures being traumatic in the future.

Coping as the Clinician

Processing trauma can be challenging for both the facilitator and the participating child. Specialists describe symptoms, including fatigue, feeling emotionally overwhelmed, and physically sick after a processing session.

> Working with traumatized individuals may take a greater toll on the practitioner than working with other types of clients. In all cases, helping professionals, caregivers, and family of traumatized individuals are most at risk for compassion fatigue or secondary trauma reactions.
>
> (Steele & Malchiodi, 2012, p. 164)

Bearing witness to a trauma story is a powerful experience; therefore, it must come with protections for you as a professional. Goelitz and Stewart-Kahn (2013) explain,

> One way to prevent this is to be clear about our thoughts, emotions, and physical states prior to meeting with survivors. While tuning in, it can also help to think about losses, anticipating the possibility of these feelings coming up.
>
> (p. 34)

Find ways to ground yourself prior to the intervention, protect yourself during the intervention, and let the experiences go after the intervention. Know your limits. For example, avoid processing with more than one patient a day, or working with a case that brings up personal emotional memories for you. Sometimes the best option is to refer them to another professional for support. When processing sessions are complete, especially particularly intense sessions, find a colleague to help debrief the intervention. It is important to have an opportunity to process the experience yourself, while maintaining boundaries and not bringing the stories home.

Educating Others

Pediatric medical traumatic stress is "a set of psychological and physiological responses of children and their families to pain, injury, serious illness, medical procedures, and invasive or frightening treatment experiences" (Rzucidlo & Campbell, 2009, p. 131). "A child may find the stress of multiple painful or frightening medical procedures as tolerable if they are in a supportive environment with nurturing relationships" (Oral et al., 2015, p. 1). Educating medical caregivers and family members on supporting traumatized children can ensure that both the environment and relationships are supportive. Perry and Szalavitz (2006) eloquently state, "Fire can warm or consume, water can quench or drown, wind can caress or cut. And so it is with human relationships: we can both create and destroy, nurture and terrorize, traumatize and heal each other" (p. 5). The provision of medical care can result in the cure of an illness along with subsequent damage to the spirit. When specialists share stories of what children hear, misunderstand, and experience with medical professionals, they can positively impact medical practices and ensure that the medical team is honoring children's emotional safety while healing their physical bodies.

Informing parents and caregivers of the same information can better place them in a position to advocate for and support their children. Upon reflection of years of patient stories, it is clear that many of the traumas endured by children could have been avoided with proactive education, patience, and the right support. Educating others on ways to ensure the emotional safety of patients is as crucial as the therapeutic interventions themselves.

Reflection

Clinicians can often have a feeling of helplessness when working with traumatized patients. Regardless of the toys provided, basic play sessions, and expressive activities, specialists still feel at a loss, as if those interventions were not enough. Although those interventions hold value, medically traumatized patients need more. The child life specialist's repertoire has always included the skillset to process medical trauma. Medical play interventions are instinctual, for example, after a painful IV, following a particularly frightening MRI, or when a child is struggling to cope with the medical environment. These children are utilizing medical play to process their experiences. In contrast, it appears that processing is rarely being offered to children who are facing extreme medical traumas. When children face these experiences, medical professionals are unsure where to begin helping or believe 'this is their new normal.' Therefore, trauma processing is sometimes labeled as unnecessary. Children's reactions to processing directly contradict this unfounded premise. Children demonstrate an increase in coping and understanding after they play out their stories. The look of relief on caregivers' faces, the newly engaged and communicating patient, and the satisfaction of the professional after supporting a child with the trauma all tell us that we can make a difference. Children have stories to tell; it is our job to help them. "Using creative activities to tell their crisis stories offers them (children) an opportunity to begin to give form to raw experiences, gain some sense of cognitive mastery over the crisis, and make important discoveries about possible resolutions" (Echterling & Stewart, 2008, p. 198). As we develop our knowledge of medical trauma and its effect on children, the complexity of our interventions must develop as well. It is no longer acceptable to ignore these traumas. Healing the emotional self and providing a means to communicate trauma stories must be the normal standard of care, not the exception. Only then can clinicians guide children into finding their power in otherwise overwhelming situations.

REFERENCES

Echterling, L. G., & Stewart, S. (2008). Creative crisis intervention techniques with children and families. In C. Malchiodi (Ed.), *Creative interventions with traumatized children* (pp. 189–210). New York: The Guilford Press.

Forgey, M., & Bursch, B. (2013). Assessment and management of pediatric iatrogenic medical trauma. *Current Psychiatry Reports, 15*(2), 1–9. https://doi.org/10.1007/s11920-012-0340-5

Goelitz, A., & Stewart-Kahn, A. (2013). *From trauma to healing: A social worker's guide to working with survivors.* New York: Taylor & Francis.

Hosier, D. (February 24, 2014). *Childhood trauma: Reaction to trauma according to age.* Retrieved from: http://childhoodtraumarecovery.com/2014/02/24/childhood-trauma-reactions-to-trauma-according-to-age/

Jones, R., & Peterson, L. W. (2012). PTSD in children: A healthcare perspective. In W. Steele & C. A. Malchiodi (Eds.), *Trauma-informed practices with children and adolescents* (pp. 14–15). New York: Taylor & Francis.

Kisiel, C., Lyons, J. S., Blaustein, M., Fehrenbach, T., Griffin, G., Germain, J., . . . National Child Traumatic Stress Network. (2010). *Child and adolescent needs and strengths (CANS) manual: The NCTSN CANS comprehensive—Trauma version: A comprehensive information integration tool for children and adolescents exposed to traumatic events.* Chicago: Praed Foundation/Los Angeles, CA and Durham, NC: NCTSN.

Levine, P. A., & Kline, M. (2006). *Trauma through a child's eyes: Awakening the ordinary miracle of healing: Infancy through adolescence.* Berkeley, CA: North Atlantic Books.

Levine, P. A., & Kline, M. (2012). Five principles to guide children's play toward resolution. In W. Steele & C. A. Malchiodi (Eds.), *Trauma-informed practices with children and adolescents* (pp. 202–205). New York: Taylor & Francis.

Marsac, M. L., Kassam-Adams, N., Delahanty, D. L., Widaman, K. F., & Barakat, L. P. (2014). Posttraumatic stress following acute medical trauma in children: A proposed model of bio-psycho-social processes during the peri-trauma period. *Clinical Child and Family Psychology Review, 17*(4), 399–411.

Oral, R., Ramirez, M., Coohey, C., Nakada, S., Walz, A., Kuntz, A., . . . Peek-Asa, C. (2015). Adverse childhood experiences and trauma informed care: The future of health care. *Pediatric Research, 79,* 227–233. https://doi.org/10.1038/pr.2015.197

Parson, J. A. (2014). Holistic mental health care and play therapy for hospitalized chronically ill children. In E. J. Green & A. C. Myrick (Eds.), *Play therapy with vulnerable populations: No child forgotten* (pp. 125–136). Lanham, MD: Rowman & Littlefield.

Perry, B. (2009). Examining child maltreatment through a neurodevelopmental lens: Clinical applications of the neurosequential model of therapeutics. *Journal of Loss and Trauma, 14,* 240–254. https://doi.org/10.1080/15325020903004350

Perry, B. D., & Szalavitz, M. (2006). *The boy who was raised as a dog and other stories from a child's psychiatrist's notebook: What traumatized children can teach us about loss, love, and healing.* New York: Basic Books.

Rzucidlo, S. E., & Campbell, M. (2009). Beyond the physical injuries: Child and parent coping with medical traumatic stress after pediatric trauma. *Journal of Trauma Nursing, 16*(3), 130–135. https://doi.org/10.1097/JTN.0b013e3181b9e078

Shemesh, E., Newcorn, J. H., Rockmore, L., Shneider, B. L., Emre, S., Gelb, B. D., . . . Yehuda, R. (2005). Comparison of parent and child reports of emotional trauma symptoms in pediatric outpatient settings. *Pediatrics, 115*, 582–589. https://doi.org/10.1542/2004-2201

Shonkoff, J. P., Garner, A. S., Siegel, B. S., Dobbins, M. I., Earls, M. F., McGuinn, L., . . . Wegner, L. M. (2012). The lifelong effects of early childhood adversity and toxic stress. *Pediatrics, 129*(1), 2011–2663. https://doi.org/10.1542/peds.

Steele, W., & Malchiodi, C. A. (2008). Interventions for parents of traumatized children. In C. Malchiodi (Ed.), *Creative interventions with traumatized children* (pp. 264–281). New York: The Guilford Press.

Steele, W., & Malchiodi, C. A. (2012). *Trauma-informed practices with children and adolescents*. New York: Taylor & Francis.

Ward-Begnoche, W. (2007). Posttraumatic stress symptoms in the pediatric intensive care unit. *Journal for Specialists in Pediatric Nursing, 12*(2), 84–92. https://doi.org/10.1111/j.1744-6155.2007.00097.x

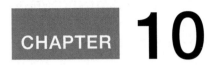

CHAPTER 10

Regaining Control

Utilizing Directive Play Therapy to Help Teens With Chronic Health Conditions

Mistie Barnes

> Although the world is full of suffering, it is also full of the overcoming of it.
> —Helen Keller, "Optimism"

Chronic health complications can be not only physically but also emotionally challenging for teens. For teens, facing the 'here and now' of a chronic illness can be devastating; coping with the potential lifetime impact of a chronic illness may seem overwhelming. The combination of general teenage challenges, such as puberty, developing independence, and interactions with peers (Broderick & Blewitt, 2010) coupled with a chronic health condition may breed insecurity, fears about the future, decreased self-esteem, increased medical complications, and increased non-compliance with medical protocol (University of Rochester Medical Center, 2017). This chapter will discuss the benefits of utilizing creative interventions and play therapy with teens, as well as explore the difference between directive and non-directive play therapy. There will also be an examination of common chronic health conditions faced by teens, a discussion of challenges faced by teens with chronic health conditions, potential responses, and creative ways to incorporate directive play therapy into the process of healing, acceptance, and growth. Directive play therapy approaches utilized clinically with teens living with chronic health conditions to combat some of their more common challenges will be shared and discussed.

LIVING WITH CHRONIC HEALTH CONDITIONS AS A TEEN

Being a teenager is challenging. Navigating the teen years can be stressful as one struggles to traverse the emotional, physical, social, and developmental landscape and move into adulthood (Wirrell, Cheung, & Spier, 2006). However, when a teen is living with a chronic health condition, the challenges escalate (Neinstein, 2001). According to the U.S. Department of Health & Human Services, Office of Adolescent Health (2016), in 2013, approximately 9% of children ages 5–17 were living with limitations due to chronic health complications. A chronic health condition is a condition that is ongoing, does not end, or continues to come back (Palo Alto Medical Foundation, 2015). Therefore, living with a chronic health condition brings ongoing illness, hospitalizations, surgeries, and treatment, which all intensify the impact of the physical, mental, social, and emotional changes teens experience. Similarly, as teens struggle to gain their independence, living with a chronic health condition impedes this process, increasing their dependence on adults for assistance with medication, physical needs, and monitoring (Rich, Goncalves, Guardiani, O'Donnell, & Strzelecki, 2014; University of Rochester Medical Center, 2017).

Common Chronic Health Conditions of the Teenage Years

The U.S. Department of Health & Human Services, Office of Adolescent Health (2016) reported that in 2012, as many as 31% of teens experienced a chronic health condition, with 28% of adolescents receiving mental health services (Otting & Prosek, 2016). These chronic health conditions include physical and mental health, such as attention deficit hyperactivity disorder, depression, and asthma. According to Neinstein (2001), additional common chronic health conditions for teens include heart disease, chronic respiratory tract diseases, diabetes, musculoskeletal disorders, hearing, visual, and speech impairments, along with a variety of mental health complications. The Palo Alto Medical Foundation (2015) reported that chronic health conditions experienced by teens also include arthritis, allergies, celiac disease, chronic fatigue syndrome (CFS), sickle cell disease, scoliosis, obesity, epilepsy, eating disorders, lupus, and cerebral palsy.

Teens are not exempt from chronic health conditions, although how they are experienced may vary greatly. In many cases, adolescents are more prone to develop specific chronic health conditions. Some illnesses, such as certain mental health disorders and Crohn's disease, for example, may first show symptoms in adolescence (Crohn's & Colitis, 2016). Whether diagnosed during childhood or during adolescence, living with a chronic health condition produces unique challenges for the teens who are living this experience.

Challenges Facing Teens Living With a Chronic Health Condition

On the surface, clinicians working with teems affected by chronic health conditions may consider their chronic health condition their primary, if not their only, challenge. However, living with compromised health as an adolescent brings about many additional concerns. First, the care of a chronic health condition often requires ongoing or repetitive health care treatment, surgeries, or hospitalizations. This leads to missed school and a potential drop in academic standing (U.S. Department of Health & Human Services, Office of Adolescent Health, 2016). For some, excessive absences may result in repeating an academic year. Additionally, many teens living with a chronic illness often experience additional illnesses. According to the U.S. Department of Health & Human Services, Office of Adolescent Health (2016), nearly one-fourth of teens living with a chronic health condition have at least one medical need that is not being addressed or treated.

A third challenge facing teens living with a chronic health condition relates to their physical development. Adolescence is a time when teens experience physical changes; it is a time of growth and development (Smith-Adcock & Tucker, 2016; Sloan, Sawyer, Warner, & Jones, 2014). This time period often brings about intense insecurity as these changes occur; bodies, feelings, and social environments are all in transition. Experiencing a chronic health condition during this time may intensify normal developmental issues related to physical development and feelings of adequacy (Mogtader & Leff, 1986; Rich, Goncalves, Guardiani, O'Donnell, & Strzelecki, 2014; University of Rochester Medical Center, 2017). Teens with a chronic health condition may experience physical illness, may have visible scars from treatment, may experience a change in their looks, or may be unable to/required to wear certain clothing or medical devices due to their health condition (Neinstein, 2001). These physical manifestations of a chronic illness, along with the normal physical challenges of adolescence, may increase feelings of inadequacy and self-consciousness.

Developing autonomy is another area that deserves special consideration for teens who are experiencing a chronic health condition. The teen years are a time of remarkable growth in the independence of adolescents (Erikson, 1950). This is a time when teens begin to figure out who they are, develop their own identity, and begin to differentiate from their family unit (Erikson, 1950; Koltz & Tarabochia, 2014; Rich et al., 2014; University of Rochester Medical Center, 2017; Wirrell et al., 2006). However, the presence of a chronic medical condition may impede this process. While most teens are exhilarated with every aspect of exploring the newfound freedom that comes with age, teens living with a chronic medical condition may have a different experience. There may be mixed messages in regards to this freedom: is it a curse or is it a luxury? For teens in general, leaving the safe cocoon of parental protection to explore an unknown world, while exciting, may produce anxiety. This anxiety is amplified when there are health concerns (University of Rochester Medical Center, 2017). Additionally, pushing a teen to finding their footing as they grow into adulthood, after protecting them throughout their health struggles, may be a battle of nerves for many parents, particularly when the adolescent may still be experiencing health complications. While both teen and parent work toward the developmental task of gaining autonomy, the chronic health complications may make this process a bit more frightening and uncomfortable.

The next task confronting teens living with a chronic illness is that of socialization. As individuals move from being children to teens, their focus developmentally moves from the family group to the peer group (Broderick & Blewitt, 2010; Smith-Adcock & Tucker, 2016), with the peer group becoming teens' primary social system and support. However, a chronic health condition may involve ongoing medical treatment, time spent in the hospital, and missed days at school (U.S. Department of Health & Human Services, Office of Adolescent Health, 2016), all of which interfere with a teen's ability to make and/or maintain peer relationships and develop peer support. This lack of peer support may increase self-esteem concerns, as the teen struggles to find acceptance by peers and of oneself (Mogtader & Leff, 1986; Neinstein, 2001; University of Rochester Medical Center, 2017; Wirrell et al., 2006).

A final, yet significant, complication faced by teens living with a chronic health condition is medical non-compliance. This issue is one of the more complicated issues faced by adolescents living with a chronic health condition. Teens are in a very tricky position when it comes to maintaining medical compliance. Developmentally, adolescents are beginning to gain autonomy. Therefore, responsibility for the management of a portion of their illness is one area where many teens are often given responsibility (University of Rochester Medical Center, 2017), whether in the form of medication management, monitoring their illness, or some other form of treatment management. There are challenges to this necessary developmental milestone, however. Developmentally, many teens may not yet have reached the level of dependability or responsibility necessary to be in charge of a potentially life-altering illness; they are still learning. Additionally, teens may engage in rash, unwise decision making. They may not yet be responsible enough to adequately manage their illness, they may choose to alter their recommended treatment if they dislike a certain aspect of the treatment, or they may choose to forgo their treatment altogether (University of Rochester Medical Center, 2017). For many teens, the realization they will have a lifetime of illness may be overwhelming. Feelings of anger, resentment, or self-consciousness regarding their condition, coupled with ongoing illness and medical treatment, along with the common feelings of invincibility many teens developmentally experience may overwhelm a teen's coping skills, leading to medical non-compliance. This medical non-compliance can have serious ramifications for a teen with a life-threatening chronic health condition (University of Rochester Medical Center, 2017). Refusing to manage their meds, making poor dietary choices, and skipping or altering other areas of treatment may lead to coma, serious illness, or in some cases, death.

Teen Responses to Living With a Chronic Health Condition

There are many responses a teen living with a chronic health condition might have. These responses range from concerns about their health, concerns about school, their self-esteem, peer interactions, or issues with the long-term implications of having a chronic health condition.

First, an emotional response is an expected reaction to living with a chronic health condition. An emotional response might be a mixture of sadness, frustration, or anger related to the stressful situation (Slyter, 2012).

Additionally, teens might express concern with how they may look due to the impact of their medical condition, or how their peers might respond to the changes in their body. As well, teens might experience grief over the loss of activities, such as sports, which might accompany a chronic health condition. Some teens might also worry about missing school and how that might impact their academic standing (American Academy of Pediatrics, 2017).

Finally, teens may also experience fear regarding their medical status. When living with a chronic medical condition, there may be ongoing medical treatment, long-term care, surgeries, and recurrent hospitalizations. The medical condition and the related treatments may result in fear in regard to specific upcoming procedures, as well as their medical future. An additional response for many teens may be fear and frustration related to misperceptions about their medical condition (American Academy of Pediatrics, 2017). It is not uncommon for parents and, at times, medical professionals to attempt to protect teens from what might be considered a harsh truth in regard to their medical condition and prognosis, or to consider the medical information too complicated to explain. However, the lack of knowledge, or more specifically, the imagined truth a youth might envision, may be far more devastating than honest discourse regarding their medical status.

THE THERAPEUTIC RELATIONSHIP WITH A CHRONICALLY ILL TEEN

Most clinicians view the therapeutic relationship as the primary indicator of success in the clinical relationship (Gladding, 2012). The therapeutic relationship has been acknowledged as being as or more important in the healing/recovery process than any other therapeutic factor (Gladding, 2012; van Grieken et al., 2016). According to Clark Moustakas (1973), a clinician respects their young clients for who they are and where they are, with no expectation. Therapeutically, there is no greater gift, particularly for a chronically ill teen who may be struggling not only with natural developmental milestones, but also with increased challenges related to their illness, such as loss of control of their environment and their bodies, real or perceived alienation from peers, and decreased self-esteem related to their illness. This gift will form the foundation of a healing therapeutic relationship.

INCORPORATING PLAY THERAPY

Incorporating play into therapy in the treatment of children with chronic health conditions may serve multiple purposes. Levine and Kline (2007) indicate that play allows children to communicate in a language that is natural to them, sharing with adults experiences that they have not yet mastered nor resolved (Muro, Ray, Schottelkorb, Smith, & Blanco, 2006). The sharing of what they have experienced, as well as the act of retelling through play, allows the opportunity for healing as the child or adolescent gains a sense of mastery in the retelling through play. Play therapy, as well, provides an opportunity for a client and clinician to make contact (Axline, 1964; Giordano, Landreth, & Jones, 2005; Landreth, 2012), and to begin moving past the anticipated relationship of a 'judgmental adult' who has an expectation to a more open and permissive relationship (O'Conner, 2001). The therapeutic process, often involving exploring and working toward resolution of difficult experiences, can also be made more enjoyable through the use of play therapy (O'Conner, 2001). Play therapy serves as a source of observation, provides pathway for understanding, and a means of gaining more data (Landreth, 2012), while improving the potential of meaningful communication taking place between the clinician and the child (Axline, 1964; O'Conner, 2001).

Additionally, play allows for the reenactment of traumatic experiences, often releasing negative emotions, such as pain and tension, which are associated with the trauma. Play, in the therapeutic environment, allows a client to work through feelings, to more fully express feelings, belief systems, fears, and concerns, and as a way to rehearse behaviors for use in the real world (Landreth, 2012). Play also provides an opportunity to practice "newly developed emotional, cognitive, social, and life skills" (O'Conner, 2001, p. 34). Utilizing play can be a safe way to explore past experiences and express related emotions (Kagan & Landreth, 2009), as the situation, emotion, or target is oftentimes disguised within the play (Axline, 1969; Kottman, 2001; O'Conner, 2000).

Play therapy encourages children to work within their most natural and normal communication styles; they are not forced to communicate as adults. Therefore, play therapy may be beneficial in treating a range of issues (Burns, 2005; Landreth, 2012; Muro et al., 2006). Children have the experience of working with an adult who encourages them to communicate in their most natural language, play, and work toward resolution of challenging symptomology using play (Axline, 1964; Findling, Bratton, & Henson, 2006; Landreth, 2012; Muro et al., 2006; O'Conner, 2000). "Children experience much in life they find difficult to express in language, and so they use play to formulate and assimilate what they experience" (Oaklander, 2001, p. 45). The use of adult treatment approaches, attempting to use more verbal styles as opposed to play, oftentimes results in a lack of progress in treatment. "Play, like young children, is preoperational. It is therefore incompatible with the concrete formal operations of adult therapy" (Sweeney & Landreth, 1993, p. 352). As with adults, not every play therapy theory or method will work or be suitable for every child. The method should be based on the theoretical orientation of the clinician, how a clinician perceives change taking place (Kottman, 2001), as well as the symptoms, needs, and developmental level of the child (Giordano et al., 2005; Landreth, 2012).

DIRECTIVE VERSUS NON-DIRECTIVE PLAY THERAPY

As with most types of treatment, play therapy draws upon multiple theories and models, utilizing numerous techniques. When engaging in play therapy, two primary formats may be utilized: non-directive/non-structured play therapy or directive/structured play therapy (Gil, 1991; Kottman, 2001; Landreth, 1991; O'Conner, 2000). Within each of these two formats of play therapy, there are multiple theories that a clinician can choose to personalize the treatment to the specific needs of their individual clients.

Non-Directive Play Therapy

Non-directive or child-/client-centered play therapy is a non-structured and non-intrusive form of play therapy. It is a shared experience through which a clinician encourages a child to direct the session, believing the child will work toward healing, growth, and self-actualization. This belief in a child's ability to heal focuses on providing acceptance, non-interference, and understanding (Landreth, 1993). Based upon the work of Carl Rogers, Virginia Axline further developed the client-centered play therapy approach. Children can choose their tools of therapy (toys), as well as how they are used (themes) (Gil, 1991). Non-directive play therapy has been found to effectively address a myriad of childhood disorders (Landreth, 2012), and is not based on interpretations, rather on allowing the child to perform as the expert, working toward mastery and resolution of challenges in their own time through their own choices with support, guidance, and attention from the clinician (Gil, 1991; Kottman, 2001).

Directive Play Therapy

Directive, or structured play therapy, oftentimes considered a form of expressive arts, incorporates clinical work rooted in pre-designed or pre-scripted, clinician-driven play-based activities or techniques (Kottman, 2001), as opposed to play that is child-directed. According to Gil (1991), clinicians who engage in directive play therapy

> structure and create the play situation, attempting to elicit, stimulate, and intrude upon the child's unconscious, hidden processes or overt behavior by challenging the child's defensive mechanisms and encouraging or leading the child in directions that are seen as beneficial.
>
> (p. 36)

Directive play therapy focuses on the child and specific symptomology and is often time-limited in its scope (Gil, 1991). Directive play therapy serves as an umbrella encompassing a host of creative/expressive arts techniques, including music, drama, play, art, bibliotherapy, puppet play, and therapeutic games, to name a few (Gil, 1991; Gladding, 2016; Green & Drewes, 2014). Directive play therapy also encompasses several therapy types, such as family therapy and Filial Therapy (Gil, 1991).

Using and Incorporating Creative Interventions and Directive Play Therapy With Teens

The needs of the chronically ill teenager are unique from other populations. They are in transition from childhood to adulthood (Broderick & Blewitt, 2010), therefore they may be too young to play, but not always ready or cognitively capable of sitting down to discuss their feelings, their experiences, or their needs. They are experiencing a life-altering event, a chronic illness, which sets them apart from a majority of their peers. Therefore, a treatment method different from the traditional talk therapy is often utilized, such as creative interventions. According to Gladding (2016), incorporating some form of creative interventions, or expressive arts, produces a multitude of benefits, helping clients heal both physically and mentally. The use of creativity in the healing process decreases acting out, improves self-esteem, develops awareness of emotions related to specific events, improves motor coordination, increases relaxation, and teaches the ability to cope with stressful situations, aiding in the recovery from traumatic experiences, such as medical procedures and treatment.

According to Bratton, Taylor, and Akay (2014), the integration of humanistic play therapy and expressive arts has been effective with young adolescents. Utilizing expressive arts in the counseling process with teens experiencing a chronic health condition emphasizes the view that directive play therapies incorporating music, movement, drama, poetry, art, and play can be a successful treatment approach (Sawyer & Willis, 2011). As teens seek out avenues to explore their identity and adequately express themselves, creative interventions become a natural medium for treatment (Perryman, Moss, & Cochran, 2015).

There has been an increase in the use of the creative arts in the counseling process (Gladding, 2016) for several reasons. First, integrating creative arts into the helping process is a means to aid clients in becoming more connected and integrated. Second, the creative arts have a focus on energy and process. The creative arts, in most situations, require participation and generate emotion and behaviors. Participating in creative interventions often creates new energy and the feeling of accomplishment, as there is a tangible outcome to the process. Third, creativity in the helping process allows a client to have a more visible and focused outcome; they can see where they are going and how to get there (Gladding, 2016). Fourth, utilizing creativity in the helping process allows for the incorporation of creative expression, enriching the experience for those engaged. The fifth rationale for incorporating creativity involves establishing a new sense of self and finding a new perspective on life. This is especially important for those who are experiencing or recovering from an adverse experience, such as a chronic illness. Another reason Gladding suggests incorporating creativity into counseling is due to the concrete nature of the experience. Clients can replicate creative experiences that are beneficial, as well as producing a historical timeline of their process and progress. Seventh, client and clinician both may find added insight in the clinical experience when incorporating creativity. Research has also found that incorporating the use of the creative arts clinically has resulted in improved socialization and cooperation. Finally, the expressive arts are multicultural. Clinicians provide a variety of tools and allow clients to utilize the tools that best suit them and their current, specific needs (Gladding, 2016).

It has been established that youths benefit from the opportunity to play and express themselves creatively, as it is the "reservoir and wellspring of a child's fundamental capacity to assimilate and adapt creatively to life experiences" (Wojtasik & Sanborn, 1991, p. 295). While the hospital setting for teens receiving treatment may limit their potential for social exploration, the opportunity to play and freely express themselves creatively opens the potential of the healing power of play, "for diversion, for instruction, as preparation for frightening or painful medical procedures, and as a means of mastering feelings of anger and helplessness" (Wojtasik & Sanborn, 1991, p. 295).

Based on the literature, incorporating creativity, or directive play therapy, into the therapeutic experience would seem to be the most appropriate approach for the chronically ill teen. "Chronically ill children often feel helpless, and in play therapy can experience being in control of their play and in charge of the outcome, thus returning to a state of feeling in control," (Landreth, Homeyer, Glover, & Sweeney, 1996, p. 61). Allowing a freedom of expression of their, at times, challenging experiences, directive play therapy will provide an opportunity for healing, acceptance, and growth.

CASE STUDY—THE EXPERIENCE OF A CHRONIC ILLNESS

Penny was diagnosed with an autoimmune digestive disease at 8 years of age. Medically, she had experienced illness since she was a toddler, going from doctor to doctor, with her parents most often being told she had yet another stomach virus. These were no simple viruses, however; Penny would spend days with severe stomach cramps, nausea, vomiting, and an upset stomach. At one point, Penny's mom asked a physician, "Will you please send her to a specialist? She just keeps getting sick." Offended, the physician shoved a medical supply tray and told Penny's mom to go elsewhere if she wanted a referral. One doctor, however, told Penny's mom that no child contracted the same virus time and time again, and made a referral.

Just before her eighth birthday, Penny met with a gastroenterologist at a large children's hospital. The day of her first appointment, a Friday, the doctor began testing. After the initial testing, the doctor sent them home with instructions to return on Monday and to be prepared to stay. Upon returning Monday, Penny underwent painful and exhausting testing. After a particularly painful biopsy, Penny's parents were given the news; she was diagnosed with an autoimmune digestive disease. The gastroenterologist gave her parents some very stern words to guide the entire family. He told her parents,

> Penny will most likely be on medicine for the rest of her life. She's old enough now to take it herself. You can also choose to make her independent or make her an invalid. The choice is yours. Always send her to school. Even if you have to go get her in an hour, send her to school. If you keep her at home, in a few minutes, she may feel better, and she will have lost an entire day, so send her.

Treatment began immediately, while Penny was still in the hospital, but the outlook was grim. Penny's parents began going to support group meetings. However, at the time, Penny was one of the youngest children to be diagnosed with this particular disease in the area, so resources were limited. For the next six to eight months, Penny endured hospitalizations every month due to her illness.

Treatment and life changes to address the chronic illness for Penny disrupted her entire life. She began taking medication, up to 30 pills per day. She had an allergic reaction to one medication, while the steroid was taken in such high doses that she became so swollen with fluid, she could no longer sleep lying down. Her physical appearance changed, and she was teased and called 'cabbage patch' (for the doll) due to the swelling. She underwent frequent testing and treatments, including frequent stays in the hospital. At times, some of the treatments to address the illness caused complications almost as challenging as the disease itself. Due to the potential damage to her bones caused by high doses of steroids, Penny was no longer allowed to participate in physical activities; she could no longer participate in soccer, softball, gymnastics, baton, tap dancing, ballet, or other activities. The steroids also caused repeated bouts of kidney stones, which were agonizing and resulted in repeated stays in the hospital. The intensity of the disease itself increased, as well, and began to act throughout her body. Penny experienced severe migraines with vomiting, necessitating trips to the emergency room for treatment. During one visit, her blood pressure rose so high, she was held in the emergency room at stroke level. Juvenile arthritis also developed, leaving Penny unable to walk at times, and being carried by family members. Ear infections were on the growing list of illnesses that required frequent hospitalizations for Penny during this time period.

Penny had several supports in place throughout this process. Penny had a very supportive school system that educated her classmates about her illness, and prepared them for her return to the school setting whenever there was a hospitalization early in her illness. As a young teen, one teacher volunteered to provide extra assistance in Penny's education, as she experienced multiple hospitalizations; the teacher dropped homework in her parents' mailbox every night for her father to pick up and take to the hospital, and upon her release from the hospital, the teacher would visit her home to ensure she was caught up to her class. This extra attention, however, did not mitigate the damage caused by repeated absences, a lack of interaction with peers, and unavoidable interaction with peers who were uneducated about Penny's illness and the impact it was having on her body. At one point, the school system was also a source of conflict, as the school attendance officer became involved due to Penny's excessive absences as a result of repeated hospitalizations.

Penny had a supportive family, both nuclear and extended. Penny's parents and siblings accommodated her illness as much as possible, with her parents enrolling her in art and music classes to compensate for the missing extracurricular activities Penny had to stop when she was first diagnosed.

At one time, as an adolescent, Penny asked her mother, "Why can't I be like other kids? Why am I always sick?" Asked with the genuineness and innocence of youth, to her mother, these questions were heartbreaking. To Penny, it was an expression of isolation and an awareness of the uniqueness her chronic illness had created.

Through Penny's music and art, she found she could express herself. She could safely re-create her experiences through a creative medium that was accessible even with her illness. She created pictures depicting freedom and beauty, scenes of nature and the outdoors at times when she was homebound. As Penny grew and her illness waxed and waned, she held on to her love for creativity and the freedom of expression this medium provided.

As a child, and then an adolescent with a chronic health condition, Penny found creative expression an invaluable tool in living with an autoimmune digestive disease. Facing typical teen challenges, along with many of the challenges commonly experienced by teens living with a chronic health condition such as peer isolation, developing autonomy, self-esteem concerns, and anxiety, a more structured approach to implementing creative expression would be beneficial in Penny's growth, healing, and development. In the following section, I will discuss directive play therapy approaches to use with Penny and other children who are living with chronic health conditions.

DIRECTIVE PLAY THERAPY APPROACHES WITH PENNY AND/OR ADOLESCENTS LIKE HER

Working with chronically ill teens, particularly those experiencing some of the issues that confronted Penny, offers an opportunity to incorporate a variety of directive techniques from which to choose. For this section, I will share examples of directive play therapy activities I have developed to address five common areas of concern for teens like Penny living with a chronic health condition.

Stress/Anxiety

Rationale for Penny: Living with a chronic health condition can be stressful, given ongoing medical procedures, hospitalizations, and concerns with health, as well as the increased anxiety resulting from puberty, social situations, and developing independence. For Penny, living with an autoimmune digestive disease impacted her in multiple ways physically, as well as creating challenges for her socially, as she spent much time in the hospital, away from friends, school, and extracurricular activities. Addressing the stress resulting from these challenges would allow Penny the opportunity to identify, express, and release the stress in a safe, contained environment.

Title: The Monster in Me

Overview: With "The Monster in Me," teens are encouraged to create a tangible representation of their stressor so they can take control and manage their anxiety.

Treatment Goals

- Identify a specific situation/event/scenario that is creating stress or anxiety
- Tangibly create a representation of the stressor
- Identify how to control the stressor.

Materials Needed

- Play-Doh

Description

- Teen is given a variety of colors of Play-Doh.
- Teens are encouraged to consider what issues they have experienced or are concerned may arise at present.
- Teens are directed to create a symbol using the Play-Doh, representing the monster they are facing that is or may cause them difficulties. These symbols can be literal or abstract, and can be created in whatever way the counselor feels best represents their concern.
- Alternatively, teens may alter their creation when asked how they can alter it to create a figure that no longer causes the same level of stress.
- Alternatively, at the end, teens may choose to symbolically vanquish their creation as they learn to discuss how to move past this issue.

Processing Questions

- What name might you give your creation?
- What does your monster represent to you?

- How might your monster hinder you?
- How has it hindered you in the past?
- What could you do to alter the monster so that it no longer hinders you?
- How has it impacted other areas of your life?
- What plans could you make to change how it impacts you?

Self-Esteem

Rationale for Penny: Living with a chronic health condition can have a negative impact on the self-esteem of teens. The chronic health condition itself may result in changes to the body, while the treatment of the condition may also result in changes other teens do not experience. The teen living with a chronic health condition lives a life unlike other teens, with doctor's visits, hospitalizations, and medications—all things that set them apart and make them different from their peers and can take a toll on how they value themselves. For Penny, spending weeks in the hospital, no longer being allowed to participate in extracurricular activities, and taking up to 30 pills a day began to negatively alter her self-perception. Having the opportunity to explore her own identity and develop a deeper understanding of who she is and who she is in relation to others in the world would allow Penny to begin to rebuild her self-esteem, and with it, her perception of self.

Title: Who Am I?

Overview: For teens and pre-teens, developing an understanding of who they are, who they want to be, and how to get to that point can be a challenge. Their bodies, their identity, and their ideas are ever-changing. In "Who Am I?," the goal is to help participants improve their self-esteem by looking at themselves in a different way, explore their own self-concept, and develop a deeper understanding of their own personal identity.

Treatment Goals

- Improve self-esteem by seeing oneself in a different way
- Explore self-concept
- Develop a deeper understanding of personal identity.

Materials Needed

- "Who Am I?" writing prompts.

Description

- Provide each participant with "Who Am I?" writing prompts.
- Encourage each participant to complete each prompt with the first answer that comes to mind, leaving no prompt blank. Share that the goal for this writing exercise is to help clients dig deep, explore who they are, and develop an understanding of what things mean to them.

- Upon completion, participants are encouraged to share out loud what they have written.
- Discuss responses.
- Note: the "Who Am I" writing prompts are only starters. Prompts that are more specific to each participant may be added, or participants may add their own prompts.

"Who Am I?" Writing Prompts

1. When you were younger, what did you want to be when you grew up? Is this still true for you?
2. What has been your most significant relationship? How did it shape you?
3. What is your favorite memory from childhood/when you were younger?
4. What is your least favorite memory from childhood/when you were younger?
5. What is your favorite holiday and why?
6. What is the one dream you look the most forward to having come true?
7. In five years, if you can live anywhere, where will it be? Why?
8. What is the one most valuable lesson, positive or negative, that you have learned from your parents?
9. Who do you least want to be like?
10. Who do you most want to be like?
11. What is one personal characteristic you want to develop?
12. What is one personal characteristic you have of which you are most proud?
13. What is one personal characteristic you have that you think you could improve?
14. What is one thing you feel you missed out on when you were younger?
15. For what are you most thankful?

Feelings Expression

Rationale for Penny: Living with a chronic health condition, for many, is often an emotionally charged experience. For teens, this may result in feelings of sadness, frustration, anger, or confusion. For Penny, having the opportunity to process these feelings openly in a safe, neutral, and nurturing environment would allow her to begin to process her feelings about her illness, living with her illness, and how her illness will impact her life.

Title: Two-Faced

Overview: "Two-Faced" encourages participants to explore two sides. They are encouraged to explore the side of themselves shared with others, as well as the side of themselves typically not shared with others; participants explore what is hidden and the meaning this might have for them.

Treatment Goals

- Identify what emotions are most often hidden from others
- Explore three ways to make the feelings we present more congruent with how we truly feel.

Materials Needed

- A drawing of a mask/face divided down the middle
- (Alternative: plastic masks and paint/crayons/markers).

Description

- Clinician discusses that sometimes we all wear masks, similar to what we wear at Halloween. These masks are used to hide our true faces from others—our true faces that show how we feel about ourselves, about others, about what might be going on around us.
- Participants are asked to complete the "Two-Faced" sheet. On the left, they will draw the face (mask) presented to others in a given situation, and on the right, the face behind the mask, their true selves.
  - After completing the drawings, participants will identify three ways they can alter their mask to be more congruent with their true selves.
- Note: this can be an 'in general' format or regarding a specific situation.

Processing Questions (optional)

- What are the differences in the mask and what is beneath the mask?
- Is it difficult to maintain the mask? What makes it difficult?
- Is maintaining a mask necessary? What makes it necessary?
- If you could wear a different mask, what would it be?
- Because it is difficult to express the feelings being hidden by the mask, what are some additional ways to express those feelings?

Coping Skills

Rationale for Penny: Living with a chronic health condition may be an isolating experience for many teens. They may be physically cut off from peers due to hospitalizations and treatments, and emotionally separated due to a lack of understanding and fear. As well, teens may have difficulty connecting with and reaching out to parents, siblings, or others who may wish to offer support—those who are not in a position to understand their challenges. This may leave a teen feeling isolated and alone. Thus, being able to develop coping skills and identify with whom a teen can connect and depend upon, as well as in what way, may be crucial to their journey through the medical process. For Penny, being separated from her peers and family due to repeated hospitalizations, as well as the social disconnect that may occur with a chronic health condition, Penny would benefit from an opportunity to consciously identify a support system she can count on, and explore in what ways those individuals are able to be a support.

Title: Pieces of Me

Overview: In this activity, we are able to identify individuals who are a support, as well as identify a values system through the use of this activity. Even the youngest of children can identify people who contribute to who they are, people that are important to them. Some, however, especially teens, may list poor role models, or individuals that you feel may not be a good role model. It is important to explore with your client what characteristics about this person got them onto the list, while reiterating that all people have positive, as well as not positive things about them, and to be selective in the qualities they value—in other words, just because someone has one positive quality, it doesn't mean they all are.

Materials Needed

- A drawing of a heart with lines drawn throughout the heart, dissecting it into a puzzle.

Treatment Goals

- Identify support system
- Identify personal values
- Assess growth of support system over time.

Description

- Discuss that similar to how the food we eat makes our bodies grow, the people who are important to us all become a part of us and help us grow. So, we want to figure out who the important people in our world are.
- Instruct clients to identify all the people you feel help you become who you are, people who support you, who you trust, and you can go to when you need help—in essence, your support system.
- Clients then utilize the "Pieces of Me" worksheet to identify people important to them and who contribute to who they are.
- Clients are then asked to look at all of the people who make them who they are, and identify one thing about each person that makes them important, a quality that contributed to their addition to the sheet. In this way, clients are also identifying a values system, as qualities likely to appear are trust, honesty, friendship, and so forth, and we are able to assess what qualities and values are most important to them.

Processing Questions (optional)

- What quality got each person onto the list?
- Was it difficult to identify people to put on the list?
- Let's talk about some of the characteristics that you value in people that makes them important to you, and why you want them to be a part of who you are.
- What qualities, of the ones you identified, are ones that you have?
- Are there any of the qualities you do not have, but would like to develop?

Special Considerations

Some clients, especially teens, may list poor role models, or individuals you feel may not be someone they should go to. Explore with your client what about this person got them onto the list, and reiterate that all people have positive and not so positive qualities, and how we can incorporate the positive qualities. Some clients may have difficulty identifying a support system, such as those who have been in foster care, have poor social skills, have experienced abuse, or who have demonstrated trust issues.

Peer Relationships

Rationale for Penny: Peer relationships are a frequent casualty when a teen faces a chronic health condition. Frequent hospitalizations and an inability to socialize due to illness leaves many teens isolated and lagging behind in social skills development. For Penny, spending time in the hospital, not having an opportunity to engage in extra-curricular activities, and frequently missing school, it would be beneficial to have an opportunity to interact with peers and family in a positive way to not only experience constructive methods of empathy and having a positive social interaction, but to also have an interaction that is conducive to building esteem.

Title: What I Like About You!

Overview: Participants are encouraged to enhance their ability to display empathy and to increase their ability to find positives in others. Through doing so, other participants in a group or family session will have an opportunity to receive positive feedback from family/group members. "What I Like About You!" encourages positive peer/family interaction and enhanced empathy development.

Treatment Goals

- Improve empathy for others
- Increase ability to identify positive characteristics in others
- Improve self-esteem as related to positive peer reinforcement
- Engage in positive peer/family interaction.

Materials Needed

- Empty gift boxes with a removable lid and an opening in the top (may be created in session)
- Blank slips of paper.

Description

- Discuss the importance of not only receiving, but giving. For this activity, we are going to give presents rather than receive them. These presents are going to be presents that are very special—they are going to be gifts of positivity!

- Present each member with a gift box. Alternatively, members may create their own unique gift boxes during session.
- Give each participant a slip of paper for every other participant present, including themselves, instructing them to write a positive for every participant present—this can be about a positive experience they have shared, a positive behavior, a physical attribute, and so forth. Participants may have extra slips if they would like to write more than one thing about other members.
- Instruct participants to put their slips of paper into the box of the appropriate participant. Go around, allowing participants to choose one slip from their box to share with the group. Participants are then encouraged to go around a second time, time permitting.
- After session:
  - Participants are encouraged to add to their gift box every week and to ask family/friends to add to their box.
  - Participants are encouraged to pull a slip from the box whenever a stressful situation arises, as a coping activity. The member is to read the slip they pull from the box, and take it with them for the day, if needed.

CONCLUSION

With the high number of adolescents living with chronic health conditions, understanding chronic health conditions, the challenges inherent in living with a chronic illness, and how to work with teens living a chronic illness is crucial. Living with a chronic health condition leads to a plethora of complications. While there is literature available on different forms of treatment for teens, as well literature on chronic illness, clinicians continue to strive to find the most appropriate treatment for adolescents living with a chronic health condition. Based on the challenges faced by these teens, both those related to chronic health conditions and those that are developmental, directive/structured play therapy shows promise of producing positive outcomes, both mentally and physically.

REFERENCES

American Academy of Pediatrics. (2017). *The stresses faced by teenagers who are chronically ill or disabled*. Retrieved from: www.healthychildren.org/English/health-issues/conditions/chronic/Pages/The-Stresses-Faced-By-Teenagers-Who-Are-Chronically-Ill-or-Disabled.aspx

Axline, V.M. (1964). *Dibs in search of self* (rev. ed.). New York: Ballantine Books.

Axline, V.M. (1969). *Play therapy* (rev. ed.). New York: Ballantine Books.

Bratton, S.C., Taylor, D.D., & Akay, S. (2014). Integrating play and expressive art therapy into small group counseling with preadolescents: A humanistic approach. In E.J. Green & A.A. Drewes (Eds.), *Integrating expressive arts and play therapy with children and adolescents* (pp. 253–282). Hoboken, NJ: Wiley.

Broderick, P.C., & Blewitt, P. (2010). *The life span: Human development for helping professionals* (3rd ed.). Upper Saddle River, NJ: Pearson.

Burns, G.W. (2005). *101 Healing stories for kids and teens: Using metaphors in therapy*. Hoboken, NJ: John Wiley & Sons.

Crohn's & Colitis. (2016). *Understanding Crohn's disease.* Retrieved from: www.crohn-sandcolitis.com/crohns?{unescapedlpurl}&cid=ppc_ppd_msft_cd_da_chrons_diseas_Phrase_64Z1867745

Erikson, E. (1950). *Childhood and society.* New York: W. W. Norton.

Findling, J. H., Bratton, S. C., & Henson, R. K. (2006). Development of the trauma play scale: An observation-based assessment of the impact of trauma on the play behaviors of young children. *International Journal of Play Therapy, 15,* 7–36.

Gil, E. (1991). *The healing power of play: Working with abused children.* New York: The Guilford Press.

Giordano, M., Landreth, G., & Jones, L. (2005). *A practical handbook for building the play therapy relationship.* Northvale, NJ: Jason Aronson.

Gladding, S. T. (2012). *Counseling: A comprehensive profession* (7th ed.). Upper Saddle River, NJ: Pearson.

Gladding, S. T. (2016). *The creative arts in counseling* (5th ed.). Alexandria, VA: American Counseling Association.

Green, E. J., & Drewes, A. A. (Eds.). (2014). *Integrating expressive arts and play therapy with children and adolescents.* Hoboken, NJ: John Wiley & Sons.

Kagan, S., & Landreth, G. L. (2009). Short-term child-centered play therapy training with Israeli school counselors and teachers. *International Journal of Play Therapy, 18*(4), 207–217.

Koltz, R. L., & Tarabochia, D. S. (2014). Technology: Using it as a means to creatively connect with adolescents. *Journal of Creativity in Mental Health, 9*(3), 380–398.

Kottman, T. (2001). *Play therapy: Basics and beyond.* Alexandria, VA: American Counseling Association.

Landreth, G. L. (1991). *Play therapy: The art of the relationship.* Florence, KY: Accelerated Development.

Landreth, G. L. (1993). Child centered play therapy. *Elementary School Guidance & Counseling, 38*(1), 17–30.

Landreth, G. L. (2012). *Play therapy: The art of the relationship* (3rd ed.). New York: Routledge.

Landreth, G. L., Homeyer, L. E., Glover, G., & Sweeney, D. S. (1996). *Play therapy interventions with children's problems.* Northvale, NJ: Jason Aronson.

Levine, P. A., & Kline, M. (2007). *Trauma through a child's eyes.* Berkeley, CA: North Atlantic Books.

Mogtader, E. M., & Leff, P. T. (1986). 'Young healers': Chronically adolescents as child life assistants. *Care of Children's Health, 14*(3), 174–177.

Moustakas, C. (1973). *Children in play therapy.* New York: Jason Aronson.

Muro, J., Ray, D., Schottelkorb, A., Smith, M. R., & Blanco, P. J. (2006). Quantitative analysis of Long-term child-centered play therapy. *International Journal of Play Therapy, 15*(2), 35–58.

Neinstein, L. S. (2001). The treatment of adolescents with a chronic illness. *Western Journal of Medicine, 175*(5), 293–295. Retrieved from www.ncbi.nlm.nih.gov/pmc/articles/PMC1071594/

Oaklander, V. (2001). Gestalt play therapy. *International Journal of Play Therapy, 10*(2), 45–55.

O'Conner, K. J. (2000). *The play therapy primer: An integration of theories and techniques* (2nd ed.). New York: John Wiley & Sons.

O'Conner, K. J. (2001). Ecosystemic play therapy. *International Journal of Play Therapy, 10*(2), 33–44.

Otting, T. L., & Prosek, E. A. (2016). Integrating feminist therapy and expressive arts with adolescent clients. *Journal of Creativity in Mental Health, 11*(1), 78–89.

Palo Alto Medical Foundation. (2015). *Chronic diseases and conditions.* Retrieved from: www.pamf.org/teen/health/diseases/chronic.html

Perryman, K. L., Moss, R., & Cochran, K. (2015). Child-centered expressive arts and play therapy: School groups for at-risk adolescent girls. *International Journal of Play Therapy, 25*(4), 205–220.

Rich, C., Goncalves, A., Guardiani, M., O'Donnell, E., & Strzelecki, J. (2014). Teen advisory committee: Lessons learned by adolescents, facilitators, and hospital staff. *Pediatric Nursing*, 40(6), 289–296.

Sawyer, C. B., & Willis, J. M. (2011). Introducing digital storytelling to influence the behavior of children and adolescents. *Journal of Creativity in Mental Health*, 6(4), 274–283.

Sloan, E. D., Sawyer, C., Warner, T. D., & Jones, L. A. (2014). Creativity in the cinema: Adolescent entertainment or violence training? The Hunger Games. *Journal of Creativity in Mental Health*, 9(3), 427–435.

Slyter, M. (2012). Creative counseling interventions for grieving adolescents. *Journal of Creativity in Mental Health*, 7(1), 17–34.

Smith-Adcock, S., & Tucker, C. (2016). *Counseling children and adolescents: Connecting theory, development, and diversity*. Thousand Oaks, CA: Sage.

Sweeney, D. S., & Landreth, G. (1993). Healing a child's spirit through play therapy: A scriptural approach to treating children. *Journal of Psychology and Christianity*, 12(4), 351–356.

University of Rochester Medical Center. (2017). *Psychological complications of chronic illness*. Retrieved from: www.urmc.rochester.edu/encyclopedia/content.aspx?ContentTypeID=90&ContentID=P01658

U.S. Department of Health & Human Services/Office of Adolescent Health. (2016). *Physical health: Chronic conditions*. Retrieved from: www.hhs.gov/ash/oah/adolescent-health-topics/physical-health-and-nutrition/chronic-conditions.html#

van Grieken, R. A., Verburg, H. F., Koeter, M. W. J., Stricker, J., Nabitz, U. W., & Schene, A. H. (2016). Helpful factors in the treatment of depression from the patient's, carer's and professional's perspective: A concept map study. *PLoS ONE*, 11(12), 1–14. https://doi.org/10.1371/journal.pone.0167719

Wirrell, E., Cheung, C., & Spier, S. (2006). How do teens view the physical and social impact of asthma compared to other chronic diseases? *Journal of Asthma*, 43, 155–160.

Wojtasik, S., & Sanborn, S. (1991). The crisis of acute hospitalization: Case of Seth, age 7. In N. B. Webb (Ed.), *Play therapy with children in crisis: A casebook for practitioners* (pp. 295–309). New York: Guildford.

PART IV

The Use of Medical Play With Terminal Illness in Children

CHAPTER 11

Child-Centered Play Therapy With Children Who Are Dying

Kristie Opiola and Dee C. Ray

We are multifarious creatures, forever becoming more of who we might be.
—Haugh (2012)

Even in the face of death, children work toward safety, health, creativity, and relationship. Children who confront life-limiting circumstances may suffer from physical and psychological pain, yet they maintain the biological motivation to enhance their understanding and ways of being. We, as therapists, can trust that children who are dying strive to move toward greater functioning even under such challenging conditions. Like the bloom of the flowers in the desert, a hospitalized child encountering death and dying struggles to break through austere realities to experience the healthiest version of life and peace in death. The therapist's responsibility is to provide a relationship that fosters and supports the child's struggle, allowing the child to access the biological force to enhance self in the midst of what may be considered the harshest of life's conditions.

Child-centered play therapy (CCPT) is recognized in the medical community as an intervention that meets a child's developmental needs while facilitating the child's natural progression toward self-acceptance and enhancement. Children naturally communicate through play, therefore "play therapy is a developmentally and culturally responsive intervention particularly suited to treat young children's social, emotional, and behavioral problems" (Bratton, 2013, p. 30). Specifically, CCPT identifies the safe and trusting relationship between child and therapist as vital to the healing process. CCPT is a therapeutic approach that relies on the interpersonal relationship between a child and trained play therapist that utilizes the child's natural medium of communication—play—to facilitate the development of a safe environment for the child to fully express and explore his or her feelings, thoughts, experiences, and behaviors (Landreth, 2012). In this chapter, we present CCPT as a responsive approach for terminally ill and dying children. In the medical setting, where children are likely to lose a sense of autonomy and control over their actions and bodies, CCPT offers a child the experience to feel fully capable to direct his or her process of grief, loss, and pain. Children who encounter imminent death have little control over their biological processes, but they maintain the ability to direct how to cope with their losses in self-enhancing ways.

REALITIES OF CHILDREN WHO ARE DYING

The death of a child is an uncommon, difficult, and painful event (Doka, 1995). Approximately 400,000 children die each year in the United States (Heron, 2016), with over 20% of deaths due to complications or progression of complex chronic conditions (Niswander, Cromwell, Chirico, Gupton, & Korones, 2014). The leading causes of disease-related deaths for children under the age of 15 are chromosomal and congenital abnormalities, malignant neoplasms, heart disease, respiratory distress, influenza, cerebrovascular disease, and neurodegenerative diseases. The death of a child can be sudden, such as in accidental or homicidal deaths, or can occur from a chronic illness, such as cancer. Although on the decline, cancer is the leading cause of death by disease in the United States. Dying children who enter the terminal phase of a chronic or life-threatening illness no longer receive aggressive treatment options and the focus turns from curative to palliative or hospice care (Pearson, 2005). At this point in care, the emphasis is on optimizing quality of life and managing pain and disease symptomology (Friebert & Williams, 2015). For other children, diagnoses may be terminal, such as spinal muscular atrophy (SMA), and the child's care focuses on quality of life instead of curative treatment (Hynson, 2012). Palliative care services are a complementary service and address the holistic needs of dying children, their family members, and the community through a multidisciplinary medical team. The foci of palliative care providers are the physical, emotional, intellectual, and spiritual needs of dying children and their families (Pearson, 2005). Friebert and Williams (2015) noted that the National Hospice and Palliative Care Organization (NHPCO) reported most children die in hospitals, but there is an increased trend of planned at-home deaths for children. Feudtner and colleagues (2011) affirmed NHPCO's report by noting that an increasing number of children with complex chronic conditions planned to die in a home setting instead of a hospital setting over the past 15 years.

Impact on Child

Early life experiences can impact the child's ability to cope with and overcome challenging situations. Children who experience medical challenges early in life can have behavioral, emotional, cognitive, and social problems. Children at end of life have many concerns and need help to process through their fears and curiosity (Pearson, 2009). Children with a terminal or life-ending illness often suffer from associated and easily understandable emotional disorders, such as anxiety and depression (Aldridge & Sourkes, 2012). According to Weaver and her colleagues (2016), children's anxieties are heightened when children's fears about treatment and illness are not addressed. Anxiety can intensify as the terminally ill child slowly worsens and lives with the uncertainty of life and death (Aldridge & Sourkes, 2012). Children also experience heightened anxiety due to their concrete and literal cognitive abilities. When caregivers do not openly communicate treatment related information to children, they "are left to wonder, interpret and imagine what is happening to them" (Orloff & Jones, 2011, p. 212), potentially causing greater fears and misunderstandings. Therefore, children need open communication about diagnosis, treatment, and prognosis. Children benefit from small amounts of information explained on a developmentally appropriate level. Children who have battled chronic illness for a period of time often comprehend more about illness and health than their same-aged peers. Terminally ill children are often perceptive and instinctively read nonverbal cues from their parents and health care providers. They are able to notice changes in the parent's affect and behaviors that indicate changes in their care and often understand changes in their health care before a parent tells them.

Developmental Understanding

A child's response to death is impacted by overall developmental cognitive under-standing based on the child's age and cognitive functioning (Pearson, 2009). Cognitive understanding of death progresses across age ranges. Researchers confirm that by the age of 4, children have a considerable understanding of some concepts related to death, such as finality of life and non-functionality of being dead, yet other concepts such as causality and universality of death are grasped later, around the ages of 7 to 10 (Bonoti, Leondari, & Mastora, 2013; Rosengren, Gutierrez, & Schein, 2014) Children's previous experiences, family communication style, and culture can also con-tribute to and influence a child's understanding of death and dying. Children who have previous experience with death understand death at earlier ages and with a greater sense of maturity, specifically the concept of causality (Bonoti et al., 2013). Because causality is a later-embraced concept for children, their egocentricity may contribute to them believing that their actions led to the progression of their illness or impending death. At early ages, children are concerned and develop understanding regarding the biology of death, aligning with their more concrete cognitive abilities. At later ages (over 7), children embrace more spiritual and religious conceptualizations of death and grow in their beliefs regarding life continuity beyond death (Rosengren et al., 2014) indicating strong cultural and religious influences on understanding of death for mid-dle childhood. Children's understanding of death is influenced by parents' willingness and openness to discuss death. Parents often operate under the myth that because children cannot developmentally comprehend death as a concept, the subject is best avoided. However, children's curiosity regarding death and their cognitive abilities to understand aspects of death indicate that open discussion is useful and at times nec-essary in order to avoid sending the message that death is not an embraceable topic. As school-age children mature, they find it challenging to speak about death directly, perhaps due to family and cultural messages that death is a scary and avoidable topic. Children may subtly ask questions or externalize their discussions about death to avoid direct discussion. Providing both verbal and non-verbal methods of approaching the subject of death is critical for parents, caregivers, and therapists.

Loneliness and Isolation

Two common emotions expressed by terminally ill children are loneliness and isolation (Aldridge & Sourkes, 2012). These children spend a large amount of time away from home and their peers. As the child's disease progresses, the child often stops attending school due to frequent hospitalization and specialty medical visits or due to pain management issues (Orloff & Jones, 2011). They are less involved in social activities and events and have fewer interactions with their same-aged peers. They spend substantial time with adults instead of same-aged peers. Due to long hospital stays and potentially needing to travel for services, terminally ill children often spend less time with the siblings as well, increasing their loneliness. Many terminally ill children seek control over their environments (Aasgaard, 2006) to keep loved ones near and avoid separation or seek protection from parents and caregivers (Hynson, 2012). Control is often manifested through excessive demands and commanding others to bring about a sense of safety in the environment.

Loss

Terminally ill children experience a multitude of losses in relation to their illness (Aldridge & Sourkes, 2012), particularly that of normalcy. Illness is unpredictable and the child's predictable and safe world changes as his or her disease progresses. The child also experiences a loss of one's ability as the disease progresses. For instance, a school-aged child may lose the ability to control his or her bowels and along with it, the trust and confidence in his or her body to function normally. As the child physically deteriorates, the child's autonomy is also lost. The child becomes more dependent on others for daily care. Strong emotions often accompany loss. Children may feel sadness, frustration, resignation, or anger toward the changes. Anticipatory grief is a common reaction to loss and entails the process of grieving in advance when a person knows loss is inevitable (Wolfelt, 1996). According to Wolfelt, grief is a natural and necessary process of coping. Grief and loss are two sides of the same coin and often accompany one another. Children express their grief and reaction to loss in multiple ways, with young children typically processing through their grief through the use of play (Pearson, 2009).

Preparing for Death

In preparing for death, Sourkes (2006) highlighted children's preoccupation with time. They appear eager to complete tasks to accomplish important projects. For instance, one 9-year-old child created a list of her favorite items and identified to whom she planned to give the items. A 12-year-old female made and decorated picture frames with her signature drawings for each of her family members as a legacy project. A 10-year-old child began to ask his mother to read to him. The child's request created alone time for him and his mother. The child appeared to create meaningful interactions with his mother. Each of these activities was an important step for the child so they felt prepared to die. As a child nears death, the children may turn inward and pull away from their external world (Aldridge & Sourkes, 2012). They may talk less and retreat from interacting with others. During this time, children still enjoy the presence of a safe person.

Communication

Children and parents may hide their feelings to protect each other. Aldridge and Sourkes (2012) highlight the importance of emotional support. Children seek support from a variety of people. They may seek emotional support from a parent, caregiver, medical personnel, or psychosocial team member. Children tend to test the acceptance and emotional readiness of providers as they seek support. When children identify a person as safe, they may share their concerns, fears, and questions. Children are curious and may ask many questions (Pearson, 2005). It is not uncommon for the child to repeat the question several times or ask several people the same questions as they seek understanding and to increase their trust that others are telling them the truth and not protecting them. A child's ability to cope with difficult emotions is improved when they have a safe person with whom they can share their concerns (Sourkes, 2006). Early and prompt referrals to mental health professionals can alleviate long-term emotional suffering for children (Weaver et al., 2016).

Impact on Families

Families whose children have a life-threatening diagnosis experience a multitude of transitions. Each family member experiences these transitions of illness-related identities in unique ways (Hynson, 2012), and this process typically begins immediately upon time of diagnosis. The child who is sick is diagnosed, then transitions from health to illness. The child also makes a transition from child to patient, while the parent transitions from 'typical' parent to a parent of a sick child. Over time, additional transitions occur. Parents take on a greater role in providing medical care at home and transition from parent to temporary nurse. Families may transition from spending most time at home to frequent visits to the hospital or doctor's offices. For children with chronic and potentially life-threatening illnesses like cancer, they may experience a transition from diagnosis to cure to incurable prognosis. No matter the transition, the families experience an array of psychosocial needs.

The effects of chronic and terminal illnesses on a family can be vast and devastating. The loss of a child is uncommon and parents frequently experience long periods of emotional distress and chaos (Pearson, 2005). According to Doka (1995), parents often experience shock, disbelief, helplessness, panic, fear, anger, emptiness, withdrawal, and longing. Parents' emotions come in phases of predictable or unpredictable (Hynson, Aroni, Bauld & Sawyer, 2006). Parents reported predictable emotions are easier to handle and they experience less anxiety when they know how they will feel. Unpredictable emotions are difficult for parents to manage and cause higher anxiety for parents. Foreman, Willis, and Goodenough (2005) discussed parents' expressions of sadness and isolation, as they did not feel that they could share their emotions with their extended family and friends because they do not feel understood or their extended support systems are not empathic to their needs or difficulties. For instance, parents of children with cancer are inundated with many stressors that place them at risk for emotional difficulties (Streisand, Kazak, & Tercyak, 2003). Initially, parents receive significant support from friends and family. Unfortunately, as treatment persists, support often decreases and families feel like they are fighting the battle alone (McGrath, 2001). According to Hynson and colleagues (2006) and Weaver and colleagues (2016), parents desire social support and wish more opportunities existed for support groups with other parents experiencing similar losses. Providing parents with resources and connecting them with trained parent partners may alleviate their feelings of isolation.

Some of the key losses for parents of terminally ill children are the loss of identity, security, and way of life. The parent's role of protector and nurturer is challenged by a child's illness (Hynson et al., 2006). Their long-term dreams, hopes, and desires for their dying children are forever changed and often lost. Parents struggle with anxiety and the unpredictable nature of death while trying to comfort and support their child (Best, Streisand, Catania, & Kazak, 2001; Manne et al., 1996). Their daily routines are altered, and they experience increased emotional and physical demands.

Parents who care for dying children experience an increased demand on their time, efforts, finances, and coping skills (Robinson et al., 2006). Parents of terminally ill children are forced into many different roles (Orloff & Jones, 2011). Frequent in-home medical visits, administration of medications, monitoring appropriate and healthy diets and fluid levels, and management of the stressors and demands of daily family life add to a parent's stress level. Parents fear the strain of multiple roles and demands placed on them due to their child's terminal illness prevents them from appropriately attending to other responsibilities and causes them to feel as if they are failures (Weaver et al., 2016). As their terminally ill child deteriorates, parents' focus streamlines to the needs of the ill child and they may struggle to meet the needs of other children (Orloff & Jones, 2011). Marital relationships may become strained as the parent is more focused on their parenting role than nurturing their spousal role. Commonly, parents feel guilty as they are unable to respond to everyone's needs.

Siblings often become forgotten within the family (Orloff & Jones, 2011). According to Houtzager and colleagues (2004), siblings often experience feelings of isolation, anxiety, uncertainty, jealousy, guilt, anger, and loneliness. The family structure and routine can be permanently altered when a parent's focus is on the dying child. Siblings may be forced to give up extracurricular activities because family times are allocated to taking care of the dying sibling (Pearson, 2005). Within the family structure, siblings are not typically involved in the treatment process—they often stand by and witness their dying sibling's suffering (Orloff & Jones, 2011). Changes in mood, such as withdrawal, attention-seeking behavior, and mood swings can indicate negative coping strategies, which are common in siblings (Wolfelt, 1996). Often, siblings feel unimportant as parents may or may not be physically present at activities (Orloff & Jones, 2011). Siblings may feel confused by their parent's emotional distance and misinterpret the reason for the change in behavior. In addition, parents may employ extended family and close friends to care for siblings, increasing unpredictability in who will pick the child up from school or where the child may sleep that night. Siblings, in particular girls and older siblings, take on more responsibility to help parents, and therefore suffer more from restrictions on their daily lives and overall development.

Because parents and siblings are dealing with their own grief and unreasonable stress, they may often be limited in their presence and full acceptance of the emotional needs of a child who is dying. The child who is ill may need someone to sit quietly or someone who will simply play with him or her without discussion. The child who is dying may need to openly play out or discuss the details of death, or the realness of pain and struggle. When family members are focused on helping the child feel better and maintain hope regarding a cure, the child may feel misunderstood and disconnected, thereby increasing a sense of isolation and belief that something is unacceptable about how he feels or thinks. The therapist is in the position of being able to provide a safe environment that allows full expression for both a terminally ill child and family members.

MENTAL HEALTH PROVIDERS

Children who are dying receive services from medical and psychosocial professionals. Each professional has a unique role in supporting the dying child and his or her family. Psychosocial team members include social workers, child life specialists, psychiatrists, psychologists, and counselors. A collaborative, team approach to care services is the best approach (Weaver et al., 2016). Many of the providers function from a medical model and attempt to cure or resolve the child's grief. In the medical model, the responsibility to create change or cure the patient is placed on the professional. The most common approach to mental health services in the health care setting is cognitive therapies (Orloff & Jones, 2011). Sourkes (2006) identified that many dying children begin therapy services because of the stress related to their illness. The professional may utilize prescriptive cognitive activities to help the child grieve and cope with pending losses. Psychosocial care is not formulaic and requires flexibility (Aldridge & Sourkes, 2012). Wolfelt (1996) expressed concern for formulaic and prescriptive approaches, as he believes grieving children need a safe space to mourn with a companion. He believes that prescriptive models underestimate a child's ability to grow and heal. In addition, prescriptive and cognitive activities have a specific focus and limit the professional's opportunity to learn the child's experience and fully hear and understand the child's perspective.

Aldridge and Sourkes (2012) encourage mental health professionals to follow the child's lead in the therapeutic relationship. Mental health services should provide children with a space where they can process their feelings, fears, and uncertainty (Orloff & Jones, 2011). Bluebond-Langner (1978) encouraged mental health professionals to provide a safe relationship where children can openly talk or play about their illness and prognosis. The professional maintains the child's need for privacy and desire to protect their parents from difficult conversations. Counseling offers the child a safe space to gain awareness of one's feelings and make sense of the intangible parts of grief and loss (Orloff & Jones, 2011). Glazer and Landreth (1993) encouraged counselors to provide a warm and accepting environment where children can resolve their fear, pain, and guilt about death.

CHILD-CENTERED PLAY THERAPY

Child-centered play therapy (CCPT) is a developmentally responsive therapeutic approach to help children with an array of emotional, behavioral, and social concerns (Axline, 1969; Ray & Landreth, 2015), and one of the most widely utilized therapeutic approaches for play therapists when working with children (Lambert et al., 2007). CCPT therapists believe in the power of the child-therapist relationship as a catalyst for therapeutic change for terminally ill children processing through and coping with challenging feelings, experiences, thoughts, and behaviors related to their impending death. CCPT is based on the work of Carl Rogers, who believed people are predisposed to strive toward growth and fulfilment of their potential when in a nurturing and supportive environment (Rogers, 1951). The central concept of CCPT in the context of working with children who are terminally ill is the actualizing tendency. The actualizing tendency is the biological force universal to all humans and unique to each individual that moves the person in a constructive and growth-enhancing direction (Bozarth, 1998; Haugh, 2012; Wilkins, 2010). When a child encounters adverse environments and circumstances, the actualizing tendency can be stunted or distorted, seeking to continue growth but in a way that can be self- or other-destructive. In the case of a child facing a chronic, life-limiting condition, she will naturally seek to enhance life as it is. However, if the child encounters interactions or circumstances that send the message that her natural ways of responding are unacceptable, she will develop coping skills that are incongruent with the actualizing tendency. For example, if a child attempts to talk about being scared to die and the parent responds by telling the child that he will be okay and there is no need to worry, the child receives the message that there is something wrong with the way he feels or thinks. Or, if a child plays out a funeral scene and the parent immediately changes the play to something more fun, the child may begin to think that she cannot trust her natural way to communicate to the parent. In response, the child feels less control, a lack of trust in self and others, and may respond by engaging in behaviors that send these messages.

In response to the child's need to work in alignment with this actualizing tendency, the therapist provides an environment in which the child's direction is valued as the road to healing. The CCPT therapist presents as a person who is genuine, open to self-experiences and the experiences of others, and capable of transparently sharing herself (Ray, 2011). The therapist experiences and communicates unconditional positive regard to the child, assured in the belief that the child has what is needed within himself to move toward healthy functioning and the importance of honoring the perception of the child. Finally, the therapist communicates empathic understanding to the child so that the child feels fully understood and accepted in the moment. It is through relationship and realization of full acceptance that the child is able to let go of negative behaviors developed from being disconnected with the self-actualizing tendency and initiate changes that are aligned with the actualizing tendency and lead to self-enhancing behaviors.

The Focus of CCPT

The focus of CCPT is on the child, not the child's problematic behaviors or challenging experiences (Landreth, 2012). According to Rogers, "the best vantage point" to

" *best vantage point* "

understand the child is from the child's internal frame of reference (Rogers, 1992) because children, when truly allowed and encouraged, are naturally the experts of their own lives, feelings, and concerns (Breemen, 2009), which is often expressed through their play (Landreth, 2012). In CCPT, play is recognized as the manner in which children communicate and express themselves (Axline, 1969; Landreth, 2012), no matter their spoken language, cultural background, and developmental processes (Sweeney & Skurja, 2001). Play is an essential component of childhood and a determining factor in children's overall mental health and well-being (Elkind, 2007; Ginsburg, 2007). Developmentally, young children struggle to verbalize their concerns and feelings to others. Play offers children a physical way to 'talk out' their difficulties and experiences (Axline, 1969). Because death is an abstract concept that involves multiple subconcepts, children who are dying need both non-verbal and verbal ways to connect their concrete experiences with the idea of death. CCPT is typically intended for children 3 to 10 years of age. In play therapy, children are provided opportunities to express, share, communicate, explore, and create meaning of themselves and their worlds; to master their inner struggles, feelings, desires, and perceptions to gain a fuller understanding of their internal experiences (VanFleet, Sywulak, & Sniscak, 2010). Development and health are enhanced when children are in an environment with an affectionate, empathic, and non-judgmental adult who relates to the child through play (Ginsburg, 2007; Ray & Landreth, 2015). Therefore, the relationship is the catalyst for therapeutic change.

The CCPT Therapist's Role

The primary role of the play therapist is to create an accepting, caring, and trusting relationship with the child so that the child feels safe to explore and express their concerns (Wilson & Ryan, 2005). The therapist believes in the child's ability to direct play where it needs to go for self-enhancement and follows the child's lead in the play session (Landreth, 2012). The therapist is patient, understanding, and accepting of the child's discovery of his or her inner self (VanFleet et al., 2010). Play therapists are very active and attuned to the deepest level of each child's needs, feelings, and experiences, and genuinely respond and convey unconditional positive regard and empathy to the child (Rogers, 1992). Landreth describes the therapist's attitude as one of expectancy and "anticipation as the vulnerable inner person of the child emerges" (p. 81). The therapist provides a permissive environment free from threat, judgment, or evaluation, so the child's actualizing tendency moves toward self-realization (Axline, 1969). A non-threatening and permissive environment provides children with opportunities to direct and explore their worlds through play. The playroom is set up with carefully selected play materials (Landreth, 2012) including nurturing, aggressive, real-life, and expressive toys and materials. The child is in the lead and is free to play with any toy he or she would like, sending a message that the entire child is welcome and accepted in this special space (Ray & Landreth, 2015). Children are not rushed or prompted to talk about particular experiences, feelings, or behaviors. Instead they are given time to learn, practice, grow, and heal (VanFleet et al., 2010). Given the time and space needed, a child can play out and bring a variety of feelings to the surface, helping them relax and gain mastery over oneself. Once the child's feelings and experiences are out in the open, the child can "face them, learn to control them, or abandon them" (Axline,

1969). According to Landreth (2012), "the permissive environment with an accepting and caring therapist allows the child the freedom to explore, test boundaries, share frightening parts of their lives, or change" (p. 70).

In the context of children who are chronically or terminally ill, CCPT structure is adjusted to fit the needs of the child. Although traditional CCPT is provided in a play-room with specific materials and space (Landreth, 2012; Ray, 2011), toys and materials may be limited to a travelling bag or box for use in a hospital room or home. Dying children and their families often require flexibility regarding the location for therapeutic services. A traditional office setting may not meet the needs of the child. Play therapy services may not follow the traditional therapeutic hour due to the dying child's stamina (Aldridge & Sourkes, 2012). Sometimes, 20 minutes may suffice for a child who is in pain or experiences fatigue. Setting weekly appointment times may not work appropriately for this population. Calling ahead and checking to see if the child is awake may prevent unproductive clinical time, as fatigue and lethargy may cause children to sleep during a scheduled session. The most important feature of CCPT is providing a relationship in which the child feels fully accepted and able to express all feelings and thoughts; other structural components can be modified to meet the child's needs.

CASE STUDY: LINA

The following case study is drawn from the clinical experience of the first author (KO) and exemplifies ways therapists can incorporate child-centered play therapy and parent consultation into their work with terminally ill children and their families. This case study is a compilation of several children in order to maintain confidentiality and is placed in hospital and clinic setting.

Medical Background

Lina, a 7-year-old Latina American female, was diagnosed with a brain tumor at the age of 5. For the past two years, Lina received a mixture of aggressive chemotherapy and radiation, as well as surgery, which caused her to lose her hair and left a large scar on the left side of her head. Lina typically spent a week at the hospital once a month for medical treatment. Her aggressive treatment was mildly effective, but Lina's tumor became unresponsive to medical treatment and was growing. Lina's doctors informed her parents that there were no more treatment options to cure Lina's cancer. The medical team and her parents decided to transition Lina to palliative care. Her parents stated they were open to trial studies if Lina met study criteria. Her parents did not want the doctors to tell Lina about the change in her condition out of fear she would give up hope and stop fighting her disease.

Background Information About Lina

Lina was an active child who enjoyed playing with dolls with her friends and siblings. The medical team often described Lina as a positive and outgoing spirit who brightened the medical unit. She was very playful and enjoyed when the medical staff engaged with her in play. Lina loved music and was often seen dancing in her room or around the hospital. It was not uncommon to see Lina at the nurses' station sharing her most recent dance moves with the nursing staff. Lina also liked to play 'tricks' on the medical staff.

Lina's immediate family consisted of her parents and two siblings. They lived approximately two hours from the hospital, and her siblings were not able to visit her as often as they would have liked because of the distance. Lina's mother was a stay-at-home mother and typically accompanied her to clinic visits and hospital stays. Lina's father worked for a large company and spent substantial time at work to compensate for their increased medical bills. Lina's father had stated his company and co-workers were very kind and donated their sick leave so he could be at the hospital as much as possible. Lina's younger brother and older sister were very close to Lina and struggled when she was away from home. They often called the hospital and checked in with how she was doing. Periodically, the siblings were able to come to the hospital and play with Lina. In addition, Lina had a large extended family that provided support and watched Lina's siblings when Lina was in the hospital. Lina was very close to her maternal grandparents and a paternal aunt, who occasionally stayed with her at the hospital so her parents could spend time at home with her siblings.

Cause for Referral to Play Therapy

Lina had told her medical team that she was very tired. She received encouragement to take a nap, and she had been assured that if she was struggling to sleep, they could prescribe medication to help her sleep. Lina looked disappointed when her parents and medical team responded in this way, and she became verbally aggressive toward those who tried to console her. The nurses observed her getting angry with her mother and lashing out at her when she tried to help her. In addition, Lina struggled when her parents left, and the medical staff described her as clingy. Her nurses and parents were worried because these emerging behaviors were out of character for Lina. Her parents told the medical staff that they were all tired and were hoping for more time at home, but Lina's pain was best controlled in the hospital. I was first contacted by Lina's nurse practitioner to provide services to Lina to help with her bursts of anger toward her parents and the nursing staff. Initially Lina came to the playroom. When Lina's disease progressed, I brought my traveling toys to her bedside. I had three goals for her time in play therapy. First, I hoped our time together would provide Lina with a safe and accepting space where she could share, freely emote, and express her fears, worries, and needs. I wanted to provide Lina with companionship as she explored difficult feelings and experiences in hope that she did not feel alone or unaccepted. Last, I hoped to convey my belief and trust in her to lead her play where she needed it to go.

Lina in Play Therapy

I introduced the playroom to Lina by saying, "In here is the playroom and you can play with the toys in lots of the ways you like." Initially, Lina was skeptical of play therapy and hesitantly played with a variety of toys in the playroom. She played briefly and then looked at the play therapist and watched as she reflected and responded to her play. Lina asked a fair number of questions and asked if it was OK for her to play with certain toys. Lina initially played in the sandbox, and would scoop sand and attempt to build castles and mountains. She became frustrated when her creations would not hold together, telling the play therapist the sand was stupid. Lina slowly began to talk and share more about herself. She would ask if I knew she had a sister or brother and if I knew her favorite toys. She also wanted to know why she was coming to play therapy. Lina's questions indicated her uncertainty about me and my role in her life. I reflected Lina's curiosity of coming to play therapy by responding, "You're curious about me and unsure about this space." I did not give her specifics of why she was referred to play therapy because I did not believe it was necessary for her growth and healing. Instead, I connected with Lina's emotions and uncertainty about me and our relationship, reflecting her desire to understand her situation.

Lina's play shifted from the sand to the kitchen area, and she created a variety of meals to eat. Eating was a big issue for Lina because her medication caused large sores in her mouth. The nurses shared that she would always order huge meals, but after trying them she would rarely eat much. Lina started to share how close she was to her family and did not like being so far away from them. She stated that her mother made delicious dinners and she missed her cooking most of all when they were in the hospital. Lina continued to cook meals for three sessions and then created the meal and would call her siblings on the phone while she pretended to eat. She would role-play discussing the day and what her siblings were up to during the day. In parent consultation, I shared Lina's theme of connectedness with her mother and how she was missing mealtime traditions. Her mother shared that family mealtime was very important to the family and they all missed the opportunity to talk while Lina was in the hospital. Her mother and I brainstormed ways to recreate a similar tradition while Lina was hospitalized. With the help of the child life specialist, I provided Lina with a speaker phone for her room and meal delivery times with her family's dinner schedule to foster greater support for Lina while she was in the hospital or frequent stays for clinic visits.

Lina began playing out battle scenes in the sand with wrestling figurines. Lina shared that the soldiers were feeling tired and struggling to be so strong. I reflected the soldiers' hard fight and how exhausting it was constantly being strong. I also reflected that the soldiers were exhausted and battle weary. Lina continued this play over several sessions. After the ninth session, Lina began personalizing this message, stating she was tired of fighting. Lina then began to bury the soldiers after they lost their battles. She slowly began to add figures and animals to the sand and would bury them. She reflected they were lost and animals would search to find their family member. Around this time, Lina became too sick to visit the playroom and play therapy sessions were moved to her clinic or hospital room.

I shared Lina's theme of strength and battle with her parents and how she appeared to understand that she may not be strong enough to win her fight with cancer. Her mother was very tearful but felt that she did know, even though she tried hard to shield her from this knowledge. She shared she did not feel strong enough to start a conversation about her dying, but if she asked she would discuss it with her. I reflected her mother's distress and emotionally supported her. I asked her mother a few questions about what information she needed and about her fears about these conversations. I did not push the mother to take any specific action and instead focused on supporting and encouraging her.

Lina began to bury the figures in her bedsheets. She would state that the figures were gone and the family members would have to move on and forget about the buried figure. She was often sleeping during the daytime so play therapy was put on hold. Lina's primary nurse shared that Lina was playful at night and she was often unsure how to respond to her play as she felt she was "working hard" to make sense of her impending death. I shared some reflective listening skills and emotionally supported the nurse as she processed through her experiences. Lina rarely spoke of her impending death with her parents and often appeared to protect them from her emotions. One evening while her mother took a break, Lina played with her primary evening nurse. She played out a funeral scene for the buried toy. Her nurse sat with her as she role-played the family's eulogy for their loved figurine. The nurse reported to the child life specialist and me in the morning. She played this scene out with her two more times.

Shortly after this moment, Lina was suddenly more awake during the day. Her nurse would call me when she was awake and I would come down to see her in her room. On the first visit, Lina asked to make a music video. She shared how she wanted the video to go and together we planned out a way to make her vision come to life. She practiced with her nurses at night and two days later we recorded her video. Lina planned a variety of dance moves for herself and her backup dancers (nurses) as she sang along with one of her favorite songs. At this same time, she began to talk more freely with her mother about her impending death. Although she wanted to protect her, Lina's mother listened and shared her sadness with her daughter. They met with the hospital chaplain. She asked to plan her funeral and shared details of how she wanted the day to go. Lina died a week later.

Parent Consultation

While working with Lina, I also met with her mother every few days to check in with her and answer questions she had. I also shared general themes from Lina's sessions. Initially, the main focus of the parent consultations was emotional support for Lina's parents, as her mother and father were struggling with her changed behaviors and impending death. I worked closely with Lina's social worker and child life specialist to provide support for all family members. I also shared the importance of sharing information with other team members to ensure that Lina's mother was receiving the support she needed and helping the child life specialist know additional areas of support.

Over time, the focus of the parent consultations shifted to ways her parents could provide an emotionally safe environment so that Lina was free to discuss her thoughts and feelings around her death. I spent the majority of time listening and reflecting emotions. I rarely provided advice as Lina's mother was keenly aware of how to best support her daughter. It appeared she doubted herself and I provided her with reassurance as well as a person with whom she could share this difficult journey. Periodically, I shared some developmental tidbits, such as developmental understanding of death and common misunderstandings about death to help her mother comprehend her behaviors and understanding, and to normalize her experiences and her behaviors. In addition, the child life specialist provided Lina's mother with similar information and support as well as information for Lina's siblings.

Theoretical Understanding

The environment in which a child grows mediates how he or she develops his or her self-concept and self-worth (Axline, 1969). Children have a desire to feel prized, capable, and valued by important loved ones, especially parents and other primary caregivers. When a children's concept of self matches their experiences, they are in a state of congruence. On the other hand, when a child is criticized and judged, the child feels threatened and will deny or alter his or her concept of self in exchange for love and acceptance from others. To maintain the acceptance of others, children rely on others' evaluation and acceptance, believing they are worthy when they meet the expectations and demands of their caregiver, referred to as conditions of worth. Internal divisions between the child's experiences and child's concept of self, known as incongruence, continue and cause the child to feel vulnerable and anxious. Children express their incongruence in their behaviors and emotions (Ray & Landreth, 2015).

In the context of this theoretical discussion, Lina struggled with the issues common to children who are dying. She was lonely, missing her siblings, peers, and time with other family members. She missed traditions and rituals, such as mealtimes, that gave structure and meaning to her life. Meals also seemed to be a way that her mother shared her nurturing and how she received such nurturing. Her loneliness was exacerbated when she could no longer interact physically with the nursing staff as she had done earlier in her hospitalization. And her inability to share her thoughts and play regarding death with her mother and family additionally furthered her sense of isolation. She was frustrated from a lack of control over her body and her situation, which led to her intensity in reaction to frustrating experiences such as not being able to sleep. Advice, reassurance, and pain relief were psychologically inadequate to meet Lina's emotional needs as she faced her death. In CCPT, Lina could experience an environment in which she was in control. The play sessions allowed Lina to experience control so that she would have less of a need to exert control that interfered with her medical condition (VanFleet et al., 2010). In relationship with the play therapist, Lina could have someone be with her who had no negative reaction to her play of missing her family, thinking about her death, and being frustrated with her situation. The play therapist provided her with her complete acceptance and understanding of her anger, sadness, and confusion. She made no attempt to fix things or "make Lina feel better. By understanding and accepting that she knew what she needed to express and that all of her feelings and thoughts were valid, Lina was able to experience that she was acceptable in all of these feelings. She could further experience strength in her abilities to confront what was ahead of her, the release of the actualizing tendency. Through her experiences with the play therapist and with her night nurse, Lina was also able to practice how she might express her reaction to death with her closest caretaker, her mother. It was through her relationships with her play therapist and nurse that she developed the capacity to engage her mother in what she knew intrinsically would be difficult for both of them. Ironically, it was an 7-year-old girl who helped her mother come to accept the death of her daughter.

The play therapist's work with Lina's parents and nurse were also invaluable components of the CCPT process. In CCPT, the therapist came to understand what was most important to Lina and could share these understandings with the parents. Through consultation, the therapist helped the parents figure out ways to respond to Lina in the ways she most needed and not in the ways they believed she needed. It was also through the therapist's acceptance and support of Lina's mother that she was able to provide more readily for Lina. As the play therapist accepted the mother's feelings and hesitancies, restraining from giving advice and guidance, Lina's mother felt understood and not judged; hence, she could respond more empathically to Lina on her terms. The play therapist's work with the nurse was one of the unique features of CCPT in action. The skills of genuineness, unconditional positive regard, and empathic understanding are teachable skills to any layperson. The play therapist taught these skills to the nurse so that the nurse could serve as a therapeutic agent for Lina. In the end, Lina was engaged in multiple relationships in which she felt understood, and her way of dealing with her death was affirmed and valued.

Therapist's Self-Reflection

Both as a CCLS and play therapist, I learned substantially from my experiences in working with Lina and other children who are terminally ill. Several themes come to mind when reflecting back on this specific experience. First, patience is very important when therapeutically working with children who are terminally ill. My anxiety and desire to help her work by rushing her processing and gaining understanding of her illness was unhelpful and not needed. Early in my relationship with Lina, I learned she had incredible inner strength and was able to work toward healing at her pace. She would appease me in moments when I interrupted her process by giving me a sly look and then continuing on her journey. These moments reminded me that I was a fellow traveler and did not have the road map to where she needed to go. I did not need to prove myself or try harder. Instead I needed to slow down so I could be fully present to follow Lina to fully understand her. Lina had a keen way of reminding me that I did not know what it was like to die, and therefore I could not prescribe what she needed. My past experiences could guide me on the common needs of dying children but could prevent me from seeing Lina's unique and immediate needs. Lina's needs included acceptance, patience, understanding, freedom, and empathy. Therefore, I have learned that I need to follow the child and family and meet them with expectancy. Landreth (2012) explored the importance of meeting a child with eagerness and anticipation. In my relationship with children, I agree that is it important to approach my interactions with patience, gentleness, and anticipation as the child shares their experiences, feelings, and understanding about themselves and their world.

Through Lina's play, I learned how perceptive she was, especially at a time when many medical staff and family members tried to protect her. Lina was profoundly aware of her change in prognosis even though no one had verbally told her she was dying. I believe she observed her environment and the people around her. She saw changes in their affect as well as less urgency and intensity from the medical staff to treat her illness. Lina's play was full of insight into her knowledge about her prognosis. Lina's sand play indicated she knew she was losing her life to cancer. She attempted to understand what death was like as she buried her figurines and animals in the sand, as well as what it would be like for her family, especially her siblings. I got the sense she knew how hard it would be for her siblings to lose her as she played out animals searching for the figurines. Her attempt to console her emotional anxiety for her family was seen in her funeral scenes. Lina had a strong desire to support her family in their grief process but knew they were not ready to do so. Instead she processed it in her play. She wanted her family to be OK with her death and know it was OK to move on. Her nightshift nurse stated her eulogy was emotionally moving as she talked to her family members and shared her hopes and dreams for them. She then appeared to gain a sense of control over her impending death and appeared more comfortable and content in her knowledge that she was dying. She created a plan for ways to help her family memorialize her and remember her existence. She initiated interactions that set her plan in motion. She was gentle in her attempts to talk with her parents about her death. She asked to speak with the hospital chaplain and shared her wants for her funeral. And she created a music video to leave her loved ones with a lasting memory of her living doing something she loved, instead of her dying of cancer. I believe Lina died when she knew her family was OK with her death and when she was at peace with her prognosis.

Lina gave many subtle clues that she knew she was dying. I have learned simple statements such as "I'm tired" or comments about time may be signs the child is seeking opportunities to talk or non-verbally process about death. Children may make statements at odd times or when it is least expected. And a child may use humor, such as saying "I'm not dead yet" after waking up from a nap, to ease emotional tensions about death and conversing with their loved ones. It is important for therapists and psychosocial team members to look out for these subtle, vague statements or behaviors. They are not always easy to identify, but I have found that children will repeat the process until someone is willing to listen and understand their thoughts and feelings. I have also learned that many people misunderstand the subtle cues and the child's attempt to connect and process their understanding of their pending death. For Lina, her comments about being tired were larger than needing a nap or medication. One indication of her desire to share her emotions was her escalating anger toward others when they encouraged her to take a nap or attempted to give her medication to sleep. I have seen and heard stories of other children express similar feelings or withdraw after attempting to connect and process their experiences. Other children have made comments about not being here for their next birthday or never going back to school. Other examples from clinicians include a child who collected watches of the medical staff and the child commented, "I don't have enough time." I believe each of these statements were the child's attempt to see if their loved one or support system were ready to hear and understand their experiences.

I have also found that both parents and children function in a dance-like sequence as they attempt to protect each other and function under a state of mutual pretense. Bluebond-Langner (1978) studied dying children and their awareness and communication patterns at end of life. She defines mutual pretense as an interaction approach between dying children, their families, and those who care for them. The main goal of mutual pretense is to maintain societal roles and the relationship at a very emotionally challenging time. Under mutual pretense, children and adults attempt to protect each other by following typical societal patterns and to keep the relationship from breaking down. Lina's mother worried that disclosing her terminal prognosis would speed up her death because she felt she would quit fighting her cancer. She attempted to protect her by avoiding conversations related to her prognosis. Instead she encouraged her to continue to fight this disease and she consented to treatment and procedures that would most likely not extend her life. Lina also protected her mother and behaved in ways that protected her from difficult emotions and conversations. She would initiate arguments when she realized she was struggling to cope with her questions, or she would suddenly become fatigued and state that she needed to rest because she played so hard. In addition, Bluebond-Langner discussed providing children with a relationship in which they can safely share their thoughts and feelings with a person who can handle discussing matters of illness and death, as well as allowing them to maintain mutual pretense when needed. In this relationship, the safe person, such as a therapist, can genuinely accept and openly understand. For Lina, her night nurse, child life specialist, and play therapist provided the safe environment where she could play out and share. These relationships allowed her to process through her difficult emotions and experiences and fostered greater inner strength to slowly approach the subject with her parents.

During their illness, children need opportunities to play, especially at end of life. They may not be able to be totally independent—they may need some help. But they should always be in the lead. Never do for a child what he or she can do or tell you to do for them (Landreth, 2012). You may need to hold up a pad of paper or concoct a paint brush glove so a child can still paint. You may need to play for some children as they direct you because their bodies will not allow them to move as freely as they once could. Adaptations may be needed. I also never know what the child may need. It was important that I remain continually open to the experience that a child, Lina in this case, may ask for or lead with. Lina had a strong desire to make a movie about zombies. I believe this was related to her treatment and how she felt she was losing a battle. She would play for brief amounts of time and then comment that her life was in danger because of the sun-opening windows and pretending to die. She also played out death and funeral scenes to make sense of what was to come. In this context, Landreth (2012) indicated that the relationship between a dying child and a person willing to follow as the child leads allows the child to guide the relationship in ways the child needs and are important to the child, not what the therapist thinks is important. Time with a therapist may offer a child an 'oasis' where the child is free to direct and control their environment, something very hard to do in a hospital or medical space. This freedom contradicts the reality of the medical environment where the child is directed and controlled by others and his or her disease.

My work with Lina was both personally rewarding and emotionally challenging. Lina's fight to live and delight in her daily interactions was inspiring. I enjoyed our time together and looked forward to our interactions. Lina had a joy for life that was infectious. In the difficult moments she would treasure the smallest accomplishment or task. I remember at the end of a particularly emotional session, she looked down at her work and smiled. Her smile resonated with pride and ease for what she had achieved. She appeared lighter, as if her inner strength shined through. Lina's action was subtle and I could have easily missed her smile. I was honored to witness and journey with her at a very emotionally sensitive time. I often smile as I think of her or when a task reminds me of her.

On the other hand, I experienced an array of painful emotions—in particular, sadness. The knowledge of Lina's failing prognosis weighed heavily on my heart. I found it helpful to share my sadness with peers. Without sharing my feelings and experiences, I felt alone and watched it impact my non-professional relationships. Confidentiality is hard to maintain when loved ones are asking what is wrong and know your day was challenging. Speaking with my peers allowed me to leave the office and be prepared to engage with loved ones in a more present and authentic way (and maintain confidentiality). Watching Lina struggle to live made me think a lot about my own life and if I cherished the people and activities in which I am involved. I felt guilty that I rushed through life without appreciating each moment. Over time, I have learned that life is not fair and can end quickly. Just like the children I worked with, I must value each moment I have, treasure important people in my life, and take time to let them know how important they are to me.

I also experienced anxiety and struggled to know if I was enough for Lina. I feared she needed more than I could provide her. Although I thoroughly enjoyed my interactions with Lina, our time together was challenging. I trusted Lina to lead me and be in control of her play. But I did not always trust in myself. I struggled to be still and believe in my ability to provide her with the acceptance and understanding she deserved. I remember seeking supervision and begging an expert to come see Lina. He kindly stated that I was exactly what Lina needed. I did not trust him and felt disappointed that Lina was stuck with me. I felt compelled to 'do' something more and sought consultation from peers. They suggested activities I could provide to help her and I would think "she's already doing that on her own." I learned my need for more was my own internal struggle and discomfort with sitting still and watching someone die. Like Lina, I wanted her to live. I was deeply saddened and was grieving for our joint loss. I have learned grief is hard and everyone needs the opportunity to grieve. I found it helpful to create feeling and grief rituals to help find closure to our relationship and memorialize the children I worked with.

Death and talking about death is very uncomfortable for many people, especially pediatric medical personnel. Some physicians, nurses, and care providers become uncomfortable when trying to comfort children and their families in end of life care. I believe one's personal experiences, beliefs about death, and lack of education often make these conversations and experiences awkward for adults. For instance, I have seen doctors focus solely on life-saving measures and ignore the child's and family's end of life wishes. One doctor was so uncomfortable with the idea of not continuing treatment that the doctor stopped or diverted conversation every time the parents or child brought up palliative care options. And I have observed nurses nervous when death and end of life discussions or play begins. They often shared they were unsure what to say or how to function during these experiences, so they went into task-oriented roles to lessen their anxiety. Many medical personnel have not received training in grief and loss, and therefore function from their own experiences. In these two experiences, I found it important to listen to the team members and help them process their own grief in losing the patient. And I believe we can help medical staff find alternative ways of being in these uncomfortable situations. Our role as social and client advocates can help a family get their unique needs met at a difficult time. But we must remember to go into these conversations with an open heart and mind so we can hear all sides and perspectives. Several times I found myself seen as the 'enemy' in discussions because the medical staff member did not feel heard and understood.

Families who have children who die from chronic illness may struggle after their child dies. The hospital and medical staff become a pseudo family with whom they grew close. The sudden end to the relationship was very hard for many families I have worked with. One family shared that they still have a phone message on their answering machine from their child's primary physician from two years ago. They do not want to erase it, because it helps them remember their child and all the staff they grew close to. I believe follow-up messages are helpful for families as they grieve. Simple messages sharing a memory or 'gift' their children imparted on the medical team helps families feel their child was important to the staff and that their legacy lives on.

I found that highs and lows are common when working with this population. I experienced emotions on both extremes. Some days I felt content, peaceful, joyous, inspired, happy, proud, and honored to work with the children and families. These emotions made it easier to come back to the playroom and interact with the children. On the other hand, some days were emotionally hard. I experienced deep sadness, anger, frustration, sorrow, and exhaustion. Because I operate from a CCPT perspective, which means fully entering the child's world and seeing the world as the child sees it, the level of presence and empathy can be challenging and require significant personal resources. On bad days, I struggled to be fully present and genuine in session. I had difficulty understanding the child, as I was unaware of my own feelings. When I experienced a bad session or an overall crummy day, I recognized the need for self-care rituals to help me be more present. Unfortunately, I did not always make the time to participate in my own self-care, and instead felt obliged to attend a meeting or attempted to respond to another need. In a hospital setting, there will always be another need, so I had to learn how to care for myself. My typical and brief self-care strategies are to walk outside or grab ice cream with a colleague to help me renew my inner strength. After a child died, I participated in a grief ritual to honor that child. Grief rituals vary by person and are personal. For me, grief rituals offered quiet time to think about the child and our relationship. I enjoyed creating something that reminded me of the child. A peer planted a seed and another peer collected beads that represented the child's spirit. Overall, I found that when my bad days outweighed my good days, I was lacking in self-care and needed to take better care of myself (and a mental health day off). I found it easy to get stuck in the mundane and methodically work, but this population and environment required my full attention and health.

Over the years, I have learned several self-care habits that helped me stay present and mentally healthy. Just like therapy, self-care habits need to fit the individual, as prescribed habits tend to be unsuccessful. For me, sleeping, eating healthily, and exercise are essential for my health. Finding outside activities that refuel me are important to balancing work–home life. I enjoy time with friends and cooking, whereas a colleague enjoyed time at church and reading. No matter the preference for individual therapists, the critical piece is finding personal activities that energize and nurture the therapist. In addition, I find therapy very helpful in managing the 'burdens' of the job. Working with dying children is heavy work. Time with my therapist helped me emotionally heal from all I saw and experienced. I found that it took effort to stay healthy and I had to be mindful of what I needed in order to be fully present and therapeutic in my next relationships.

CONCLUSION

Children who face chronic and terminal illness or medical conditions require mental health support that recognizes their needs for self-direction, control, and understanding. Anxiety, depression, confusion, and pain are common experiences for terminally ill children, and often result in behaviors that can be problematic such as overt attempts at control, relationship conflict, and medical non-compliance. Caretakers are often influenced by their own responses to extreme stress and loss, and therefore have difficulty understanding their children's feelings and motivations. Problem behaviors and relational disruptions can leave a child who is dying feeling even more lonely and isolated. Yet, as all children, those who are dying have the biological drive to know what they need and how to work toward getting those needs met. In an environment where a child feels fully understood and accepted, this actualizing tendency is released and children develop self-knowledge and skills to move them toward inner peace (theoretically conceptualized as congruence) and relational accord. CCPT is a mental health intervention that provides the child a developmentally appropriate language and the relationship to facilitate a child's movement toward self-enhancement. In CCPT, a child who is dying can express fears and concerns that are most present, allowing the child to work through barriers to acceptance of a present and future that are unknown. Therapists who provide CCPT to children who are terminally ill operate in an environment of intense emotions for all people involved. When operating from a CCPT perspective, therapists need to be well-trained in play therapy, person-centered philosophy, medical settings, medical teams, terminal conditions, and human reactions to grief and loss. Perhaps most importantly, the therapist needs to engage in self-care strategies that personally nurture and energize in order to provide the level of presence and therapy needed for each child and family. In relationship with a person who can offer genuine empathy and acceptance, children who confront loss and death can engage in their multifarious abilities to continue becoming more of what they want to be.

REFERENCES

Aasgaard, T. (2006). Children expressing themselves. In A. Goldman, R. Hain & S. Liben (Eds.), *Oxford textbook of palliative care for children* (pp. 119–127). New York: Oxford University Press.

Aldridge, J., & Sourkes, B. M. (2012). Psychological impact of life-limiting conditions on children. In A. Goldman, R. Hain & S. Liben (Eds.), *Oxford textbook of palliative care for children* (2nd ed., pp. 78–89). New York: Oxford University Press.

Axline, V. M. (1969). *Play therapy.* New York: Ballantine Books.

Best, M., Streisand, R., Catania, L., & Kazak, A. E. (2001). Parental distress during pediatric leukemia and posttraumatic stress symptoms (PTSS) after treatment ends. *Journal of Pediatric Psychology, 26(5),* 299–307.

Bluebond-Langner, M. (1978). *The private worlds of dying children.* Princeton, NJ: Princeton University Press.

Bonoti, F., Leondari, A., & Mastora, A. (2013). Exploring children's understanding of death: Through drawings and the Death Concept Questionnaire. *Death Studies, 37,* 47–60.

Bozarth, J. (1998). *Person-centered therapy: A revolutionary paradigm.* Ross-on-Wye, UK: PCCS Books.

Bratton, S. (2013) Head start early mental health intervention: Effects of child-centered play therapy on disruptive behaviors. *International Journal of Play Therapy, 22(1),* 28–42.

Bratton, S. C., Ray, D. C., Rhine, T., & Jones, L. D. (2005). The efficacy of play therapy with children: A meta-analytic review of treatment outcomes. *Professional Psychology: Research and Practice, 36(4),* 376–390.

Breemen, C. V. (2009). Using play therapy in pediatric palliative care: Listening to the story and caring for the body. *International Journal of Palliative Nursing, 15(10),* 510–514.

Doka, K. (1995). *Children mourning, mourning children.* Washington, DC: Hospice Foundation of America.

Elkind, D. (2007). *The power of play: Learning what comes naturally.* Philadelphia, PA: Da Capo Press.

Feudtner, C., Kang, T. I., Hexem, K. R., Friedrichsdorf, S. J., Oseng, K., Siden, H., . . . Wolfe, J. (2011). Pediatric palliative care patients: A prospective multicentre cohort study. *Pediatrics, 127,* 1094–1101.

Foreman, T., Willis, L., Goodenough, B. (2005). Hospital-based support groups for parents of seriously unwell children: An example from pediatric oncology in Australia. *Social Work with Groups, 28(2),* 3–21.

Friebert, S., & Williams, C. (2015). *NHPCO facts and figures: Pediatric palliative and hospice care of America.* Retrieved from National Hospice and Palliative Care Organization website: www.nhpco.org/sites/default/files/public/quality/Pediatic_Facts-Figures.pdf

Ginsburg, K. R. (2007). The importance of play in promoting healthy child development and maintaining strong parent-child bonds. *Pediatrics, 119,* 182–191. https://doi.org/10.1542/peds.2006-2697

Glazer, H. R., & Landreth, G. L. (1993). When a child is dying. *The Education Digest, 59(1),* 64–67.

Haugh, S. (2012). A person-centred approach to loss and bereavement. In J. Tolan and P. Wilkins (Eds.), *Client issues in counselling and psychotherapy* (pp. 15–29). London: Sage.

Heron, M. (2016). *Deaths: Leading causes for 2014*. National Vital Statistics Reports, vol. 65 no 5. National Center for Health Statistics, Hyattsville, MD.

Houtzager, B. A., Oort, F. J., Hoekstra-Weebers, H. M., Caron, H. N., Grootenhuis, M. A., & Last, B. F. (2004). Coping and family functioning predict longitutudinal psychological adaptation of siblings of childhood cancer patients. *Journal of Pediatric Psychology*, 29(8), 591–605.

Hynson, J. L., Aroni, R., Bauld, C., & Sawyer, S. M. (2006). Research with bereaved parents: a question of how not why. *Palliative Medicine*, 20(8), 805–811.

Hynson, J.L. (2012). The child's journey: Transitions from health to ill-health. In A. Goldman, R. Hain & S. Liben (Eds.), *Oxford textbook of palliative care for children* (2nd ed., pp. 14–27). New York: Oxford University Press.

Lambert, S.F., LeBlanc, M., Mullen, J., Ray, D., Baggerly, J., White, J., & Kaplan, D. (2005). Learning more about those who play in session: The national play therapy in counseling practice project (phase I). *Journal of Counseling & Development*, 85, 42–46.

Landreth, G. L. (2012). *Play therapy: The art of the relationship* (3rd ed.). New York: Routledge.

Manne, S., Miller, D., Meyers, P., Wollner, N., Steinherz, P., & Redd, W. H. (1996). Depressive symptoms among parents of newly diagnosed children with cancer: A 6-month follow-up study. *Children's Health Care*, 25(3), 191–209.

McGrath, P. (2001). Identifying support issues of parents of children with leukemia. *Cancer Practice*, 9(4), 198–205.

Niswander, L., Cromwell, P., Chirico, J., Gupton, A., & Korones, D. (2014). End-of-life care for children enrolled in a community-based pediatric palliative care program. *Journal of Palliative Medicine*, 17, 589–591.

Orloff, S.F., & Jones, B. (2011). Psychosocial needs of the child and family. In B.S. Carter, M. Levetown & S.E. Friebert (Eds.), *Palliative care for infants, children, and adolescents: A practical handbook* (2nd ed., pp. 202–226). Baltimore, MD: Johns Hopkins University Press.

Pearson, L.J. (2005). The child who is dying. In J.A. Rollins, R. Bolig & C.C. Mahan (Eds.), *Meeting children's psychosocial needs: Across the health care continuum* (pp. 221–275). Austin, TX: Pro-Ed.

Pearson, L.J. (2009). Child life interventions in critical care and at end of life. In R.H. Thompson (Ed.), *The handbook of child life: A guide for pediatric psychosocial care* (pp. 220–237). Springfield, IL: Charles C. Thomas.

Ray, D.C. (2011). *Advanced play therapy: Essential conditions, knowledge, and skills for child practice*. New York: Routledge.

Ray, D.C., & Landreth, G.L. (2015). Child-centered play therapy. In D.A. Crenshaw & A.L. Stewart (Eds.), *Play therapy: A comprehensive guide to theory and practice* (pp. 3–16). New York: Guilford Press.

Robinson, K. E., Gerhardt, C. A., Vanatta, K., & Noll, R. B. (2006). Parent and family factors associated with child adjustment to pediatric cancer. *Journal of Pediatric Psychology*, 32(4), 400–410.

Rogers, C.R. (1951). *Client centered therapy*. Boston: Houghton Mifflin.

Rogers, C.R. (1992). The necessary and sufficient conditions of therapeutic personality change. *Journal of Consulting Psychology*, 60(6), 827–832.

Rosengren, K., Gutierrez, I., & Schein, S. (2014). Children's understanding of death: Toward a contextualized and integrated account IV: Cognitive dimensions of death in context. *Monographs of the Society for Research in Child Development*, 79, 62–82.

Sourkes, B.M. (2006). Psychological impact of life-limiting condition on the child. In A. Goldman, R. Hain & S. Liben (Eds.), *Oxford textbook of palliative care for children* (pp. 95–107). New York: Oxford University Press.

Streisand, R., Kazak, A.E., & Tercyak, K.P. (2003). Pediatic specific parenting stress and family functioning in parents of children treated for cancer. *Children's Health Care*, 32(4), 245–256.

Sweeney, D.S., & Skurja, C. (2001). Filial therapy as a cross-cultural family intervention. *Asian Journal of Counseling, 8*(2), 175–208.

VanFleet, R., Sywulak, A.E., & Sniscak, C.C. (2010). *Child-centered play therapy*. New York: Guilford Press.

Weaver, M.S., Heinze, K.E., Bell, C.J., Wiener, L., Garee, A.M., Kelly, K.P., . . . Hinds, P.S. (2016). Establishing psychosocial palliative care standards for children and adolescents with cancer and their families: An integrative review. *Palliative Medicine, 30*(3), 212–223. https://doi.org/10.1177/0269216315583446

Wilkins, P. (2010). *Person-centred therapy: 100 key points*. East Sussex, UK: Routledge.

Wilson, K., & Ryan, V. (2005). *Play therapy: A non-directive approach for children and adolescents* (2nd ed.). Burlington, MA: Bailliére Tindall.

Wolfelt, A.D. (1996). *Healing the bereaved child: Grief gardening, growth through grief and other touchstones for caregivers*. Fort Collins, CO: Companion Press.

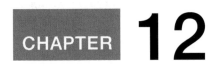

CHAPTER 12

It's All About the Living

Play-Based Experiences With Children Facing End of Life

Morgan Livingstone

> The sky's awake, so I'm awake, so we have to play.
> —Princess Anna, *Frozen* (Walt Disney Pictures, 2013)

Any child with a serious, complex, or life-threatening condition has tremendous needs during their care, from diagnosis through to palliative support. Life-prolonging treatments, medications, procedures, and skilled pain management, along with adaptive equipment to manage day-to-day tasks and facilitate movement, are important aspects of early palliative care. These medical and physical interventions focus on the *life* of that child, keeping them alive, but are not necessarily focused on the *child* that is doing the living. Often providing time and opportunity to play is minimized when parents and the medical team are so focused on managing the clinical symptoms of a child's illness and the impact of those symptoms, including pain, discomfort, and loss of abilities, on the child. Although it is often undervalued and overlooked, this is the time when play becomes the essential modality through which to enhance the child's ability to seek pleasure during difficult times, as well as process, problem solve, and seek understanding about what is happening to them and their body. Play can offer a release from pain, aid a child in communicating their needs, wants, and desires about the life they are living, and give them the ability to transport themselves in creative and imaginative ways.

This chapter will highlight the importance of play as a part of complete care for children of all ages facing end of life through diverse patient case studies that share the experiences of a community-based child life specialist. Using play adapted to the interests and abilities of the child or youth, this child life specialist shares play experiences that explore real-life struggles and uncover the range of social and emotional needs of the *living* child facing death. These playful approaches to serious matters can be adapted by other creative professionals working with children facing a life-limiting illness and end of life.

THE CRITICAL ROLE OF PLAY

Play is an essential part of life for a child. Play is such an important aspect in a child's healthy development that it has been recognized as a basic human right by the United Nations in Article 31 of the Convention on the Rights of the Child (1989). Even in the absence of toys, children are innately able to find a way to play by themselves, with others, and with their environment. It is through play that children at a very early age engage and interact in the world around them. Play allows children to create and explore a world they can master, conquering their fears while practicing adult roles, sometimes in conjunction with other children or adult caregivers (Hurwitz, 2002). As they master their world, play helps children develop new competencies that lead to enhanced confidence and the resiliency they will need to face future challenges (Pellegrini & Smith, 1998).

When a child is diagnosed with a life-threatening illness, they face many challenges and frightening experiences that can and often do overwhelm the child, parents, and those close to the family (Boucher, Downing, & Shemilt, 2014). Yet despite the devastating consequences of terminal illness, children have the unique and ever-evolving needs, desires, and rights of any other child (Amery, 2009). They *need* play.

The World Health Organization (WHO) defines palliative care as (1998):

an approach that improves the quality of life of patients and their families facing the problem associated with life-threatening illness, through the prevention and relief of suffering by means of early identification and impeccable assessment and treatment of pain and other problems, physical, psychosocial and spiritual.

- Palliative care for children is the active total care of the child's body, mind and spirit, and involves giving support to the family.
- It begins when illness is diagnosed, and continues regardless of whether a child receives treatment directed at the disease.
- Health providers must evaluate and alleviate a child's physical, psychological, and social distress.
- Effective palliative care requires a broad multidisciplinary approach that includes the family and makes use of available community resources; it can be successfully implemented even if resources are limited.
- It can be provided in tertiary care facilities, in community health centers and even in children's homes.

Palliative care as an established field of practice in medicine has grown and developed greatly over the past two decades (Feudtner, Friebert, & Jewell, 2013). Important guidelines and recommendation statements prepared by the American Academy of Pediatrics (AAP) focus on the essential aspects of the medical care provided to children and families facing end of life, and outlines the roles of the greater multidisciplinary team that is working collaboratively to provide this care. Noticeably absent in these 12 guidelines and recommendations and in the preceding WHO definition are any mentions that the child be provided with play. These important foundational documents are missing one of the most essential parts of a child's complete care: play.

There have been some developments within the medical community and the AAP that are beginning to highlight the importance of play in the general healthy development of children. The AAP clinical report on *The Importance of Play in Promoting Healthy Child Development and Maintaining Strong Parent–Child Bonds* (Ginsburg, 2007) acknowledges the benefits of play, discusses the present barriers children face in accessing adequate time for play in today's modern society, and offers advice for pediatricians that promotes strategies that will support children to be resilient and to reduce excessive stressors in their lives. This report states that because pediatricians have a unique and important role in promoting the physical, emotional, and social well-being of children, they have a natural role to serve as caring, objective child professionals in their work with parents and caregivers. These important frontline members of the medical community are beginning to understand what kids already know: play is essential to a child's life.

Seeing the lack of complete care guidelines for the rights of life-limited children, the International Children's Palliative Care Network (ICPCN) created a charter of rights for children facing life-threatening or life-limiting illnesses. Within this charter, it is clearly stated that wherever possible, life-limited children be provided with opportunities to play, access leisure opportunities, interact with siblings and friends, and participate in normal childhood activities (ICPCN, 2008). This charter still lacks the instructions for types of play—nothing specific, and no steps or guidelines for what play is recommended.

Including and supporting the parents, siblings, and extended family in play opportunities can benefit all parties, and most importantly benefits the dying child. Dying can create distance between the child and their family. This distance often happens when a child tries to protect their parents from upset by keeping their 'BIG' feelings to themselves, and they may open up about their thoughts and feelings about the dying process with only a few special people. In families that are closely involved in the care, who invite play with their child, and who participate in an open and honest approach to the dying process, this natural distancing can be less marked and the child remains close to their parents (Adams & Deveau, 1984).

At any particular moment, the medical team's goal is to cure and treat, while the child's goal is self-pleasure (Gray, 1989). Ensuring that the right balance and pacing of medical attention, procedures, and assessments with periods of play doesn't need to be a challenge, and it can be a goal for the child, family, and medical team to seek each day. And this should be done together.

CHILD LIFE PLAY PRACTICES: CHILDREN AND FAMILIES I HAVE HAD THE PRIVILEGE OF PLAYING WITH

Death is very much a part of life, but that fact doesn't make it any easier. I have been working with dying children since my initial Child Life internship in an infectious disease ward with sickle cell and hemophiliac teen patients who were victims of tainted blood transfusions. Before treatments could manage HIV/AIDS as a lifelong illness, patients were stuck in isolation in the infectious disease ward, with little contact with the outside world. They were waiting around to die. Their only freedom from illness and the disease was their time with family, friends, and their child life specialist. This continues to be a sad reality for many children and youth in developing countries. As a child life specialist new to the profession, I realized that these patients needed to focus on a whole lot of living, not the dying part. After all, they weren't dead yet! Right?

During my time in the infectious disease ward, one HIV-positive teen felt trapped in the ward, cut off from the normal experiences he needed and wanted as a young man. In our time together, naturally our play was adapted for him as a teen, and we played many video games and many rounds of high-stakes hospital poker, created our own board games and hosted tournaments with the medical staff. Through our time together, he always listened to music. I noticed that we listened to the same tracks over and over. When I asked about this, it turned out it wasn't that they were his favorite tracks, but that he had no access to any new music. After a little discussion about music preferences, I set out to solve this problem. A local DJ happily put together a variety of live music for this patient. Our music was never dull again no matter what we were playing. Something so small and simple sure can make a difference in the *life* of this teen.

And so began my journey to change the way we approach end of life child life supports, and how we play with patients and their families facing end of life. After that position, I moved into pediatric oncology and general oncology, where I was working with children with cancer and children whose parents/grandparents were facing a palliative cancer diagnosis. This is where I really learned that palliative care is about long-term complete care for ongoing life, while living with and managing symptoms before death. Sometimes the actual death takes years after the palliative diagnosis.

Play with dying children has many important purposes. Sometimes play takes place as a means to teach about the medical experience and cope during important medical procedures designed to extend the life of the child or manage the physical symptoms associated with the body's response to metastatic or progressive disease. Other times, there is no purpose to the play at all but to have fun, laugh, and explore. It may have nothing to do with the illness, the physical or psychological symptoms of dying. It is just play for play's sake. Sometimes play functions to help children explore concepts around death and dying. It allows them to learn what it is, figure out what it means to them, and what they want *before* they die and what they want *when* they die. Here I will share actual play experiences I had the honor of participating in with children of all ages who were facing life-limiting illnesses.

Gina: 2 to 4 Years

Gina, a lovely child with metastatic retinoblastoma (eye cancer) and I developed a close relationship over a period of years after her initial cancer treatment was incomplete and unsuccessful and her tumor recurred in her eye socket at the age of 2 years. Gina's family had come to Canada for specialized medical treatment from central Africa. Our work together started with medical play and preparation for immediate surgery to remove the large tumor, and preparation for 25 radiation treatments. This was a big order for a young child with no previous contact with a child life specialist, and little contact with people outside of her home community. I knew it was important that I connect with her immediately and use play as a form of communication, in addition to the phrases I had taught myself in her language. I was the first person Mom and Gina met when they arrived at the airport. I had a soft stuffed animal as a welcoming toy and transitional item into a new and strange place. Play was essential even when we met for the first time.

We played with a large cloth doll and assorted medical materials to familiarize Gina with what she would see at the hospital in preparation for her surgery. Within our playtime we also practiced placing an IV on the doll and used the mask repeatedly in preparation for sedation in the operating room. Gina enjoyed the play, methodically exploring and manipulating all the materials, following the steps I would demonstrate for the different aspects of her upcoming surgery. All the while, her mother was assisting by quietly translating English into the family's language to ensure understanding. This closeness during these play sessions also offered Gina's mother a chance to see how I explained procedures and medical experiences using play and in child-friendly language, which helped her to continue supporting this learning and exploration of what will happen with each procedure.

Simplifying information and ideas using play for very young children means being creative, thoughtful, and aware of a child's development. With Gina, it was important to offer layered learning and play opportunities, and slowly build on each topic or area of learning. Asking a 2- or 3-year-old about how they are feeling can be a challenge if they aren't aware of what feelings actually are, and are not sure how to label feelings, so I started with simple stories and materials about feelings. These included the book *My Many Colored Day* by Dr. Seuss (1996), accompanied by toy animals featured in the book and feelings faces to demonstrate different feelings using movement and faces. We practiced moving our bodies in ways that showed how we were feeling. Sometimes skipping and dancing was used when demonstrating happy or excited feelings and slow, low movements showed our sad and scared feelings. Anger popped from our bodies in bursts and BIG stomps on the floor. All these important feelings were safely being shared in a playful, fun, and safe way as we played together.

Similarly, when introducing play and preparation for 25 radiation treatments, I knew I had to be creative while still acknowledging that this was a very young child, so I used familiar and simple concepts with a little imagination to prepare her for radiation. Using the *Very Hungry Caterpillar* book by Eric Carle and a homemade felt board story set, we explored the life cycle of the caterpillar to butterfly. The cocoon stage helped me to creatively but playfully illustrate and explain what it means to stay very still, and not move at all. This would be essential to Gina completing the necessary CT scans and her 25 radiation treatments without sedation and the nausea and vomiting associated with that sedation medication. After repeatedly playing and practicing lying still like a caterpillar in a cocoon, Gina and I explored the special hard molded mask designed to keep her head still during these radiation treatments. The mask, to be fastened to the table with a top section that would clamp down around her little head, would ensure Gina could not move her head at all. These radiation masks can be a challenge even for an adult patient, so we had to rethink the mask's job as a part of the cocoon, essential to helping Gina stay still so that she could emerge from her 'cocoon' as a 'butterfly' after radiation was completed. Placing a fuzzy butterfly sticker in the nose of the mask acted as the 'special button' Gina needed to press for the magical transformation into a butterfly. This playful approach to something so challenging changed everything, and Gina would hop up on the table, touch her nose to the sticker and lie still like a caterpillar in a cocoon. Mom gave encouraging messages over the intercom from the radiation technician's control room. Emerging from a radiation treatment was followed with a set of paper wings attached to the table by the radiation technicians, and a pair of costume wings I would bring to each session. Gina, her mother and I would fly and 'flutter' down the hallway after radiation. This was fun!

When Gina's father and three sisters were finally able to make the journey overseas to join her and her mother, our play sessions expanded and extended to include them as much as possible. It was important to include Gina's siblings and model how to play with Gina throughout active treatment and into the more serious palliative stage of her illness when she began to lose some ability and mobility, and was confined to a bed or wheelchair. Using open-ended play materials and toys including puppets, dolls, and stuffed animals promoted creative storytelling between siblings and encouraged interaction. These animals and puppets often received medical attention, allowing Gina and her sisters to explore concepts and experiences that were now a part of Gina's life.

During the palliative stage of Gina's illness when she was 4, there were discussions with the medical team about whether they would return home to central Africa or remain here, because travel would only be possible while Gina was able to tolerate it without a great deal of medical attention and support. Remaining in Canada was determined to be the best plan for her care needs through the palliative care. My work with Gina focused on remembering the people and places back home that Gina missed and activities she loved and would now no longer have the chance to do again. Her love of swimming in a lake near her home became a part of our sensory play. Water play was adapted to fit in a basin on her lap while sitting in her wheelchair; we would dip our hands in the water, diving our fingers to the bottom and splashing with glee. Using small toy boats we imagined floating and fishing on that lake, together, and with her family and friends. Spending time in nature, on neighborhood walks in the community with her family, was a part of each day. It was important for the family to know that it would not only be nice to take Gina outdoors in her wheelchair each day to feel the warm sun on her skin, but also would promote more time together as a family in the community. Talking aloud about adventures and telling stories was an important way to transport Gina out of her wheelchair and she could travel anywhere in her imagination. This practice of storytelling aloud and playing out adventures became the most appropriate means to discuss her beliefs about end of life. We read picture books about death and dying, including *Lifetimes* by Mellonie and Ingpen (1983) and *The Fall of Freddie the Leaf* by Buscaglia (1982). These books facilitated questions Gina had about what would happen to her body after her death. To help her understand how the body stops functioning when a person dies, we used a large felt board body, with bones and organs we could stick on with Velcro. We discussed in simple words what each organ does, and what it stops doing when a person dies. The job of the lungs is to breathe air. When someone dies, the lungs no longer breathe. The heart's job is to pump blood through our entire body. When someone dies, their heart stops beating. These play-based learning opportunities included exploring the body and its functions, and discussing the good questions that arose, including whether Gina would need food to eat after death, and if she would need a blanket to keep her body warm after death. We created a doll to represent a person that was dying. We repeatedly practiced saying each organ that would stop working, the heart, the lungs, the brain, and on and on. We used the words "dying," "died," and "dead." We wrapped the body in fabric, placed it in a plain cardboard box representing a coffin and ceremonially buried it, sharing kind words about the doll at a mock funeral. This play was repeated many times to help Gina understand these concepts about death, and in order to ensure there were no misunderstandings or misinformation about what happens when a person dies.

Gina and her family believed in heaven, and our play naturally shifted to focus on concepts about heaven through sensory play. Soft cotton balls became fluffy white clouds, smooth white feathers represented the wings of angels. After many months of palliative care in the home, Gina died surrounded by her loving family.

Leslie: 8 Years

Leslie was from a northern, rural community surrounded by forest, rivers, and small lakes. Traveling many hours into the city for his medical care meant he and his mother were away from his father and siblings for the many months of treatment he needed. My time with Leslie began with an understanding that the type of cancer that he had was not curable, and that with the right treatments, the quality of his life could be improved and possibly extended for a short period of time. When we began to play together, Leslie was filled with energy and laughter, so we focused on gross motor activities that let us use our bodies in BIG ways. The hospital environment didn't offer many opportunities to really move, so we played 'keep it up' games using balloons and lightweight balls. I exaggerated my movements like a slapstick comic to encourage laughter and lightness in this playtime. My epic crashes as I dove across the room for the balloon became sources of great release during the stress-filled treatment days. We would often include his Mom, and occasionally we could persuade medical team members to join us, too. Including the team allowed Leslie to better connect with his radiation oncologist, neurologist, and oncologist; the play made them fun people, not just doctors dictating treatment.

When Leslie was able to join me in my playroom, we played elaborate dinosaur adventures using large plastic dinosaurs, volcanoes, toy trees, and rocks. Playing out lengthy battles between herbivores and carnivores allowed for tremendous debates about dinosaur attributes, horns, tails, teeth, and eventually led to important discussions about what happened to dinosaurs many millions of years ago. Dinosaurs were extinct. They died. Extinction. Dead. They were gone and never came back. Dinosaurs helped us talk about, and play about, life and death. These important concepts about death, dying, and the finality of death were easier to approach using dinosaurs. It was as if it wasn't actually 'death' we were talking about; it was just dinosaurs. Leslie was asking questions, exploring concepts and learning about death using and playing with dinosaurs. These were important discussions that were made fun and safe through play.

As his cancer progressed and impacted his ability to see clearly through his overly watery eyes, and some paralysis on his left side left him confined to his bed or wheelchair, we explored ways to play in bed and go on adventures without even leaving his room. Part of Leslie's life at home included hunting and fishing, and he was missing out on these experiences while sitting in the hospital bed. I created a magnetic fishing pole with laminated paper fish with paperclip lips, each one printed like the types of fish from the local lakes near Leslie's home. We fished off the end of his bed, over and over again. We fished with his Mom, his nurses, and his doctors. Discussions about medical care, planning, and how Leslie was feeling took place while we all quietly fished together off the end of his bed, making it seem more natural and less scary. We did blindfolded fishing to even the playing field when his eyes watered so much they compromised his ability to see anything clearly. To make things more competitive, we gave points to certain fish and kept a record of who caught the most fish each day, and who got the most points based on the fish. It was fun and competitive play that invited everyone's participation, while honoring a lovely family experience he so missed while in the hospital.

As Leslie's mobility was reduced due to the cancer's spreading through this brain, his ability to move and communicate was more and more limited. His voice was a whisper, heard only if you put your ear near his mouth, and his right hand the only part of his body he was able to successfully control. Watching television became a new focus because play was harder and harder to participate in. I noticed professional wrestling was a popular choice for Leslie's viewing, so I created a special wrestling card game that would allow Leslie to control the play. Leslie would turn the cards with his right hand; each card had a wrestling move printed on it, and I would make the toy wrestlers, big plastic action figures, execute each move against their opponent in an epic battle by the bedside! I would grunt and trash talk as the wrestlers I held threw each other across the bed, shaking the bed as each wrestling move was completed. Leslie's silent lopsided smile and eager hand turning the cards helped me pace the action. Playing FOR Leslie was essential to helping him cope with his limited ability.

We extended Leslie's use of his one functioning hand to include creative and expressive arts as a part of his play. By adapting finger painting activities, I would drape a mess towel over his chest area, placing slippery finger paint paper on top so Leslie could move his paint dipped hand back and forth, creating streaks of color and small handprints. Small toy cars could be dipped in paint and driven over the paper using his right hand, a rainbow of textured wheel tracks making their way across the paper. Having a warm water filled basin nearby with cloths to clean up our paint messes became a part of the games we played, as Leslie would try to get as much paint on me, my face, my hands and arms, as I tried to clean his hands off. Many days I would head out on my journey home with unnoticed blobs of green paint on the underside of my arms and in my ears. My colorful ride home made many people smile, and made Leslie's Mom laugh out loud as I told her the story the next day.

Leslie was able to go home for the very end of his life. As I prepared for them to leave the hospital for the long journey home, I gave his Mom a collection of all the art Leslie and I had completed together in a bound portfolio, and included photos of our play together. I always kept track of our art work with a small date written in the corner along with his name. Once home, Leslie's family focused on just being with him during his final days. They played with him and for him as he lived his last few days. He died in his bedroom at home wearing his Buzz Lightyear costume at the exact moment that everyone had stepped out of his room, answering the phone, making tea, having a bathroom break. It was as if he waited until everyone was ready, then died alone but surrounded by love. He was buried in that costume and with his beloved wrestling toys from our fabulous game. Play was honored as an important part of his life even after his death.

Brian: 13 Years

I met Brian by accident, not through the usual referral process from a doctor, nurse, or child life specialist. It was really a fluke the family found me. Brian had a very serious brain tumor that would be fatal within the year of diagnosis. As his family struggled with the diagnosis, and what and how to tell a young teen the truth about his tumor, Mom asked for help. The first stop was a new age psychologist who referred Brian to an alternative healer. Then, by chance, that healer knew about my oncology work in the community and gave them my contact information. This certainly was not through the normal channels, and could have been missed completely.

After talking and planning with Mom, I came to see them at their home. The initial plan for my work was to help prepare Brian for all the treatments ahead, understanding what it means to take part in a clinical trial, and eventually explain that his tumor was not survivable. For Brian's family, the task of breaking this news and telling Brian themselves was too difficult. They needed help to begin the discussion about palliative care.

Brian and I got started right away getting to know each other. I set out to get to know as much as I could about him: what he liked, what he didn't. We discussed his interests and passions such as sports, games, movies, activities, friends, family, beliefs, even dreams and hopes for his future. Like a detective, I wanted to figure out everything about him to better plan, to engage him and meet his needs in our time together. This relationship building includes trust, caring, and fun that will allow our partnership to evolve into a strong foundation as we spend more time together.

Brian's passion for video games, movies, and sports made its way into most of our sessions together. Whether we played a few rounds of games together on his Xbox or watched a movie, we made sure to balance the hard clinical work of cancer, medicine, and treatment with fun, escape, and a wicked sense of humor. Our mutual love of zombies was well supported in mainstream pop culture through endless graphic novels, video games, and new movies on a weekly basis. We enjoyed them all and debated the many qualities of each one including the all-important questions—fast-moving zombies or slow and lethargic zombies? The zombie theme offered us a total escape from his reality; it allowed us to joke about his brain tumor and theorize about what would happen if a zombie ate a brain filled with cancer. Humor helped sometimes.

Exploring Brian's feelings took place at the beginning of every session to give us a baseline about how he was feeling. We would then revisit how he was feeling as we learned new things about his body and how it was responding to treatment, and if things were changing, as they do frequently during palliative care. In the beginning of our time together, we used a stamp set of round feelings faces and would stamp each one and explore each feeling. As we spent more and more time together, the stamp set was not needed, as Brian became more skilled with the familiar routine of assessing his own feelings. An example of our feelings-focused work includes:

My Feelings

Happy—not on meds anymore, tummy feels better

Bored—but able to distract myself

Scared—What's going to happen to me? What are my options? How will this affect me? How will this affect my family?

Frustrated—the medicine didn't work

Nervous—What will happen to my body now? How will the tumor affect me?

Anger—Letting it out is important—swearing, yelling, throwing, smashing, screaming into a pillow

Optimism—the GOOD list—playing video games, watching TV/movies, friends, room makeover, sometimes school is fun.

We also worked hard on figuring out what Brian knew so far about his tumor and treatments and what questions he had for me, the doctor, and his parents about what was happening to his body and how his life would be impacted during treatment. We played with and explored my many brain toys and materials—squishy stress-ball brains, educational brain toys, puzzles, and books. While exploring these toys, we were also learning where in the brain his tumor was located and what that area of the brain does and what it controls in our bodies. This allowed us to explore and discuss the possible impact the treatments might have on him and his ability to do activities and tasks, and the impact on his body. Problem solving how to improve Brian's frequent blood draws included some medical play with butterfly needles to gain some mastery and overcome fears, finding a few preferred positive distractions he could use during these blood draws and determining how to advocate for what he needs to be and feel successful when at the clinic. These works lead us to create numerous plans for success that were meant to guide the medical team and his family in their interactions with Brian throughout the ups and downs of his care.

Amid the daily grind of treatment, checkups, diagnostic assessments, and scans, it was important for me to promote family time and normal adventures that a family might do together. Working with numerous special community agencies, I set out to provide access to free tickets to local sports teams, music concerts, and movie premieres. Although it is virtually impossible for a family to put cancer out of their minds, I wanted Brian, his parents, and his sister to at least put it aside for a few hours of pleasure, together as a family. As Brian's accessibility changed due to side effects that left him with poor balance and unclear vision at times, I adjusted these outings to include access to corporate suites that were more accessible and private.

As the treatments impacted Brian's ability to attend school, our time together at the home increased. We began working with a local wish-granting agency, and Brian and his family began to plan the coolest Star Wars–themed 'Man Cave' that would include a place for his beloved toys and collectables and act as his 'space' at home. Designers visited in consultation about colors and his preferences for furniture, characters from the movies, and his needs based on the impact of treatment. Together Brian and I created a list of toys, games, and movies he hoped to stock his new room with. We played with his action figures, re-watched the Star Wars movies, and did web-based searches for cool ideas and inspiration. This offered a positive distraction from the seriousness of treatment and helped us build anticipation and excitement for the eventual reveal of the Man Cave. This man cave became Brian's place: the place to be with him.

As Brian's cancer progressed despite the treatments, we began our discussion about the seriousness of his diagnosis and the type of tumor he had. I stuck to the facts, kept it simple and used clear language in the beginning. "What we know about this tumor is that no one has survived it. This tumor will eventually cause you to die." "We don't know when you will die because of the new medicines the doctors are using in the clinical trial." "The doctor's hope with this clinical trial is that they will learn how to better treat this tumor." "The doctors do not know if the treatments you are receiving will be able to stop this cancer, but they hope it will help to extend your life." These initial statements about the seriousness of his tumor lead to deeper important discussions about life, death, and dying and what they mean to Brian. It also allowed us a chance to plan for how Brian wanted to live now, while knowing he was dying.

Brian and I brainstormed what he wanted to focus on, on his own, with the medical team and with his family. His list was simple:

Wellness
Quality of Life
Hopeful
Optimistic
Live Life

Communicating this focus was important to the way forward. Brian wanted to focus on the positive. He was living and wanted his life to be hopeful. If a drug wasn't working, or the side effects were too great, he wanted to problem solve next steps, new treatments, and strategies. He did not want to just give up and stop treatment. This desire to try new and different approaches to continue treating Brian's cancer led to diet changes thought to improve his response to treatment and rob the tumor of fuel. Naturally, the new diet and its restrictions were not the most delicious for a young teen. So, my work shifted to include seeking out places that could make us teen food favorites in a healthy way. In my adventures around town, shaking hands and making friends with foodies led me to find a Healthy Hawaiian pizza and organic soda pop that met the dietary restrictions. Our pizza party was both teen taste buds delicious and good for us!

The side effects of treatment were frustrating for Brian. Brian was a big guy, tall and solid, so these balance issues meant he struggled with walking more and more, making walking almost impossible even with a person assisting and a walker. Eventually Brian required a wheelchair to get around. We tackled this frustration with humor again. Brian and his Mom set out to make humorous T-shirts that poked fun at his wheelchair, including one particularly hilarious one of a comic stick-man falling out of a wheelchair with a caption above that said "Oh, Crap." Brian wore these shirts proudly to every appointment he had at the hospital with the palliative team. He needed and wanted to have something funny to start the conversation, because much of the news was not good. The ability to make T-shirts expanded and extended into making shirts as gifts for family and friends. These shirts were a unique legacy-building activity of something Brian created. I still have my shirt and wear it often.

Anger was an important feeling to acknowledge as his vision was affected, causing terrible headache-inducing double vision. The medical patches were functional, covering one eye to prevent the double vision. But these bandage-like patches were far too clinical; homemade pirate patches were more Brian's style, so multiple padded patches were created in straight black, as well as neon colors. If he had to wear a patch, Brian may as well have fun with it and really stand out! As much fun as it was to have fun, it was also important to openly talk about and play out the angry feelings about the changes in his body, the deterioration of his abilities. We created pillows to safely punch out angry feelings. Releasing anger was important both to let it out and to talk about it openly. We discussed these angry feelings about all aspects of treatment, his tumor, and his body's betrayal as it succumbed to side effects of treatment and the impact of the tumor on his brain, while we made two papier-mâché monsters using recycled and colorful tissue paper. One monster represented Cancer, and the other represented Fear. The plan for these funny-looking monsters was to take out our anger on them, and smash them like a piñata, but in our deeper discussions about feelings, cancer, and fear, Brian decided that the monster Fear would be spared. Brian would keep Fear because fear is a natural part of life, even when facing death. We smashed the Cancer monster into a million little pieces. But we kept Fear.

Through these small setbacks and deterioration came the inevitable hospitalizations when things got complicated. Swallowing became a challenge. Choking on water was scary and could compromise Brian's airway, so into the hospital he would go. This was hard for Brian and his family. The hospital wasn't comfortable for him; he longed to leave and get home and play the more mature video games he wanted to play, watch the movies he wanted to watch. Food and drinking-related play was fun and frustrating. We added liquid thickeners to drinks and soups in hopes of finding the right balance of thickening without getting too gross. We played racing games doing taste samples of different drinks, soups, and blended foods, then rating how good they were or how awful they were. Brian and I laughed and cried with each new taste test, and agreed that our overall goal was to make sure no one fed him chicken noodle soup jelly. That's where we drew the line. I prepared rousing toilet paper target practice games to release angry feelings when the hospitalization got to him. We threw big wet handfuls of toilet paper at the targets representing the tumor, the hospital, and the routine procedures he could no longer stand, and the treatments that were causing extreme side effects. Throwing wet globs of paper was silly but serious fun in the hospital, and the messier it was, the better.

As things dragged on, while the medical team tested and scanned Brian's body and problem solved what to do with both treatments and managing his palliative symptoms, the hospital stays got longer and longer and Brian worried about getting home. He was especially concerned about not having the chance to hold and pet his cat, a source of distraction and calm through his peaceful moments alone at home when guests had left, community medical team members were done with their work, and family members tended to the mundane daily tasks that called them away. I knew given his age that a simple stuffed animal might not meet this strong desire to be with his cat. I also knew that he had declined the pet therapy visits at the hospital. I had heard of a special "cat immersion" project that another hospital had done for a patient that missed their cat. I collected cat photos and videos from all friends, family, and colleagues to create a slideshow of cats, and found recordings of cat sounds, meows and purrs, online. The "immersion" part involved tenting a plain white sheet above Brian's bed, making sure to allow for nurses' access, of course. Once the tent was up, I turned off the room lights and projected the cat slideshow into the sides of the tent and played the cat sounds. Total cat immersion was complete and provided the perfect distraction and restful experience!

The medical team continued to try new and different combinations of drugs when the clinical trial was not successful. These new medications had a particularly embarrassing impact on Brian. He was constipated, painfully so. More medications were given to address this problem, but things were slow to change. The discomfort and embarrassment was so significant for Brian that it was hard to play and do other activities. Frustration and panic would bubble to the surface when his tummy hurt, so we began creating guided imagery scripts to help Brian relax his muscles, control his breathing, and distract his mind from his body's pain. We took his love of sniper and first person shooter video games and turned them into elaborate narrative stories of a sniper on a mission. As I created these scripts, I made sure to focus on all the little details, like the color of the camouflage, the stillness of the sniper's body as it lay in position, the feeling of the breeze on the sniper's skin and hair, the meticulous control the sniper had over his breathing and each muscle in his body and what he was focusing on. For Brian, this allowed him to practice relaxing each part of his body, as the sniper did the same. We always started with the feet, then the legs, and made our way up the body. Depending on how much pain he was experiencing, Brian would often close his eye and imagine the images, but when he was panicked and worried about what was happening to his body and the pain he was feeling, he focused his gaze and stared right into my eyes while I said our sniper story aloud.

During what was to become his last time at home, Brian and I worked on his last wishes. These wishes were for functional actions, like who he would like to receive his beloved toys and video games, but also for important actions and interactions between the people in his life, too. His wishes were written for all his family members, instructing them to be kind to each other in his last days and after his death. His wishes for the medical and palliative care team were specific about his care, to ensure he was addressed as Brian before they touched him or did any procedures or assessments on him, and to request that at the very end of his life he be 'tube-free,' without IVs and catheters snaking out of his body. And he wanted to be dressed in his own clothes, not the hospital gowns. He wanted to be Brian, not Brian the cancer patient.

His last morning started with an ambulance ride to the hospital before the sun was up. Brought through the emergency room up into the ward, Brian's breathing was rapid, his panic causing his heart to beat fast while the medical and palliative team worked to assess him and his body. Surrounded by the family and the medical team I began our sniper guided imagery, holding his hands and speaking softly close to his face to ensure he could see me and focus if his eyes were clear enough. His body slowly relaxed and the breathing settled into a calm pattern. With his last wishes posted up around the room, the family and medical team began the process of following through on these important wishes. The tubes were slowly removed. The hospital gown was taken off and Brian was dressed in his soft blue track suit. He was Brian. Brian died with his immediate family holding him, and extended family members surrounding his bed in the hospital that day.

PERSONAL REFLECTIONS

An essential part of child life interactions with any child is establishing a relationship with them that is warm, respectful, empathic, and understanding. Working with a child who is dying requires an even closer relationship, a deep connection, one that is intimate. It is this intimacy that allows you to go to those deeply personal areas of a child's life and mind with them through their journey of living while they are dying. This intimacy often extends to the family as well. Much of my work with a dying child and their family takes place in their family home for a period, before sometimes shifting to a hospital or pediatric hospice for the end of life. All of this takes time, so I ensure that I offer a considerable amount of time to each child and family I help that is facing an end of life journey. This may be the hundredth family I have helped face a child living while dying, but for that child and their family, this is their only experience with this.

I take my role as a child life specialist for a dying child very seriously, while recognizing the need to provide some serious fun, too. I often explain to the child that I work for them. I am here to help them figure out all the answers to their questions, help them understand what is happening to them, and help them determine what they need and want to be and feel successful in their life facing a serious and life-threatening illness. I also stress that it's my job to help ensure that their voice is heard among their parent's desires and the medical team's plans and problem solving. It is my job to communicate what they need and want. I give them a voice.

While remaining professional, I deeply respect the need to gain closeness in my practice that allows for a lifetime of building friendships while serving humanity (Adams, 1993).

SUMMARY

Death and dying invite an atmosphere of great seriousness that often challenges hope, possibility, and fun. However serious the situation is, it must be balanced by play that invites pleasure, exploration, stress relief, and self-expression. All play should be welcomed and encouraged, and when a clinician trusts in their ability to use an open mind and imagination in their interactions with a child, their experiences will be fresh, exciting, and full of the unexpected (Freeman, Epston, & Lobovits, 1997). Sometimes the act of problem solving play ideas becomes the play itself when you infuse it with fun language and explore different narrative approaches to these actions. It is not enough to give toys and expect a child to play alone. It is more important to find opportunities to play with the child, and encourage and support play with family members. Time is so important to a child who is dying. Your time with them is the joyful part of their day, otherwise often spent with treatment, assessments, procedures, resting or sleeping, and general feelings of sadness and being unwell.

I have been so inspired by my own clinical experiences and adventures with patients and their families that I offer our versions of play at different ages and stages of development in hopes that you may adapt and adjust them to suit the needs and imaginations of the young people you have the privilege of playing with.

REFERENCES

Websites

Effective palliative care for children. (1998). *World Health Organization (WHO)*. Retrieved from: www.who.int/cancer/palliative/definition/en/

The ICPCN charter for the rights for life limited and life threatened children. (2008). *International Children's Palliative Care Network (ICPCN)*. Retrieved September 19, 2016 from: www.icpcn.org/icpcn-charter/

Professional Literature

Adams, D.W., & Deveau, E.J. (1984). *Coping with childhood cancer: Where do we go from here?* Reston, VA: Reston.

Adams, P. (1993). *Gesundheit: Bringing good health to you, the medical system, and society through physician service, complementary therapies, humor and joy*. Rochester, VT: Healing Arts Press.

Amery, J. (Ed.). (2009). *Children's palliative care in Africa*. Oxford: Oxford University Press.

Boucher, S., Downing, J., & Shemilt, R. (2014). The Role of play in children's palliative care. *Children, 1*, 302–317.

Feudtner, C., Friebert, S., & Jewell, J. (2013). Pediatric palliative care and hospice care commitments, guidelines, and recommendations. *American Academy of Pediatrics, 132*(5), 966–972.

Freeman, J., Epston, D., & Lobovits, D. (1997). *Playful approaches to serious problems: Narrative therapy with children and their families*. New York: W.W. Norton.

Ginsburg, K.R. (2007). The importance of play in promoting healthy child development and maintaining strong parent-child bonds. *American Academy of Pediatrics, 119*(1), 182–191.

Gray, E. (1989). The emotional and play needs of the dying child. *Issues in Comprehensive Pediatric Nursing, 22*(2/3), 207–224.

Hurwitz, S.C. (2002). For parents particularly: To be successful—Let them play! *Childhood Education, 79*(2), 101–102.

Pediatric Palliative Care and Hospice Care Commitments, Guidelines, and Recommendations: Section on hospice and palliative medicine and committee on hospital care. (2013). *American Academy of Pediatrics*, 132(5).

Pellegrini, A.D., & Smith, P.K. (1998). The Development of play during childhood: Forms and possible functions. *Child and Adolescent Mental Health*, 3(2), 51–57.

Children's Books

Buscaglia, L.F. (1982). *The Fall of Freddie the leaf: A story of life for all ages*. Thorofare, NJ: Slack.

Mellonie, B., & Ingpen, R. (1983). *Lifetimes: A beautiful way to explain death to children*. New York: Bantam.

Seuss, Dr. (1996). *My many colored day*. New York: Random House Children's Books.

PART V

Medical Play Therapy Through a Systemic Lens

What About Me? Sibling Play Therapy When a Family Has a Child With Chronic Illness

John W. Seymour

Illness does not ask. It demands.

—Marie Seren Cohen, 1999, p. 149

My body is a big bully to me!

—an 8-year-old client

Chronic illness impacts almost a third of American families, and presents a major challenge for the family to adapt and thrive (Cohen, 1999; McDaniel, Doherty, & Hepworth, 2014). Families often make unexpected discoveries of both strengths and vulnerabilities that they never imagined. They learn the benefits and hazards of when to stand firm and when to be flexible. They search for ways to embrace life and thrive while addressing the challenges of medical conditions and treatments, all the while knowing that the experience could last a lifetime. Children in these families look closely to the caretaking adults in the family and their siblings for coping with chronic illness.

Researchers and clinicians in many fields, including family therapy, psychology, counseling, social work, child life, medicine, and nursing have contributed to the professional literature on the risk and protective factors of families experiencing chronic illness (Anderson & Davis, 2011; Bellin & Kovacs, 2006; Cohen, 1999; Compas, Jaser, Dunn, & Rodriquez, 2012; Davey, Kissil, & Lynch, 2016; Martire, Lustig, Schulz, Miller, & Helgeson, 2004; Rolland, 1994; Paterson, 2001; Sharpe & Rossiter, 2002; Thorne et al., 2002; Van Riper, 2003). Much of the research has focused on the effects of the chronic illness on the caretaking relationship, either with a parent/caretaker and child with chronic illness, or a partner/caretaker and a partner with chronic illness. There has not been as much written about chronic illness and sibling relationships (O'Brien, Duffy, & Nicholl, 2009; Van Riper, 2003). In everyday family life, siblings are models and teachers to one another in developing social connections, problem solving, and developing a sense of identity. When chronic illness becomes a part of family life, siblings are both impacted and impactful (Cohen, 1999; Mulroy, Robertson, Aiberti, Leonard, & Bower, 2008; O'Brien et al., 2009; Van Riper, 2003).

These siblings can benefit from clinical interventions that can help minimize the risk of negative effects and maximize the resources of the siblings, family, and support system in coping with the long-term effects of chronic illness (Cohen, 1999; O'Brien et al., 2009; Van Riper, 2003). Interventions can be both remedial and preventive in reducing risks as well as increasing strengths and resources. Following a more detailed description of chronic illness, families, and siblings, a resilience-based approach for working with these siblings will be proposed and illustrated (Seymour, 2009, 2014, 2015; Seymour & Erdman, 1996).

CHRONIC ILLNESS AND FAMILIES

Illness and disability can enter a family's life at any time through the life cycle (Rolland, 1994). New parents face it when they are given the news that their newborn child has a condition such as cystic fibrosis (CF) or severe combined immunodeficiency (SCID). A family with several school-aged children face it when a sibling is diagnosed with a chronic condition such as rheumatoid arthritis (RA) or a life-threatening condition such as leukemia. Family members learn that a young child has an intellectual disability or other neurodevelopmental disorder. Anywhere along the child and adolescent life cycle, significant mental health conditions can be identified that turn out to be long-standing rather than a stress reaction to the ups and downs of life. While these conditions have very different causes, treatments, and prognoses, each has significant long-term impacts on every family member as well as the entire family unit. These children will look to both their parents/caretakers as well as siblings for support in dealing with the chronic illness.

Chronic Illness

Chronic illnesses are usually defined as conditions lasting from 3 to 12 months or more that result in limited activities of daily living (school for children, work for adults), higher rates of visits and use of specialized health care, and sometimes the need for adaptive equipment or accommodations (Van Cleave, Gortmaker, & Perrin, 2010). Depending on the scope of researchers' definitions of chronic illness, anywhere from 15% to 30% of U.S. families are impacted by chronic illness, with a slow but steady increase in the rate in the last 10 years (Cohen, 1999; Compas et al., 2012; McDaniel et al., 2014; Van Cleave et al., 2010; Wise, 2004).

Chronic illness in childhood includes conditions such as asthma, cystic fibrosis, diabetes, genetic diseases, developmental disabilities, child mental health issues, and those caused by environmental impacts in utero or in the child's early life (Torpy, Campbell, & Glass, 2010). While child mortality rates in the U.S. have decreased, there has been a doubling of the rate of childhood chronic illness (Wise, 2004). Children now are being more successfully treated for historically life-threatening conditions, living much longer, but often dealing with residual effects of chronic illness and disability (Compas et al., 2012; Van Cleave et al., 2010).

Family Dynamics and Chronic Illness

Most families have some experience with acute illnesses, which are typically time-limited, specific to an identified part of the body, accompanied by a predictable course of treatment and prognosis, and having less of a long-term impact on families. On the other hand, chronic illnesses, along with being long-term, can impact several interacting systems of the body, causing a wide range of patient problems, and often involving some difficulty in assessment and treatment. Symptoms can vary greatly from person to person, and interactions of these symptoms can cause unpredictable setbacks. Families dealing with chronic illness face two of the most difficult aspects of stress effects: symptoms that are intermittent and symptoms that are unpredictable. Psychological and psychosocial vigilance for intermittent and unpredictable symptoms can keep all family members at high stress levels (Jessop & Stein, 1985; Dodgson et al., 2000; Garwick, Patterson, Meschke, Bennett, & Blum, 2002). Along with the usual developmental and situational stressors, families with chronic illness have an extra layer of ongoing stress, making relational-based stress-reduction interventions especially effective in improving family function (Wood, Klebba, & Miller, 2000; Siegel, 2010, 2012, 2017).

Initial research on families with chronic illness were usually deficit-based rather than strengths-based models (McDaniel, Hepworth, & Doherty, 1992). These early models paralleled the medical model, using a symptom-focused, deficit-driven approach to assessment and treatment, and were lacking an understanding of the interpersonal dimension of chronic illness and interventions (Seymour, 2009, 2011). As Goldstein and Brooks (2006) have pointed out, "symptom relief has simply not been synonymous with changing long-term outcome" (p. 11). Early studies were often categorical, focusing on the effects of specific illnesses such as asthma or cancer on families. The focus tended to be on an individual's characteristics impacting coping, such as the roles of age, birth order, number of siblings, and developmental levels of the children.

More recently, there has been a growing consensus that interpersonal and social contextual factors have a greater impact on families coping with chronic illness, rather than specific characteristics of a disease or demographic characteristics of a specific family (Cohen, 1999; O'Brien et al., 2009; Rolland, 1994; Van Riper, 2003). Family members adjust to the demands of chronic illness, helping to minimize the effects of illness on the family. Over time, some of these adjustments can evolve into less functional patterns that can trigger additional family stressors impacting the course of the chronic illness. Rolland refers to this process as a circular "chain of influence" (1994, p. 11) between chronic illness factors and family life factors. A systemic understanding of chronic illness supports clinical interventions that are strengths-based, interactional, and grounded in principals for optimal family function (Bellin & Kovacs, 2006). Whatever the chronic illness, the family and each of the family members are affected (Davey et al., 2016). Chronic illness impacts family relationships, rules, and roles, and these family dynamics moderate the impact of chronic illness on family members (Cohen, 1999). Cohen (1999) found that the severity of the chronic illness was not as impactful on family functioning as were the concrete behavioral demands of caring for the illness, both for the ill child and family members.

Boss (1999, 2002) describes *ambiguous loss* as another part of this complex world of families and chronic illness. Chronic illness can trigger a series of losses, with grief becoming a way of life. This type of grieving is cyclical as compared to grieving a specific loss. Boss has identified the grief of chronic illness to include anticipatory grief (intense awareness of impending loss), disenfranchised grief (not well understood or shared by others), and frozen grief (loss of hope with an increasing sense of isolation). Grief of ambiguous loss is a relational-based rather than individual-based process. Caring for ambiguous loss goes beyond the individual grief process to address the chronic illnesses effects on family and community relationships. Relational-based and community-based interventions are indicated as interventions of choice in addressing ambiguous loss in families.

The *Shifting Perspectives Model of Chronic Illness* proposed by Paterson (2001) provides insight into the complex world of families dealing with chronic illness. Paterson has characterized living with chronic illness as an experience of dual citizenship between the worlds of illness and health. Effective coping with chronic illness consists of finding a balance between those two worlds. When the illness world perspective dominates, the effects of suffering and loss from the illness tend to be overwhelming. When the wellness world perspective dominates, some space is created between the persons and the effects of the illness. Opportunities can be identified for challenges and changes in life. Persons rather than the illness are restored as the primary source of identity. Effective coping strategies promote the ability to embrace both perspectives, including strategies to directly impact the effects of the illness as well as strategies to increase efforts toward health. Efforts to help families achieve this balance have been described in many family-based approaches (Boss, 2002; Cohen, 1999; Compas et al., 2012; Rolland, 1994).

Families successfully functioning with chronic illness have found ways of maintaining a careful balance of routine and flexibility (Cohen, 1999; Compas et al., 2012; Kramer, 2010; Livneh, 2001). Family meal times, family traditions around special events, and shared family leisure activities buffer the effects of uncertain and unpredictable effects of chronic illness and provide gentle reminders of the presence and support of family members. Families successfully functioning with chronic illness have also developed the art of improvisational living, finding opportunities for family life even when chronic illness disrupts the routine. Successful coping includes both a focus on the future as well as the ability to live in the present. While parents/caretakers may take the lead in creating this family balance, children make an important contribution. Children tend to have a here-and-now focus, helping to balance adult views that can become so future-focused that day-to-day routines are neglected. Children's humor, playfulness, intense experiences of emotions, and even impulsiveness provide fresh perspectives for family members to be more present and agile in their responses to chronic illness.

With all aspects of family life impacted by chronic illness, intervention approaches need to focus on the relational and social contextual dimensions. Family members will need support in managing the stress loads of chronic illness and dealing with the unpredictable ups and downs of chronic illness. Ambiguous loss becomes an important lens through which to assess and treat family members dealing with chronic illness. A balanced approach to family illness incorporating health and illness perspectives should inform care for every family member, and is relevant to sibling-based interventions.

SIBLING RELATIONSHIPS IN FAMILY LIFE

Sibling relationships played an important role in the development of Western theories of psychotherapy and our understanding of family life (Cicirelli, 1995). Sibling rivalry and differential treatment of siblings by parents were often the focus, with an emphasis on the less positive effects of sibling relationships (Milevsky, 2011). Current sibling research has described how siblings affect each other's growth and development through the entire life cycle (Feinberg, Solmeyer, & McHale, 2010; Hernandez, 1997). The sibling relationship is likely to be the most long-standing relationship a person will have, with many reporting significant relationships to and throughout adulthood (Brody, 2004; Kramer, 2010; McHale, Updegraff, & Whiteman, 2012). In the family unit, siblings often spend more time with each other than with adult members of the family (Cicirelli, 1995; Hernandez, 1997; Whiteman, McHale, & Soli, 2011). While certain family and cultural traditions ascribe a hierarchy to siblings, in many families the sibling relationship is often the first egalitarian-like relationship of life, laying the foundation for later adult relationships (Cicirelli, 1995).

The sibling relationship is distinctive in combining qualities of both parent–child relationships and peer relationships. Like the parent–child relationship, older siblings share in the attachment bonding process of younger siblings, playing a role in providing a secure base for the younger sibling. Siblings serve as early teachers and models for learning emotional regulation and mastery of developmental tasks (Dunn, 2007; Milevsky, 2011). Siblings are often confidants for one another, providing emotional support (Kim, McHale, Osgood, & Crouter, 2006). Recent findings in interpersonal neurobiology have expanded the understanding of how siblings co-regulate with each other (Wood et al., 2000; Siegel, 2010, 2012, 2017). As peers, siblings are early playmates to each other, providing early experiences of peer communication, problem solving, and striving for mastery, providing an important bridge to developing peer relationships in life beyond the family. These relational influences between siblings are circular: younger siblings impact older ones, and older siblings impact younger ones.

Sibling dyads, where there is a chronic illness or disability, do show a slightly increased risk of adjustment problems (Sharpe & Rossiter, 2002), so details of the sibling relationship should be included in assessment and planning interventions (Cohen, 1999; Strohm, 2008). The demands of chronic illness can consume the caretaking capacities of the parent/caretaker for the ill child, leaving few resources for the siblings. Resentment between siblings can grow because of this shift of attention to the chronically ill child, although siblings do show some tolerance for these differences when the reasons are understood (O'Brien et al., 2009). Specialized medical treatment is sometimes only available far from home, contributing to times of separation for the family. Financial resources of the family are often challenged, both from the cost of obtaining health care and the loss of caretaker/parent income when unable to work.

Even with these challenges, many siblings are found to display more warmth and positive affect with each other than siblings in families with no chronic illness (McHale et al., 2012). Siblings have been found to play a compensatory effect for one another when the caretaker/parent is focused on health care of the chronically ill child. Chronic illness can contribute to social isolation of children, who may be excluded because of the nature of the condition, the rigors of treatment, or cultural or family beliefs about the nature and cause of the illness. In these circumstances, siblings can play the role of peer support system to one another (Milevsky, 2011) and share their own peer relationships with each other.

This distinctive combination of parent–child and peer–peer qualities provides an understanding of the therapeutic potential within the sibling relationship as well as the process of developing a therapeutic relationship between the siblings and treating professional. In some instances, the sibling who is chronically ill (whether younger or older) may provide examples of patience, courage, cooperation, and emotional regulation that benefit the sibling who is healthy but not managing the stress of the chronic illness affecting the family. On the other hand, the healthy sibling may provide the one with chronic illness examples of encouragement and assistance, connection with peers, and maintaining a link with life beyond the effects of the chronic illness. There is no one pattern or direction of influence between siblings. Successful coping with a chronic illness will require siblings to have flexibility and an ability to shift back and forth between supportive and supported roles and between mentor and mentee. While parents have a significant role in shaping the family dynamics to be adaptive to the chronic illness, siblings play an important supportive role that can be cultivated in the family and through supportive clinical interventions. The therapeutic relationship combines elements of both parent–child and peer–peer, so a good understanding of the sibling relationship can provide important clues on conceptualizing the dynamics of sessions and cultivating the therapeutic relationship.

In an overview of recent research on sibling relationships, Kramer (2010) identified an emerging list of essential competencies for prosocial sibling relationships that suggest particular types of interventions, including the promotion of positive engagement between siblings (play and activities that accommodate the developmental levels of siblings), cohesion (emphasizing cooperation, loyalty, and trust), emotional regulation (dealing with conflicts and frustrations as well as fun shared experiences), and conflict resolution (collaborative problem solving, mediation). These natural processes of sibling relationships can provide the basis for remedial and protective interventions for siblings facing chronic illness. Goals of interventions would include both strategies for reducing the risks and enhancing resilience in the sibling relationship. From a systemic perspective, interventions with the sibling subsystem can impact the other family subsystems to maximize family functioning when dealing with chronic illness.

Social Context and Cultural Understanding

Cultural anthropologists have long studied cultural and family patterns of how humans approach illness, health, and healing processes. Cultural traditions provide a worldview that serves as a framework for families to understand the causes of illness, the sources of wellness, and human's role and efficacy to impact the healing process (Frank & Frank, 1993). At a more local level, families shape their own worldview of illness and healing (Kleinman, 1980, 1988). Cultural and family variations are influenced by gender, family, region, generation, and religious/spiritual traditions (Boss, 2002).

Family life throughout the world affirms the role of siblings in the function of families. Warm relationships between siblings promote positive family adjustment in any culture (Milevsky, 2011). Siblings are companions for one another and have a shared family and cultural history that is in part transmitted from sibling to sibling. In whatever culture, sibling relationships play an important role in the family's ability to survive and thrive when faced with challenges. Cultures that emphasize individualism often exhibit more sibling rivalry and competitiveness. Cultures that emphasize collectivism often have more specific roles and responsibilities for siblings caring for younger or chronically ill siblings (McHale et al., 2012).

Some studies have focused on family life and siblings in specific cultural groups to examine similarities within those traditions. Mexican American families often emphasize cultural values of *familismo* (putting the needs of the family over individuals) and *simpatia* (promoting harmony among family members) in defining sibling relationships (Gamble & Modry-Mandell, 2008; Killoren, Thayer, & Updegraff, 2008; Updegraff, McHale, Whiteman, Thayer, & Delgado, 2005). In African American families, positive sibling relationships have been reinforced with spirituality and ethnic identity (McHale, Whiteman, Kim, & Crouter, 2007). Whatever the cultural and ethnic factors, the context of the family will influence how well they manage stressors such as chronic illness, and find ways to maintain positive function of the family system (Boss, 2002).

For families with chronically ill children, helping professionals become an integral part of the social context, relating to both family members and one another in collaborative care. Working with a family and their chronically ill child can be both rewarding and demanding. Empathy and compassion are central features of the therapeutic relationship. Creating and maintaining an effective therapeutic relationship challenges therapists to face the anxiety, uncertainty, and sense of mortality experienced by client families, while simultaneously facing their own experience with these issues. Suggested personal themes for reflection might include exploring one's tolerance for ambiguity and loss, family of origin experiences with illness and care providers, and current health status of the therapist or therapist's family (McDaniel et al., 2014).

Psychotherapy with chronically ill children has its own challenges in creating and maintaining a therapeutic relationship. The vulnerability of young clients, particularly those with chronic illness, can make it difficult for therapists to balance their caretaking role to prevent an overinvolvement unlikely to help the child develop a better sense of personal agency (Malawista, 2004). Children and adolescents are less likely than adults to edit what they say or do in session. While some feelings may be expressed with words, it is likely that they will also be expressed in a range of behaviors, from imaginary play to physically acting out the pain with aggression (Gabel & Bemporad, 1994a, 1994b; Gil & Rubin, 2005). Gil and Rubin (2005) advise therapists to utilize self-reflection, collaboration, and supervision to address the personal impact of their clinical work to minimize any negative effects of countertransference in the therapeutic relationship. While much of the work with young clients is more action-based than word-based, Gil and Rubin recommend that self-reflection and clinical supervision incorporate elements of play, expressive arts, and sand tray work as well as traditional supervisory techniques.

INTEGRATIVE FAMILY PLAY THERAPY FOR RESILIENCE

Brooks (1994a, 1994b) has recommended there be a strong link between resilience research and clinical practice. Integrative family play therapy is informed by resilience research and builds on the therapeutic principles of medical family therapy (Rolland, 1994; McDaniel et al., 2014), family play therapy (Gil, 2015; Schaefer & Carey, 1994; Seymour & Erdman, 1996), and integrative play therapy (Drewes, Bratton, & Schaefer, 2011). Integrative Family Play Therapy (IFPT) combines these therapeutic principles into an integrative/prescriptive model that is trans-theoretical, creating a template for understanding therapeutic work within existing models of psychotherapy. IFPT focuses on the qualities of establishing and maintaining a therapeutic relationship with multimodal methods of assessment (Drewes, 2011a, 2011b). Interventions are tailored to the client's specific needs at the time, using therapeutic mechanisms common to most models of child therapy (Schaefer & Drewes, 2014; Shirk & Russell, 1996), so that interventions can be tailored to the child's specific needs at a specific time (Schaefer, 2001, 2011). Compas et al. (2012) emphasized the importance of customized interventions in addressing the unique circumstances of families dealing with chronic illness.

Rutter (1999) defines resilience as the "relative resistance to psychosocial risk experiences" (p. 119) and "a relatively good outcome for someone despite their experience of situations that have shown to carry a major risk for the development of pathology" (p. 120). Walsh (2016) refers to resilience as "the ability to withstand and rebound from serious life challenges . . . that foster positive adaptation in the context of significant adversity . . . [to] enable recovery and positive growth" (p. 4). Early resilience research was mostly exploratory, seeking to identify individual qualities of children who had been able to successfully deal with life challenges (Wright & Masten, 2006). Rutter's (1999, 2007) research evolved into an interactional model that identified eight specific protective mechanisms contributing to family resilience. Recent findings in interpersonal neurobiology (Siegel, 2010, 2012, 2017) have been incorporated into these models for more specific understandings of how these protective mechanisms work in families with chronic illness, as well as in our clinical work with them (Brooks & Goldstein, 2015). Resilience has been identified by Schaefer and Drewes (2014) as one of 20 *therapeutic powers of play*, and Rutter's (1999, 2007) eight resilience protective mechanisms have been adapted for play therapists (Seymour, 2009, 2014, 2015).

IFPT utilizes an ecosystemic perspective and is used to understand how family members respond to a chronic illness, looking at both how family members relate to each other as well as their surrounding social and cultural systems, along with direct services to family members, collaboration, and coordination with other caregivers and professionals involved with the family facing chronic illness (Rolland, 1994; McDaniel et al., 2014; Wise, 2004). As an interactional model, therapeutic conceptualizations and interventions include approaches from individual, family, and group psychotherapy. Power and Dell Orto (2004) have identified four themes incorporated into intervention plans with families dealing with chronic illness: maintaining family equilibrium between the demand of illness and everyday life; utilizing support systems that are sometimes uninformed on how to help; recognizing potential family problems that can be proactively addressed as they arise; and developing skills for tolerating stressors that can be compounded during a long period of chronic illness.

Play has been incorporated into Western psychotherapy with children since the days of Anna Freud (1936/1966) and Melanie Klein (1932). Play was understood as a developmentally natural way to relate to children, aiding in their expression of feelings and providing the therapist with an outward view of the inner child (Donaldson, 1996; O'Connor, 2000). Winnicott (1971) described play as a seamless part of the therapeutic process rather than a distinct modality. Play is a rich and developmentally natural activity of children as they practice interacting in a world that has both randomness and uncertainty. Eberle (2014) stated, "Play is an ancient, voluntary, 'emergent' process driven by pleasure that yet strengthens our muscles, instructs our social skills, tempers and deepens our positive emotions, and enables a state of balance that leaves us poised to play some more" (p. 231).

Siegel's (2010, 2012, 2017) research on interpersonal neurobiology (IPNB) has identified how resilience can be cultivated through play interactions that train the developing brain in making personal connections, regulating feelings, and problem solving. Perry's Neurosequential Model of Therapeutics (Barfield, Dobson, Gaskill, & Perry, 2012; Perry, 2006; Perry & Hambrick, 2008) gives a step-by-step process of applying the latest brain research to play-based therapeutic interventions. Experiential and expressive therapies such as play therapy, art therapy, drama therapy, and developmental therapies such as Theraplay (Jernberg & Booth, 1999; Munns, 2000, 2009) provide interventions that unify the cognitive, affective, behavioral, and relational dimensions that support resilience processes in family-based therapies (Seymour & Erdman, 1996).

Resilience research provides a lens of understanding how to conceptualize, implement, and coordinate services for children and their families dealing with chronic illness (Tedeschi & Kilmer, 2005). It gives play therapists ways of "identifying the child's strengths, family and community resources available, and the processes of joining them in reinforcing the child's immediate ability to cope and longer-term ability to be prepared for the next life challenge" (Seymour, 2009, p. 75). Resilience processes incorporate both remedial and preventative roles for supporting child development in families facing chronic illness (Masten & Coatsworth, 1998; Meichenbaum, 2009). Rutter's (1999, 2007) eight resilience processes, adapted by Seymour (2009, 2014, 2015), provide an outline for providing services to siblings in families facing chronic illness.

Resilience in Sibling Play: 1. Reducing Anxiety and Increasing Problem Solving

The first protective mechanism influences risk factors within and beyond the family life, and creates the basis for a therapeutic relationship for encouraging the other seven protective mechanisms. Siblings in families facing chronic illness bring a complex set of risk factors into the therapeutic space, with these risk factors having a cascading effect on the others (Rutter, 1999, 2007; Seymour, 2015). Siblings relationships are sources of both increasing or reducing anxiety, so addressing the anxiety-regulating aspects between siblings can help to reduce overall anxiousness in the family. Family members are dealing with what could be a life-threatening experience, causing disruption in their routine functioning, neglect of career or school obligations, and often a growing sense of anxiety and being overwhelmed. Risk factors such as poverty, geography, and social status can reduce access to medical care and sources of support available to other families. Children in families with chronic illness often experience interruptions in participating in social supports through activities such as sports, music, scouts, and faith youth groups. Parents struggle with multiple demands of time and energy in addressing the challenges of chronic illness along with the day-to-day responsibilities of family life. While a referral for sibling play therapy can make an important contribution to family resilience, it includes the challenge of coordinating one more appointment with one more provider. Families with chronic illness have often had a range of positive to negative experiences with care providers, sometimes creating a barrier to establishing a trusting, therapeutic relationship.

Working with siblings together gives them an immediate support system of one another in establishing the therapeutic relationship. The therapeutic space becomes a meeting place that combines elements of the family setting and medical care setting. Play therapy interventions that reinforce sibling connection, develop shared anxiety-reduction skills among siblings, and re-establish sibling problem-solving capabilities all contribute to reducing the overall risk of anxiety and decreasing the additive effects of multiple sources of anxiety. The Neurosequential Model of Therapeutics (Barfield et al., 2012; Perry, 2006; Perry & Hambrick, 2008) outlines a progressive approach to interventions, starting with calming and nurturing interventions to reduce anxiety from lower parts of the brain prior to initiating more upper brain interventions such as the development of problem-solving skills. Various play therapy models provide a range of non-directive to directive approaches to reducing anxiety. A positive, calm, accepting, and often less directive approach invites the siblings to discover and utilize their own play strategies for anxiety reduction, utilizing the play materials in the room. Resilience can be cultivated and reinforced in metaphors of play, such as finding ways to tame a dragon, or they may be more directly modeled through more structured play. Expressive and reflective approaches promoting the expression of feelings (Crenshaw, 2006, 2009; Green, 2014; Green & Drewes, 2013) can be utilized, as well as developmentally based approaches such as Theraplay (Jernberg & Booth, 1999; Munns, 2000, 2009). Cognitive behavioral strategies provide more structure to make the implicit learning more explicit (Drewes, 2006, 2009).

Along with these in-session approaches to anxiety reduction, there are the beyond-session sources of anxiety as families deal with multiple health care providers, community resources, and extended family supports that may or may not be reassuring. Whenever possible, coordination of care between the play therapist and other providers can often help these other relationships become more nurturing and supportive. The socioeconomic and sociopolitical forces in the larger ecosystem should also be addressed through social justice advocacy efforts that address the socioeconomic and sociopolitical forces that perpetuate the risks and anxiety systemically. Indirectly and directly, the therapeutic alliance created within the therapeutic space can have an impact on every level of risk beyond that space.

Resilience in Sibling Play: 2. Reducing Self-Blaming

Play therapy can also provide ways of addressing self-blame seen in siblings dealing with chronic illness in the family. Children have acutely tuned emotional senses that combine with cognitive skills that include magical thinking to sometimes make them feel like they have far more agency over the effects of chronic illness than they really do. This distortion of views of causality can lead to a sense of over-responsibility and self-blame (O'Connor, 2000). In session, these siblings may present at both ends of the continuum, with some taking adult-like caretaking roles for other family members far beyond their abilities, and with others being overwhelmed by the sense of responsibility to the point of hopelessness and helplessness. Those siblings who are more parentified may also try to take responsibility for the session, taking a co-therapist rather than sibling role. Sometimes, they are quite relieved in session to finally take a break from their caretaking role, and will be quick to engage in playfulness. Considering the variety of possible presentations, the therapist should consider interventions that range in the degree of directiveness, and cultivating sibling interactions that help to challenge the assumptions of self-blame.

Resilience in Sibling Play: 3. Reducing Blaming by Others

A child's self-blame sometimes originates or is reinforced by attributions made by other family members or care providers who may have their own exaggerated sense of the child's abilities to impact the effects of the chronic illness on family life (Rutter, 1999, 2007; Seymour, 2015). Sometimes siblings play a role in reinforcing the scapegoating of one another, whether the healthy child is blamed for their lack of help and support, or the child who is ill is blamed for reluctance or resistance to comply with care plans. Play therapy with siblings gives an opportunity to identify in play interactions how this may be occurring and provide creative ways of challenging the cycles of blame in the sibling subset (Seymour, 2009).

Self-blame and other-blame can be minimized with an initial interview and assessment process that is strengths-based, non-judgmental, and collaborative. Siblings (just as the parents/caretakers) can benefit from basic information about their own stage of development as well as the other siblings, to help them have realistic expectations of one another when dealing with the challenges of chronic illness. Just as parent/caretaker education helps them address the blaming patterns of adults beyond the family, such as educators, youth leaders, or care providers, siblings can be helpful in moderating the blaming patterns of peers in the extended family, neighborhood, school, or treatment setting.

Resilience in Sibling Play: 4. Reducing Isolation and Enhancing Attachment

Chronic illness can isolate family members from each other as well as from supportive relationships beyond the family. Debilitating pain, extended healing time, intensive treatments, and concerns about infection and compliance with treatment regimens can all contribute to this isolation. There may be fears of infection, or culturally rein-forced beliefs about illness and disability that limit contact. The regular routines of family life that reinforce strong attachment can be disrupted and ambivalent attach-ment bonds can be challenged. Siblings may be separated due to hospitalizations, spe-cialized treatments away from home, or the reluctance to interact due to not knowing how to be helpful and supportive. Children with the chronic illness can be protective of their siblings, not wanting to burden or worry them, while healthy siblings may not be as quick to share their successes, not wanting to make the sibling who is ill feel left out of those positive events. Competition for limited parent/caretaker time and energy can lead to jealousy for any of the siblings who see the other as having more attention and support. Fredrickson (2001, 2004) described how negative emotions from these events can lead to fight, flight, or freeze responses that can reduce siblings' abilities to take alternate views of a situation, initiate positive actions, or mobilize personal strengths.

Sibling play therapy provides an opportunity to assess and intervene with these concerns of isolation and attachment challenges (Rutter, 1999, 2007; Seymour, 2015). Initiating the therapeutic relationship with each sibling provides an immediate oppor-tunity to begin reversing patterns of isolation and restoring more nurturing relation-ships with the siblings. Therapists are given clues about these needs through developing a relationship with each child, observing the patterns of interactions in session, and informing those observations with a family history of relational patterns and chronic illness. Some children may begin with difficulty engaging with the therapist with playful interactions in session. Other children are eager to engage and can appear to be almost frantic in their play interactions. Therapists will need flexibility in responding to these different patterns by adjusting the degree of engagement and varying the play materials in the room to be able to gently engage siblings who are reluctant while providing more active and energetic play options for those with urgent needs for connection.

Crenshaw (2006) has described a two-level approach to therapeutic engagement, depending on the needs and readiness of the children. A *coping track* focuses on gentle and supportive engagement, emphasizing the safety and warmth of the session that can help children with basic self-regulation, the development of prosocial skills, and basic problem-solving skills. An *invitational track* builds on the strengths created in the coping track, giving structure and nurture for children to address more painful or traumatic aspects of their lives. The coping track will be sufficient for many siblings dealing with chronic illness, providing the necessary experiences and tools to cultivate their resilience. Some siblings have more traumatic experiences with chronic illness, having been a part of life-threatening health events, and longer-term well-being will be improved with work in the invitational track. Through therapeutic play, siblings have opportunities to help one another better self-regulate, develop basic coping skills that support resilience, and rehearse more successful ways of dealing with the trauma of chronic illness. The natural sibling role in the attachment process combines elements of both the parent–child and peer–peer relationship, giving siblings a distinct function of impacting attachment within the family as well as trusted relationships beyond the family. All of this helps to repair and improve the attachment bonds of the family, pro-viding more support for each family member.

Resilience in Sibling Play: 5. Increasing Self-Esteem and Self-Efficacy

Rutter (1999, 2007) described how resilience could not only be enhanced by breaking negative chains of risk as described in the first four processes, but also enhanced by creating positive chains of protective factors described in the remaining four processes (Seymour, 2015). Family members dealing with chronic illness have long-term challenges to sources of self-esteem and self-efficacy. Chronic illness can disrupt children's access and ability to participate in many typical childhood experiences that can cultivate self-esteem. The uncertainty and unpredictability of chronic illness can reduce the sense of self-control and self-efficacy. Sibling play therapy sessions can become the setting where the smallest of successes can be cultivated, collaborative play encouraged with the siblings, and these experiences can begin to be translated to beyond-session opportunities for developing personal initiative. In session, therapists can be encouraging of children's initiatives in play to try new activities and test new skills through imaginative, expressive role play. These small experiences build on one another to promote more positive emotions. Fredrickson (2001, 2004) described this process by suggesting that "joy sparks an urge to play, interest sparks the urge to explore, contentment sparks the urge to savor and integrate, and love sparks a recurring cycle of each of these urges within safe, close relationships" (2004, p. 1367). It is this process of developing positive emotions in relationships that "fuel psychological resilience" (2004, p. 1372).

Expressive arts in play therapy give siblings small opportunities to take a risk in personal expression or creation that can lead to larger initiatives toward a fuller expression of emotions and an openness to new perspectives. Simple games in play are ways siblings can identify their strengths in motor and cognitive skills that lead to a greater confidence in day-to-day interactions. This broadening perspective and growing flexibility in initiating new behaviors sets the stage for creative play in the sixth resilience protective mechanism described later.

Brooks (1994a, 2009; Brooks & Goldstein, 2015) for many years has emphasized the importance of identifying and encouraging *islands of competence* in children to cultivate their resilience. What are a child's special interests and abilities that can be cultivated to give experiences of self-expression and success? This therapeutic mechanism for resilience begins at intake by taking a strengths-based approach to the child's history, including details of talents, abilities, and potentials identified by the parents, keeping in mind that some of these opportunities may be currently disrupted by the effects of chronic illness. Siblings may volunteer their own interests and abilities directly in words or indirectly through showing curiosity about certain play materials, wearing their sport clothes to a session, bringing their favorite book to the waiting room, or bringing a school project to show the therapist. Siblings can be an important source of identifying and affirming islands of competence in each other. Sometimes siblings may need some therapeutic reframing to acknowledge a sibling's interests that are very different from their own, or to make a competitive relationship more supportive. Consider how parent–child play therapy strategies from filial therapy (Van Fleet, 1994, 2000) can be adapted to cultivating sibling relationships through play.

Resilience in Sibling Play: 6. Increasing Creative Play to Foster Creative Problem Solving

The success of implementing the first five resilience mechanisms leads to encouraging continued growth through creative play and identifying ways to begin to take the successes in the sibling play sessions into the day-to-day life of family, school, and community (Rutter, 1999, 2007; Seymour, 2015). As the siblings make progress, the play therapist will begin to notice a progression of in-session play activities and themes, from crisis management to growth themes. Early themes of helplessness, isolation, grief, and conflict evolve into themes of strengths, skills, and personal agency. Through the course of play therapy, siblings and their families will experience setbacks, providing opportunities to come back to session, play out alternatives, and resume progress after the setback (Seymour & Erdman, 1996). These reframing experiences provide reinforcement of the earlier five resilience mechanisms, such as anxiety reduction and promoting self-efficacy (Walsh, 2016). As a family builds more confidence, these newfound strengths can become the beginning of better advocacy efforts to address systemic sources of risk and develop these resilience processes in extended family, school, community, and public policy.

Play therapists have a variety of ways to promote creative expression and problem solving in sibling sessions (Crenshaw, 2006, 2008, 2009; Crenshaw, Brooks, & Goldstein, 2015; Green & Drewes, 2013; Malchiodi & Crenshaw, 2015; Prendiville & Howard, 2016). Play therapy rooms may include play therapy materials such as art and craft supplies, building sets, puzzles, simple games, costumes, puppets, stuffed animals, or figures for role-play, or a sand tray with miniatures. Some siblings will be drawn to the variety and readily engage with several different materials. Others may benefit from some selection or gentle direction from the therapist, based on the child's sensory and attentional needs. Siblings engaged in play provide the therapist with a better understanding of the individual needs and perspectives as well as the interactional quality between the siblings. Symbolic play has the effect of rehearsing the concerns and developing the problem-solving strategies of siblings. The beneficial results may be left for siblings to absorb indirectly on their own, or depending on theoretical model, the results may be more directly applied through insight-based and/or cognitive behavioral approaches.

Resilience in Sibling Play: 7. Enhancing Nurturing Relationships Beyond the Playroom

To sustain these resilience processes beyond the therapeutic play space, children need nurturing relationships in family and community life (Rutter, 1999, 2007; Seymour, 2015). Children dealing with chronic illness can benefit from identifying supportive nurturing adults at school, faith groups, community groups, and medical settings (Webb, 2007). Chronic illness presents family members with challenges to time and energy and causes disruptions in the family patterns of leisure, sport, interests in the fine arts, or involvement with a faith group, limiting the access of children to their usual contacts for support. Brooks (2009) has described these individuals as *charismatic adults* who can play vital roles in promoting the other resilience processes, such as challenging self-blame and encouraging the child in activities that promote self-esteem and self-efficacy.

Sibling play in early sessions may include play themes of children being lost, help-less, and unable to find helpful figures in their play. As progress is made with the earlier resilience protective mechanisms, helping themes and play characters begin to be added in play. These helping figures may remain symbolic in the play or they may begin to be identified as actual support persons in their lives, as the work in session begins to extend to the siblings' world beyond the session. Much as with the fourth resilience mechanism (reducing isolation and enhancing attachment), siblings can play an impor-tant role in bridging the world of family relationships to the larger world of supportive peers and adults. Skills in emotional regulation, cooperation, and problem solving learned in earlier play therapy sessions are taken by siblings back into their world to better deal with day-to-day challenges.

Resilience in Sibling Play: 8. Learning to Make Meaning of Life's Experiences

The eighth resilience process is a metaprocess that unifies the other seven processes into an overarching resilience narrative highlighting the underlying values of the family and reinforcing the effects of the other seven protective mechanisms (Rutter, 1999, 2007; Seymour, 2015). "Through the creation of a shared narrative, resilience as a thera-peutic power of play moves a child from a very private starting point in facing adver-sity to a more public transition point into the child's beyond session life (Seymour, 2015, p. 45). Freeman, Epston, and Lobovits (1997) demonstrated how children can turn problem-saturated narratives into strengths-based narratives, even in the face of chronic illness. Cattanach (2008) and Taylor de Faoite (2011) describe narrative strate-gies such as using collaborative storytelling, externalizing the problems, and creating new stories of strength and success in the face of difficulty. At the cellular level, Siegel (2010, 2012, 2017) has provided insight in how family members are impacted on a neural level as they not only co-regulate one another, but co-create meanings about their shared experiences. These shared narratives impact siblings at the micro level of their own brain development, as well as the macro level of values and meaning of the challenges of chronic illness and the resilience protective mechanisms that promote positive adaptation.

CONCLUSION: THE POWER OF PLAY IN PROMOTING SIBLING RESILIENCE

Families facing chronic illness experience a variety of stressors that challenge its respec-tive members' abilities to maintain nurturing relationships with the demands of cop-ing with the chronic illness. Resilience research provides an important lens to health professionals serving these families to identify both the risk factors that need to be reduced as well as the protective factors that need to be enhanced. With resilience being developed through positive nurturing relationships, interventions that maximize the quality of these relationships will have the greatest impact in improving resilience for the family and individual family members. Informed by research of natural sibling development and relationships, family-based interventions aimed specifically at the sibling subset can become a useful part of an overall plan of care for a chronic illness. Play therapy, utilizing the natural developmental powers of play, gives providers an entry into the world of the sibling subset well-suited for minimizing risk factors and maximizing protective factors that promote resilience. Siblings can face the challenge of chronic illness with greater confidence, a growing repertoire of coping skills, and stronger connections to their support systems, enhanced by improving the sibling relationship through play therapy.

REFERENCES

Anderson, T., & Davis, C. (2011). Evidence-based practice with families of chronically ill children: A critical literature review. *Journal of Evidence-Based Social Work, 8*, 416–425.

Barfield, S., Dobson, C., Gaskill, R., & Perry, B. D. (2012). Neurosequential Model of Therapeutics in a therapeutic preschool: Implications for work with children with complex neuropsychiatric problems. *International Journal of Play Therapy, 21*, 30–44.

Bellin, M. H., & Kovacs, P. J. (2006). Fostering resilience in siblings of youths with a chronic health condition: A review of the literature. *Health & Social Work, 31*, 209–216.

Boss, P. (1999). *Ambiguous loss: Learning to live with unresolved grief.* Cambridge, MA: Harvard University Press.

Boss, P. (2002). *Family stress management: A contextual approach* (2nd ed.). Thousand Oaks, CA: Sage.

Brody, G. H. (2004). Siblings' direct and indirect contributions to child development. *Current Directions in Psychological Science, 13*, 124–126.

Brooks, R. B. (1994a). Children at risk: Fostering resilience and hope. *American Journal of Orthopsychiatry, 64*, 545–553.

Brooks, R. B. (1994b). Diagnostic issues and therapeutic interventions for children at risk. *American Journal of Orthopsychiatry, 64*, 508–509.

Brooks, R. B. (2009). The power of mind-sets: A personal journey to nurture dignity, hope, and resilience in children. In D. A. Crenshaw (Ed.), *Reverence in the healing process: Honoring strengths without trivializing suffering* (pp. 19–40). Lanham, MD: Jason Aronson.

Brooks, R. B., & Goldstein, S. (2015). The power of mindsets: Guideposts for a resilience-based treatment approach. In D. A. Crenshaw, R. B. Brooks & S. Goldstein (Eds.), *Fostering resilience through play therapy* (pp. 3–31). New York: Guilford Press.

Cattanach, A. (2008). *Narrative approaches in play with children.* London: Jessica Kingsley.

Cicirelli, V. G. (1995). *Sibling relationships across the life span.* New York: Plenum Press.

Cohen, S. M. (1999). Families coping with childhood chronic illness: A research review. *Family Systems & Health, 17*, 149–164.

Compas, B. E., Jaser, S. S., Dunn, M. J., & Rodriquez, E. M. (2012). Coping with chronic illness in childhood and adolescence. *Annual Review of Clinical Psychology, 8*, 455–480.

Crenshaw, D. A. (2006). *Evocative strategies in child and adolescent psychotherapy.* New York: Jason Aronson.

Crenshaw, D. A. (2008). *Therapeutic engagement of children and adolescents: Play symbol, drawing, and storytelling strategies.* Lanham, MD: Jason Aronson.

Crenshaw, D. A. (Ed.). (2009). *Reverence in the healing process: Honoring strengths without trivializing suffering.* Lanham, MD: Jason Aronson.

Crenshaw, D. A., Brooks, R. B., & Goldstein, S. (Eds.). (2015). *Fostering resilience through play therapy*. New York: Guilford Press.

Davey, M., Kissil, K., & Lynch, L. (Eds.). (2016). *Helping children and families cope with parental illness: A clinician's guide*. New York: Routledge.

Dodgson, J. E., Garwick, A. W., Blozis, S. A., Patterson, J. M., Bennett, F. C., & Blum, R. W. (2000). Uncertainty in childhood chronic conditions and family distress in families of young children. *Journal of Family Nursing, 6*, 252–266.

Donaldson, G. (1996). Between practice and theory: Melanie Klein, Anna Freud, and the development of child analysis. *Journal of the History of the Behavioral Sciences, 32*, 160–176.

Drewes, A. A. (2006). Play-based interventions. *Journal of Early Childhood and Infant Psychology, 2*, 139–156.

Drewes, A. A. (2009). *Blending play therapy with cognitive behavioral therapy: Evidence-based and other effective treatments and techniques*. New York: John Wiley.

Drewes, A. A. (2011a). Integrative play therapy. In C. E. Schaefer (Ed.), *Foundations of play therapy* (2nd ed., pp. 349–364). Hoboken, NJ: John Wiley.

Drewes, A. A. (2011b). Integrating play therapy theories into practice. In A. A. Drewes, S. C. Bratton & C. E. Schaefer (Eds.), *Integrative play therapy* (pp. 21–35). Hoboken, NJ: John Wiley.

Drewes, A. A., Bratton, S. C., & Schaefer, C. E. (Eds.). (2011). *Integrative play therapy*. New York: John Wiley.

Dunn, J. (2007). Siblings and socialization. In J. E. Grusec & P. D. Hastings (Eds.), *Handbook of socialization: Theory and research* (pp. 309–327). New York: Guilford.

Eberle, S. G. (2014). The elements of play: Toward a philosophy and a definition of play. *American Journal of Play, 6*, 214–233.

Feinberg, M. E., Solmeyer, A. R., & McHale, S. M. (2010). The third rail of family systems: Sibling relationships, mental and behavioral health, and preventive intervention in childhood and adolescence. *Clinical Child and Family Psychology Review, 15*, 43–57.

Frank, J. D., & Frank, J. B. (1993). *Persuasion and healing* (3rd ed.). Baltimore, MD: Johns Hopkins University.

Fredrickson, B. L. (2001). The role of positive emotions in positive psychology: The broaden-and-build theory of positive emotions. *American Psychologist, 56*, 218–226.

Fredrickson, B. L. (2004). The broaden-and-build theory of positive emotions. *Philosophical Transactions of the Royal Society of London: Biological Sciences, 359*, 1367–1377.

Freeman, J., Epston, D., & Lobovits, D. (1997). *Playful approaches to serious problems: Narrative therapy with children and their families*. New York: W. W. Norton.

Freud, A. (1966/trans. 1946/1936). *The ego and the mechanisms of defense* (rev. ed.). New York: International Universities Press.

Gabel, S., & Bemporad, J. (1994a). An expanded concept of countertransference. *Journal of the American Academy of Child and Adolescent Psychiatry, 33*, 140–142.

Gabel, S., & Bemporad, J. (1994b). Variations in countertransference reactions in psychotherapy with children. *American Journal of Psychotherapy, 48*, 111–119.

Gamble, W. C., & Modry-Mandell, K. (2008). Family relations and the adjustment of young children of Mexican descent: Do family cultural values moderate these associations? *Social Development, 17*, 358–397.

Garwick, A. W., Patterson, J. M., Meschke, L. L., Bennett, F. C., & Blum, R. W. (2002). The uncertainty of preadolescents' chronic health conditions and family distress. *Journal of Family Nursing, 8*, 11–31.

Gil, E. (2014). *Play in family therapy* (2nd ed.). New York: Guilford.

Gil, E., & Rubin, L. (2005). Countertransference play: Informing and enhancing therapist self-awareness through play. *International Journal of Play Therapy, 14*, 87–102.

Goldstein, S., & Brooks, R. B. (Eds.). (2006). *Handbook of resilience in children*. New York: Springer.

Green, E.J. (2014). *The handbook of Jungian play therapy with children and adolescents*. Baltimore, MD: Johns Hopkins University Press.

Green, E.J., & Drewes, A. (Eds.). (2013). *Integrating expressive arts and play therapy with children: A guidebook for clinicians and educators*. Hoboken, NJ: John Wiley.

Hernandez, D.J. (1997). Child development and social demography of childhood. *Child Development, 68,* 149–169.

Jernberg, A., & Booth, P. (1999). *Theraplay* (2nd ed.). San Francisco: Jossey-Bass.

Jessop, D.J., & Stein, R.E.K. (1985). Uncertainty and its relation to the psychological and social correlates of chronic illness in children. *Social Science and Medicine, 20,* 993–999.

Killoren, S.E., Thayer, S.M., & Updegraff, K.A. (2008). Conflict resolution between Mexican origin adolescent siblings. *Journal of Marriage and Family, 70,* 1200–1212.

Kim, J., McHale, S.M., Osgood, D.W., & Crouter, A.C. (2006). Longitudinal course and family correlates of sibling relationships from childhood through adolescence. *Child Development, 77,* 1746–1761.

Klein, M. (1932). *The psycho-analysis of children*. London: Hogarth Press.

Kleinman, A.M. (1980). *Patients and healers in the context of culture*. Berkeley: University of California Press.

Kleinman, A.M. (1988). *The illness narratives: Suffering, healing, and the human condition*. New York: Basic Books.

Kramer, L. (2010). The essential ingredients of successful sibling relationships: An emerging framework for advancing theory and practice. *Child Development Perspectives, 4,* 80–86.

Livneh, H. (2001). Psychosocial adaptation to chronic illness and disability: A conceptual framework. *Rehabilitation Counseling Bulletin, 44,* 151–160.

Malawista, K.L. (2004). Rescue fantasies in child therapy: Countertransference/transference enactments. *Child & Adolescent Social Work Journal, 21,* 373–386.

Malchiodi, C.A., & Crenshaw, D.A. (Eds.). (2015). *Play and creative arts therapy for attachment trauma*. New York: Guilford Press.

Martire, L.M., Lustig, A.P., Schulz, R., Miller, G.E., & Helgeson, V.S. (2004). Is it beneficial to involve a family member? A meta-analysis of psychosocial interventions for chronic illness. *Health Psychology, 23,* 599–611.

Masten, A.S., & Coatsworth, J.D. (1998). The development of competence in favorable and unfavorable environments: Lessons from research on successful children. *American Psychologist, 53,* 205–220.

McDaniel, S.H., Doherty, W.J., & Hepworth, J. (2014). *Medical family therapy and integrated care* (2nd ed.). Washington, DC: American Psychological Association.

McDaniel, S.H., Hepworth, J., & Doherty, W.J. (1992). *Medical family therapy: A biopsychosocial approach to families with health problems* (1st ed.). Washington, DC: American Psychological Association.

McHale, S.M., Updegraff, K.A., & Whiteman, S.D. (2012). Sibling relationships and influences in childhood and adolescence. *Journal of Marriage and Family, 74,* 913–930.

McHale, S.M., Whiteman, S.D., Kim, J., & Crouter, A.C. (2007). Characteristics and correlates of sibling relationships in two-parent African American families. *Journal of Family Psychology, 21,* 227–235.

Meichenbaum, D. (2009). Bolstering resilience: Benefiting from lessons learned. In D. Brom, R. Pat-Horenczyk & J.D. Ford (Eds.), *Treating traumatized children: Risk, resilience and recovery* (pp. 183–191). New York: Routledge.

Milevsky, A. (2011). *Sibling relationships in childhood and adolescence: Predictors and outcomes*. New York: Columbia University Press.

Munns, E. (2000). *Theraplay: Innovations in attachment-enhancing play therapy*. Northvale, NJ: Jason Aronson.

Munns, E. (Ed.). (2009). *Applications of family and group Theraplay*. Lanham, MD: Jason Aronson.

Mulroy, S., Robertson, L., Aiberti, K., Leonard, H., & Bower, C. (2008). The impact of having a sibling with an intellectual disability: parental perspectives in two disorders. *Journal of Intellectual Disability Research*, *52*(3), 216–229.

O'Brien, I., Duffy, A., & Nicholl, H. (2009). Impact of childhood chronic illnesses on siblings: A literature review. *British Journal of Nursing*, *18*, 1358–1365.

O'Connor, K. J. (2000). *Play therapy primer* (2nd ed.). New York: John Wiley.

Paterson, B. L. (2001). The shifting perspectives model of chronic illness. *Journal of Nursing Scholarship*, *33*, 21–26.

Perry, B. D. (2006). The Neurosequential Model of Therapeutics: Applying principles of neuroscience to clinical work with traumatized and maltreated children. In N. B. Webb (Ed.), *Working with traumatized youth in child welfare* (pp. 27–52). New York: Guilford Press.

Perry, B. D., & Hambrick, E. P. (2008). The neurosequential model of therapeutics. *Reclaiming Children and Youth*, *17*, 38–43.

Power, P. W., & Dell Orto, A. E. (2004). *Families living with chronic illness and disability: Interventions, challenges, and opportunities*. New York: Springer.

Prendiville, E., & Howard, J. (Eds.). (2016). *Creative psychotherapy: Applying the principles of neurobiology to play and expressive art-based practice*. New York: Routledge.

Rolland, J. S. (1994). *Families, illness, and disability: An integrative treatment model*. New York: Basic Books.

Rutter, M. E. (1999). Resilience concepts and findings: Implications for family therapy. *Journal of Family Therapy*, *21*, 119–144.

Rutter, M. E. (2007). Resilience, competence, and coping. *Child Abuse & Neglect*, *31*, 205–209.

Schaefer, C. E. (2001). Prescriptive play therapy. *International Journal of Play Therapy*, *10*, 57–73.

Schaefer, C. E. (2011). Prescriptive play therapy. In C. E. Schaefer (Ed.), *Foundations of play therapy* (2nd ed., pp. 365–378). New York: John Wiley.

Schaefer, C. E., & Carey, L. J. (Eds.). (1994). *Family play therapy*. Northvale, NJ: Jason Aronson.

Schaefer, C. E., & Drewes, A. (Eds.). (2014). *The therapeutic powers of play: 20 core agents of change* (2nd ed.). New York: John Wiley.

Seymour, J. W. (2009). Resiliency-based approaches and the healing process in play therapy. In D. A. Crenshaw (Ed.), *Reverence in the healing process: Honoring strengths without trivializing suffering* (pp. 71–84). Lanham, MD: Jason Aronson.

Seymour, J. W. (2011). History of psychotherapy integration and related research. In A. A. Drewes, S. C. Bratton, & C. E. Schaefer (Eds.), Integrative play therapy (pp. 3–19). New York: John Wiley.

Seymour, J. W. (2014). Resiliency as a therapeutic power of play. In C. E. Schaefer & A. A. Drewes (Eds.), *The therapeutic powers of play: 20 core agents of change* (2nd ed., pp. 241–263). New York: John Wiley.

Seymour, J. W. (2015). Resilience enhancing factors in play therapy. In D. A. Crenshaw, R. B. Brooks & S. Goldstein (Eds.), *Fostering resilience through play therapy* (pp. 32–50). New York: Guilford Press.

Seymour, J. W., & Erdman, P. E. (1996). Family play therapy using a resiliency model. *International Journal of Play Therapy*, *5*, 19–30.

Sharpe, D., & Rossiter, L. (2002). Siblings of children with a chronic illness: A meta-analysis. *Journal of Pediatric Psychology*, *27*, 699–710.

Shirk, S. R., & Russell, R. L. (1996). *Change processes in child psychotherapy: Revitalizing treatment and research*. New York: Guilford Press.

Siegel, D. J. (2010). *Mindsight: The new science of personal transformation*. New York: Random House.

Siegel, D. J. (2012). *The developing mind: How relationships and the brain interact to shape who we are* (2nd ed.). New York: Guilford Press.

Siegel, D. J. (2017). *Mind: A journey to the heart of being human*. New York: W. W. Norton.

Strohm, K.E. (2008). Too important to ignore: Siblings of children with special needs. *Australian eJournal for the Advancement of Mental Health*, 7, 1–6.

Taylor de Faoite, A. (Ed.). (2011). *Narrative play therapy: Theory and practice*. London: Jessica Kingsley.

Tedeschi, R.G., & Kilmer, R.P. (2005). Assessing strengths, resilience, and growth to guide clinical interventions. *Professional Psychology: Research and Practice*, 36, 230–237.

Thorne, S., Paterson, B.L., Acorn, S., Canam, C., Joachim, G., & Jillings, C. (2002). Chronic illness experience: Insights from a metastudy. *Qualitative Health Research*, 12, 437–452.

Torpy, J.M., Campbell, A., & Glass, R.M. (2010). Chronic diseases of children. *Journal of the American Medical Association (JAMA)*, 303, 682.

Updegraff, K.A., McHale, S.M., Whiteman, S.D., Thayer, S.M., & Delgado, M.Y. (2005). Adolescent sibling relationships in Mexican American families: Exploring the role of familism. *Journal of Family Psychology*, 19, 512–522.

Van Cleave, J., Gortmaker, S.L., & Perrin, J.M. (2010). Dynamics of obesity and chronic health conditions among children and youth. *Journal of the American Medical Association (JAMA)*, 303, 623–630.

Van Fleet, R. (1994). *Filial therapy: Strengthening parent-child relationships through play*. Sarasota, FL: Professional Resource Press.

Van Fleet, R. (2000). *A parent's handbook of filial therapy: Building strong families with play*. Boiling Springs, PA: Play Therapy Press.

Van Riper, M. (2003). The sibling experience of living with childhood chronic illness and disability. *Annual Review of Nursing Research*, 21, 279–302.

Walsh, F. (Ed.). (2016). *Strengthening family resilience* (3rd ed.). New York: Guilford.

Webb, N.B. (Ed.). (2007). *Play therapy with children in crisis: A casebook for practitioners* (3rd ed.). New York: Guilford Press.

Whiteman, S.D., McHale, S.M., & Soli, A. (2011). Theoretical perspectives on sibling relationships. *Journal of Family Theory & Review*, 3, 134–139.

Winnicott, D.W. (1971). *Playing and reality*. London: Tavistock.

Wise, P.H. (2004). The transformation of child health in the United States. *Health Affairs*, 23, 9–25.

Wood, B.L., Klebba, K.B., & Miller, B.D. (2000). Evolving the biobehavioral family model: The fit of attachment. *Family Process*, 39, 319–344.

Wright, M.O., & Masten, A.S. (2006). Resilience processes in development. In S. Goldstein & R.B. Brooks (Eds.), *Handbook of resilience in children* (pp. 17–38). New York: Springer.

CHAPTER 14

Family-Oriented Treatment of Childhood Chronic Medical Illness

The Power of Play in Filial Therapy

Risë VanFleet

I thought I was never going to get to play again!
—a 7-year-old girl with cancer (after a play session in Filial Therapy)

Jack was 8 years old when he was diagnosed with diabetes. The early days of getting his blood glucose levels stabilized and learning to do insulin injections and the finger sticks for blood glucose testing were traumatic for him and his parents, Tim and Rena. He screamed and fought back as they tried to follow the doctors' orders, knowing that his life was at stake. The happy, well-adjusted boy that Tim and Rena had known had disappeared, replaced by a sullen, oppositional child who seemed to fight them at every turn. The worst seemed to be the glucose testing, which was needed several times each day, but he also resisted the dietary restrictions and had begun sneaking forbidden sweet things to his room. Jack's parents had learned that better diabetic control in the early years of the disease lowered his risk for the many complications of diabetes later, and they were adamant that he follow the regimen strictly. They were extremely worried about him and watched everything he did to ensure that he did not have elevated blood sugar levels or fall into insulin shock.

From Jack's point of view, life had changed dramatically, too. He had enjoyed an active life, with many outdoor activities and a fair amount of freedom riding his bike in their safe, rural community. Suddenly, he had to see doctors who frightened him, his parents were struggling with him to prick his fingers and give him injections, and they were restricting him from eating the sweets that he loved. Even at his good friend's birthday party, his mother had come along and prevented him from eating any birthday cake. His world seemed to be closing in on him. He knew he had something wrong with him and that he didn't feel well all the time, but he didn't understand the need for all the scrutiny and discomfort.

Rena and Tim had consulted with the pediatrician about his increasingly challenging behavior difficulties, and the pediatrician referred the family to me. At this time, the family had been dealing with the aftermath of the diagnosis for 8 months, and they were all stressed.

After I did my usual assessment, I recommended Filial Therapy (FT) to them. I thought it would help with the loss of control that Jack was feeling and help the entire family understand the complex emotions that were playing a role for all family members. I could provide support for Rena and Tim while showing them how to provide support for Jack. They all needed to feel more in control of what was happening, and they had to find ways to cope with Jack's diabetes and its management. I knew that FT could help the entire family make a better adjustment.

And it did. After just a few parent–child play sessions, Jack's old happy self began to re-emerge, and his parents were able to see the situation from his point of view, too. They began reconnecting after the traumatic months following his diagnosis.

BACKGROUND

Advances in medicine have significantly reduced child mortality from illness, and many diseases that previously carried a death sentence are now considered chronic illnesses because treatment has improved and lives have been spared or extended. While estimates vary, there are indications that as many as 26% of children in the United States are believed to have chronic illnesses that require lifestyle adaptations or ongoing medical care and management (Cleave, Gortmaker, & Perrin, 2010). When developmental and mental health issues are included, as many as 43% of children in the United States live with one of 20 common chronic conditions, the most common being asthma, diabetes, cystic fibrosis, malnutrition, developmental disabilities, and others (Cantrell & Kelly, 2015). Chronic childhood medical conditions put additional strains on families in a variety of ways.

For the purposes of this chapter, the term *chronic illness* is used to refer to "a long-lasting illness that requires ongoing medical supervision or treatment and/or results in physical debilitation or life-style alteration" (VanFleet, 2003, p. 65). The focus here will be on medical illnesses rather than developmental or mental health conditions, and includes childhood cancer, diabetes, asthma, cystic fibrosis, renal disease, heart disease, AIDS, and sickle cell disease.

When children are diagnosed with serious and chronic medical conditions, it can disrupt the entire family. Not only does the child have emotional and behavioral reactions, but the process of caring for and raising a child with a chronic illness can add stress for parents, siblings, and the family as a whole. The demands on families include management of the illness at home, medical treatments, occasional hospitalizations, eating restrictions, financial pressures, time for many medical appointments, and the discomfort and anxiety that is often attached. Many families learn to cope with these demands quite well, but the additional stresses can put them at risk for adjustment or psychosocial problems. This chapter briefly discusses the strains on families coping with a chronically ill child, followed by the use of FT to assist all family members with the social, emotional, and behavioral sequelae of chronic illness.

THE IMPACT OF CHILDHOOD CHRONIC ILLNESS ON FAMILIES

Chronic illness impacts families directly through the illness itself and its treatment or management, as well as through a range of family lifestyle disruptions. Detailed descriptions of family life with childhood chronic illness are found elsewhere (Bigbee, 1992; Cantrell & Kelly, 2015; Donoghue & Kraft, 2009; Eddy, 2013; Eisenberg, Sutkin, & Jansen, 1984; Graziano et al., 2016; Hauenstein, 1990; Hobbs, Perrin, & Ireys 1985; Shuman, 1996; VanFleet, 1985, 1992). The following brief descriptions are drawn from these sources as well as the author's 35 years of researching and working with children with chronic illnesses and their families.

Impact of the Illness

Chronic illnesses often are accompanied by discomfort and pain. Sometimes they drain the child's energy, hinder movement, or restrict diet. The illness can affect mood and behavior directly, and it can alter physical appearances. Emotions of all family members can be affected by worry or anger or a sense of loss. In most cases, the illness represents a loss of control with restrictions on normal activities.

All family members can feel confused about the illness and require information to understand it as fully as possible. Young children, in particular, might struggle to understand what is happening to them. Because family attentions often must center on the ill child, siblings can feel left out, resentful, or even guilty. Parents must learn complex medical information and make decisions in the context of confusing or changing medical information. Emotional reactions of all family members can create distress within the family, which can be difficult to resolve because of the omnipresence of the illness.

Childhood chronic illness can also have an impact on family members' social interactions with each other, as well as with extended family members, friends, neighbors, teachers, and employers (VanFleet, 1985). Children with the illness often report feeling 'different,' as do siblings of chronically ill children. Life changes with the first symptoms, and then the diagnosis, and it is not likely to return to what had been 'normal' up to that point. While a 'new normal' is possible, much adaptation is required first. In my dissertation research (VanFleet, 1985), and subsequent psychotherapy and play therapy practice in this area, there have been many stories presented by children with chronic illness, siblings, and parents about the numerous and large hurdles they had to surmount.

For example, a 9-year-old girl with diabetes was pleased to win a prize at a neighborhood Halloween costume contest. The prize was a chocolate candy bar. Almost immediately, a neighbor woman involved with the contest came up to the girl and loudly announced, "Oh! You can't have that! You've got sugar!" while snatching the candy from the girl's hands. The girl had planned to give the candy bar to her brothers, but she first wanted her photo taken with it to show the prize she had won. She was devastated, and her mother regretted long afterward that they didn't retrieve the candy bar from the woman for the girl.

Family roles often change with a diagnosis of childhood chronic illness. Siblings of ill children may become caregivers and protectors. If they are old enough, parents often trust them with childcare duties more than anyone they might hire, simply because the siblings know the medical processes and daily routines. Role strain occurs, and family recreational activities don't happen as often as before (Hauenstein, 1990; Quittner, Opipari, Espelage, Carter, & Eid, 1998).

Impact of the Treatment

"The treatment is worse than the illness!" is a phrase often heard from families dealing with chronic illness in a child. Treatment procedures can be painful, scary, intrusive, and traumatizing. Medical testing equipment can be frightening to adults, not to mention children. Dietary restrictions are difficult for parents to impose and for children to comply with. Multiple injections, chemotherapy, dialysis, and medication side effects represent daily reminders of discomfort, pain, and stress. When hospitalizations occur, they separate family members when they could most use the support from each other. Even when parents try their best to maintain supportive relationships, the intrusion of medical treatments into their daily lives can interfere with healthy attachment relationships.

For example, I worked for a couple of years in a medical center that served many children with cystic fibrosis. The families came from a wide geographic area, and often, one parent would stay with the hospitalized child while the other parent and siblings stayed at home. Parents on both sides of this divide reported feeling isolated and alone, despite frequent phone contacts. Those who remained at home worried in between updates about their absent family members.

Because so much medical management now takes place at home, family members often must learn and implement complex procedures. If the child with the chronic illness balks at the treatment, it can be frustrating for parents or lead to even more discord in the family. It is hard for parents to find the right balance between enacting the treatment plan and providing choices for their children to help maintain a healthy sense of control. There is a considerable sense of helplessness against the disease that can occur, and sometimes medical professionals can exacerbate this by putting even more pressure on parents to get compliance from the child. In one case, a doctor told a mother to watch her son "like a hawk" so he does everything right. The mother did that, fearing for her son's good health, and the son rebelled strongly against the constant surveillance and correction of his behavior. It is hard to find a balance when a life is threatened by illness.

Family Lifestyle Disruptions

There are many other ways that the experience of chronic illness in a child can disrupt family life, beyond what the illness itself and its treatment do. The management of time, finances, education, extended family, and friends all can be altered for these families (VanFleet, 2003). In general, having a child with a chronic illness requires several additional hours of parental attention each day, and this, of course, has an impact on how life is lived. Leisure time is reduced, as is employment in some cases. Reduced employment seems to affect mothers more than fathers, but it has a financial impact on the entire family (Hatzmann, Peek, Heymans, Maurice-Stam, & Grootenhuis, 2014). Some have shown a higher incidence of post-traumatic stress disorder in mothers, and especially in African American mothers (Greening, Stoppelbein, & Cheek, 2016). While many families adapt quite well, there are some who struggle with determining optimum levels of protection, control, and warmth, struggling to build mutually rewarding parent–child relationships (Pinquart, 2013). In my own study (VanFleet, 1985), parents reported feeling distressed that the family lifestyle changes impacted their children who were not ill, and they also reported feeling deprived of 'normal' life experiences themselves. In one parent support meeting for parents of children with type 1 diabetes that I attended to recruit people for my study, the attendees rather sheepishly asked me at the end of the meeting if I would like to stay for ice cream. They explained that they felt guilty having ice cream when their diabetic child could not, but that it was one of the few indulgences they had for themselves.

Education can also pose challenges. Some illnesses interfere with school attendance, or the child needs special arrangements or attention in the school setting. This seems to occur frequently (Donoghue & Kraft, 2009; Rynard, Chambers, Klinck, & Gray, 1998; VanFleet, 1985). Children with a chronic illness report that they dislike being pulled aside for these needs, siblings report feeling protective of the ill child when they are teased or bullied, and parents report that their own ability to relax when their children are at school depends heavily on their trust in the teacher and school nurse in dealing with medical management issues that arise.

Families also report strained relationships, at least at times, with extended family members and neighbors. The biggest complaint parents have with extended family members is when they disregard the medical management of the illness against the parents' instructions. A commonly cited example is when grandparents offer sweets to the child, overriding parents' objections with "It's okay. Just this once. What can it hurt?" While the grandparents mean well, parents have reported an increase in behavioral struggles with diet after such instances. In another example, a teenage boy in remission from cancer who painted houses during the summer was immediately told by one of his customers that she no longer needed his services because she "didn't want the responsibility of it all" when she learned of his diagnosis.

All of these factors complicate family life. Many families adapt and cope with these added challenges (Drotar, 1997; VanFleet, 1985), but some struggle with the medical system, the school system, making ends meet, and developing healthy relationships within the family. Some parents divorce under the strain of it. Most families report a loss of spontaneity in their lives, and at least some elevation of stress in the family. Furthermore, parent stress and child stress in the face of chronic illness seem to be associated with each other (Robinson, Gerhardt, Vannatta, & Noll, 2007).

FAMILY INTERVENTION: FILIAL THERAPY

The prior section's description of the stresses facing families of children with chronic illnesses might be depressing to some readers. It does demonstrate how many facets of childhood chronic illness are potentially problematic for all members of the family.

At the same time, families can be highly resilient in the face of tremendous challenges (Crenshaw, Brooks, & Goldstein, 2015; VanFleet & Mochi, 2015). For those who are not, individual and family therapeutic intervention can help build coping strategies and family cohesiveness in the face of chronic illness.

Because the entire family system is impacted in multiple ways by childhood chronic illness, it seems that the core intervention needs to involve the entire family. Because the most developmentally appropriate way to work with children, including those with illnesses and their siblings, is to use the language of play, it seems that a play-based approach is also indicated. Filial Therapy (FT), which is a theoretically integrative approach that combines family therapy with play therapy, offers considerable assistance to these families. FT can also be used as a preventive approach for families before they experience significant problems, or it can be used to intervene in highly complex and multifaceted problems. I have had experience conducting FT groups with families who seem to be coping well, or who have just recently been diagnosed, as well as with families who have extremely challenging problems triggered by or surrounding the child's illness. Family feedback has been universally very positive, and some parents have even returned to graduate school to learn to conduct it and assist other families. The sections that follow describe FT briefly, discuss its relevance to this population, highlight research and required training, and offer a case study to illustrate.

What Is Filial Therapy?

FT was developed by Drs. Bernard and Louise Guerney starting in the late 1950s and extending throughout their careers (Guerney, 1964; Guerney, 1983; Guerney & Ryan, 2013; VanFleet, 2014; VanFleet & Guerney, 2003). At this writing, they remain involved in the field. FT combines play therapy and family therapy in a psychoeducational model that has been shown to be highly effective. It is very beneficial for families experiencing chronic illness (VanFleet, 1983, 1992, 2003).

In FT, the therapist trains and supervises parents as they conduct special half-hour child-centered play sessions with their own children. The principles and skills that parents learn are drawn directly from child-centered play therapy (VanFleet, Sywulak, & Sniscak, 2010), but the parents are not considered 'therapists.' They simply learn the skills as a means of enhancing their attachment and relationships with their children. The FT practitioner remains in the therapist role, teaching, guiding, and coaching parents as they learn to use the skills and run the play sessions, and then processing dynamic material in the form of play themes and parent reactions to the sessions. With appropriate training and supervisory support, parents are eventually able to conduct these special play sessions at home without the therapist's direct supervision, although they still review them with the therapist.

The goals of FT are to help parents create a safe, accepting climate in which their children can express their feelings, learn to understand their world, solve a wide range of problems, and develop confidence in themselves and their parents. FT is designed to help parents become fully responsive to their children's feelings and problems, to improve their abilities to solve child- and family-related problems in a more child-attuned manner, and to become more skillful as parents. Families who take part in FT develop better communication skills, problem-solving skills, healthier attachments, coping capabilities, and greater family cohesion. Families also learn to have fun together.

FT is a theoretically integrative form of therapy. It draws from psychodynamic, humanistic, behavioral, interpersonal, cognitive, developmental/attachment, and family systems theories. Principles and methods from these foundations are blended in a unique psychoeducational approach in which the therapist serves as both clinician and educator. The theoretical contributions are described fully in Guerney and Ryan (2013) and in VanFleet (2014).

There are several features that make FT unique, the essential characteristics that must be present to consider an intervention to be FT. These are described in VanFleet (2014), and are also listed on my website (www.play-therapy.com/professionals.html). There are additional formats of FT that may not meet all of the essential features, but are inspired by FT and serve as valuable interventions in their own right. The most notable of these is Landreth and Bratton's (2015) Child-Parent Relationship Therapy, a 10-week parent education group format that has been effectively used with parents of ill children, too.

Benefits of FT for Families of Children With Chronic Illnesses

When considering the many needs of families with chronically ill children, there are a number of ways that FT is beneficial:

1. FT is designed specifically to strengthen family relationships. Because these can be strained by the presence of childhood chronic illness, FT can provide positive experiences that counteract the many stresses families are facing. It provides an avenue for family members to support each other fully.
2. FT gives parents something they can do that truly helps their children. This is vital for parents who feel helpless in the face of the child's illness and all that entails. It provides a bit of a respite, too, from the intensity of medical treatment and the unrelenting rigors of daily illness management.
3. FT allows children an opportunity to express their many mixed emotions and be understood by those who matter most—their parents. Too often, parents focus on getting medical compliance from the child and can experience child feelings as an annoyance or something that gets in the way. FT helps put those feelings center-stage, so they can be expressed and processed.
4. FT also allows siblings to regain some attention that they may have lost from the family in the midst of the medical appointments or processes. Parents have finite amounts of energy, and at times, siblings live in the shadow of the illness, expected to grow up and be understanding, even when their own needs might be neglected. FT gives these children a dedicated time with their parents where they can be heard and feel supported, too.

5. FT helps parents provide a generally supportive atmosphere for all of their children, and even of each other, as they learn how to traverse the difficult emotional landscape of chronic illness.

6. In the parent-child play sessions of FT, children have considerable control over the toys and how they wish to use them. They can express any feeling and have their parents accept it. Only behaviors that pose risk or destructiveness are limited, and the therapist helps parents understand the more difficult feelings children might express, such as anger, frustration, sadness, and anxiety. Because of the control permitted in the play sessions, children, too, have a way to counteract the helplessness that the illness imposes. They learn that there are still things in life that are pleasurable and over which they have some power.

7. FT provides parents with specific skills as well as how to use them in various contexts. This gives them tools to use to manage some of the difficult interactions surrounding the illness and its treatment.

8. Parents have strong feelings, too, of grief, loss, anger, frustration, anxiety, and uncertainty. These are sometimes triggered during the FT play sessions. The therapist is there to provide support and understanding, to reframe the meaning of the play, to help parents gain perspective on the challenges in their lives. FT offers hope that life can regain a sense of normalcy, even if it's a different 'normal' than what they had before. FT supports the parents as they support their children.

FT sessions are held with one parent and one child at a time. This allows all the children to have their own special times in which they can play out the things they have on their minds. Each parent plays with each child, however, so they also are able to build their own unique attachments with each child. Many times, the parents are encouraged to watch each other's play sessions with the therapist so they can eventually support each other at home. Parents learn a common set of skills and attitudes, and this seems to help them be more consistent with each other as parents.

FT is a time-limited approach with a great deal of flexibility. Families with mild to moderate problems typically require 17 to 20 1-hour sessions. More severe problems might take longer. Families with chronically ill children often have more demands on their time from their medical involvement, so sometimes they benefit from a shorter FT format, such as the 10-session, 11-hour version described in VanFleet (2003). The fact that families eventually conduct the play sessions on their own at home reduces the overall number of sessions needed. In some cases, families of ill children have found FT to offer such support to them as a whole that they prefer to continue for a longer period of time. FT offers the flexibility of many different options.

The FT Process

The sequence and methods of FT are provided in detail in other resources (Guerney & Ryan, 2013; VanFleet, 2014). They will be described briefly.

First, the therapist listens carefully to the needs that parents express, empathically responding to show or clarify understanding and to convey acceptance. The therapist also asks the parents to explain how the illness and its treatment has impacted them on multiple levels—as individuals, partners, parents, each of their children, with extended family, neighbors, and friends, at school, in the community at large and financially. The therapist also asks what their experiences have been like with the medical community—what has gone well and what has been frustrating. Again, the therapist listens carefully and empathically.

Second, the therapist uses a Family Play Observation (VanFleet, 2014) to understand family dynamics better. This involves the entire family coming to play in the playroom for approximately 20 minutes. The therapist does not provide much structure and observes the various interactions as the family spends this time together. The therapist then meets with parents alone at the end of this period, asking them to reflect on what aspects of the Family Play Observation are similar or dissimilar to what happens at home. The therapist empathically listens once again, building trust and acceptance. At the end of this session, the therapist usually makes recommendations for treatment. When FT is recommended, the therapist provides a description, a rationale based on the needs expressed and observed, and outlines the rest of the process, answering any questions that parents have.

Third, the therapist demonstrates the child-centered play sessions with each of the children in the family while the parents observe. The therapist then meets with the parents alone after that to answer questions and to further explain how this type of intervention is likely to benefit them. Specific behaviors and emotions expressed by the children are also discussed.

Fourth, the therapist holds two or three sessions to train the parents in the play session skills: structuring, empathic listening, child-centered imaginary play, and limit setting. This is done in a graduated and supportive way that is designed to ensure parent success. Each parent participates in two mock play sessions in which the therapist pretends to be a child and plays in a manner that allows each parent to practice the skills at whatever level is appropriate for him or her. The therapist provides coaching feedback along the way, and then the mock play session is stopped so that more in-depth feedback can be covered. The mock sessions are difficult for therapists to learn to conduct properly, but they enhance the learning experience for parents and allow them to learn quickly how to conduct the sessions.

Fifth, the parents begin to conduct the child-centered, non-directive play sessions with their own children, under the supervision of the therapist. The play sessions are held with one parent and one child at a time for 20 to 30 minutes each. At the end of each parent–child play session, the therapist discusses it fully with the parent, giving positive and specific feedback about the things the parent has done well and making one or two suggestions for improvement. As parents gain confidence and competence in conducting the sessions, the therapist focuses more on the child and family dynamic issues expressed during the sessions, helping parents understand and accept children's play themes, discussing parent emotional reactions, and guiding parents as they problem-solve matters at home that need immediate attention. Almost inevitably, the play session themes reflect some of the difficulties that parents have discussed during the first meetings, and the therapist discusses this in the context of obstacles or progress toward treatment goals.

Sixth, after the therapist directly observes parents conducting four to six play or until parents feel comfortable playing with each of their children in this special manner,

plans are made to shift the play sessions to the home environment without direct therapist supervision. Ideally, parents hold a half-hour play session with each child each
week, but adjustments are often needed to work this in around medical appointments
or treatment protocols. Often, families with children with chronic illnesses alternate
the children they are playing with, so that each parent conducts one or two sessions
per week, but the children each receive at least one play session. The parents continue
to meet weekly or biweekly with the therapist to discuss the home play sessions, play
themes, and their own reactions, as well as real-world dilemmas they are facing.

Seventh, if all goes well with the transfer to the home sessions, the therapist helps
parents generalize the skills from the play sessions to broader life situations. The play
sessions continue, but the parents now have additional tools to employ when dealing
with everyday situations. The generalization of the skills occurs at the end of FT in
most cases because parents have mastered them and are more likely to have success
using them in the greater complexity of daily life.

FT Adaptations for Families With a Child With Chronic Illness

In many cases, FT can be conducted as described, with scheduling flexibility when
needed if medical situations intervene. Time is devoted at each session to review medical developments or setbacks with the parents, and in some cases, additional plans are
developed collaboratively with parents for situations that require them. For example,
if a child has an MRI coming up and was frightened before, the therapist might work
separately from the FT sessions to provide a play-based intervention to assist with that.
The therapist might hold an individual session or a family session to allow the child
to 'play MRI' with one of the dolls in the playroom, or to be a doctor performing an
MRI on a stuffed animal. The therapist could use a variety of additional play therapy
methods to help the child learn better relaxation techniques.

For children whose illnesses require frequent hospitalizations, the therapist can
help parents establish a 'traveling toy kit' that they can take with them to the hospital
and use for actual FT sessions there. Some parents have held play sessions with a doll
house and figurines on the tray table, and a variety of other toys in a long, low plastic
storage box across part of the bed. Such adaptations should be cleared with hospital
personnel, especially in units where everything must be sterilized.

Sometimes a normal length of FT isn't possible because of the demands on the family. In those cases, a shorter approach might be appropriate (VanFleet, 2003; Landreth
& Bratton, 2015).

FT can easily be supplemented with children's books, storytelling, and many other
forms of play therapy to meet specific goals. Most practitioners who use FT look for
ways to involve parents as partners in nearly every aspect of treatment, however.

FT Research

Research on FT began at its inception, and has continued to the present. It is on the evidence-based therapy list in the United States (http://nrepp.samhsa.gov/ProgramProfile.
aspx?id=80). Guerney and Ryan (2013) and VanFleet (2014) provide descriptions of

the research, and key studies have been reviewed in VanFleet, Ryan, and Smith (2005). A meta-analysis of play therapy research showed a very strong effect size for FT (Bratton, Ray, Rhine, & Jones, 2005). A study of predictors of outcomes in FT showed that higher levels of parent distress and lower levels of child emotion regulation were predictive of significant reductions in child behavior problems in FT, and poorer emotion regulation in parents at the start was predictive of significant increases in parental acceptance across treatment (Topham, Wampler, Titus, & Rolling, 2011).

Some research has been conducted on the usefulness of FT with families with chronically ill children. VanFleet (1983) evaluated parent satisfaction and child behavior change after a short-term group FT pilot program with families of pediatric cardiology patients. Parents were extremely satisfied with results and showed significantly more acceptance of their children's feelings. They also reported less parental stress and improved child behaviors from pre-test to post-test. Two studies have since looked at the FT-inspired Child-Parent Relationship Therapy (CPRT) program (Landreth & Bratton, 2015), a short-term group model. A small study (Glazer-Waldman, Zimmerman, Landreth, & Norton, 1992) suggested that parents were able to more accurately judge their children's anxiety after the program and were able to differentiate themselves from their children better. A controlled study (Tew, Landreth, Joiner, & Solt, 2002) showed that children in the experimental group (CPRT) scored significantly lower than controls on measures of behavior problems, depression, and anxiety. Parents in the CPRT group showed significant increases in their acceptance of their children and decreases in their stress levels as compared with controls.

More research is needed to definitively state that FT is effective for families of children with chronic illnesses, but these studies are consistent with the clinical findings where parents report large improvements in child behavior problems and their own abilities to attune to their children. Reports from referring pediatricians have also borne this out in over 65 cases conducted by the author during the 1990s. Follow-up surveys to the 12 pediatricians who had referred cases of chronically ill children and their families to the author for FT showed that all of the physicians reported "very good" to "excellent" results in terms of reduced parent complaints about medical management at home and behavior issues. Three pediatricians who had referred 20 diabetic children ranging in age from 3 to 10 years of age reported that medical measures of glycemic control were consistently improved after the FT intervention took place. These are informal data, but they suggest that further study of this intervention is warranted. The empirical strength of FT as an intervention that builds healthy parent–child relationships, coupled with this handful of studies specific to childhood chronic illness and the informal pediatrician and client reports, suggests that FT is a viable approach worthy of wider clinical practice and more rigorous research with this population.

Competence in FT

I have often said that FT is deceptively simple. In reality, it is a complex form of family intervention that requires significant understanding of family therapy, play therapy, cognitive-behavioral therapies, client-centered therapy, and a solid grounding in child development, attachment theory, and family development. Therapists need a considerable amount of training in the FT method itself in order to internalize the values and principles as well as to develop skills for working with distraught parents and children with a wide range of problems. Scope of practice issues attend, as reading a book or watching a video is far from sufficient preparation. The many subtleties of the approach require more than one or two days of training. Ideally, training should be conducted using the FT model in the same manner in which therapists eventually use it with clients—with empathy, positive and specific feedback, and a focus on empowerment. Therapists must learn how to teach parents how to conduct the sessions as well as how to process the dynamic issues contained within play themes and parent reactions to the sessions. The best way to achieve this is to obtain training and supervision. I recommend learning the other formats and related interventions such as CPRT, as they offer empirically demonstrated benefits to clients, but to work with many of the challenges faced by families of children with chronic illness, it is also important to be fully trained in the original, full family therapy form of FT (Guerney & Ryan, 2013; VanFleet, 2014). More information on training and supervision is available at www.play-therapy.com, with articles there for parents and professionals.

Case Illustration of FT With a Medically Involved Child

The identifying information in the following case illustration has been changed to protect the privacy of the clients. The elements of the case remain unaffected by this, and the case represents a typical use of FT with a family with a chronically ill child.

Background

Leah had cystic fibrosis (CF), a genetic and progressive disease that affects various organs, but most notably the lungs and pancreas. Sticky mucus interferes with breathing and digestion, attracts bacterial infections, and eventually the disease leads to respiratory failure. Leah was referred to me by her CF physician when she was 6 years old. She was dangerously underweight and malnourished, and she had been refusing to eat much and resisting the daily treatments involving airway clearance techniques (including cupping and clapping on the chest by a caregiver), and using a nebulizer to help thin the mucus. She was therefore uncomfortable, had trouble breathing, and had experienced several infections requiring hospitalization in recent months.

Her mother, Maxi, was a single mother. Leah had no contact with her father. Maxi described an increasingly difficult path in Leah's treatment, with emotional refusals and fights when Leah wanted to avoid the treatments. Maxi told me that she probably was coming on too strong in trying to get Leah to comply, but she was desperately afraid for Leah's life. Leah's doctor had confirmed that she was on thin ice, medically speaking. Much of their daily life was consumed by arguments about eating, using her nebulizer, and providing the airway clearance techniques, which her mother had to perform. Some days were better than others.

Maxi reported that her relationship with Leah had deteriorated as Leah became more and more resistant. Leah avoided her mother when she came home from school, and the school reported that she was avoiding other children and teachers, especially during snack breaks and lunch. She had been quite outgoing prior to moving into first grade.

Family Play Observation and Recommendation of FT

When I met Leah, she was quiet and nodded her head to answer the few questions that I asked. I invited her and her mother to go into the playroom for a Family Play Observation. Leah was excited by the toys and explored the room. She showed several items to her mother, and then turned her back toward her mother to play with a couple of them. When her mother suggested they play together, Leah ignored her, and when Maxi took a toy over to Leah, she first looked and then returned to the toys she had in her lap. There were very short periods where Leah interacted pleasantly with Maxi, but most of the time she did not include her in her play. At the end, Leah went to play with Maxi's sister in the waiting area and I met with Maxi. When I discussed this with Maxi alone afterward, she teared up and told me that she was trying so hard to help Leah, but that Leah just rejected everything she did. She worried they would never get back to the pleasant mother–daughter relationship they had enjoyed when Leah was younger. I listened empathically, and after we finished our discussion, I made my recommendation for FT.

I explained how it seemed that Leah's CF and its treatment had taken over their lives, and the seriousness of her condition had led to this battle for control. Leah had lost control of her life and Maxi had lost control of Leah as well as her own life. With Maxi's permission, I had already spoken with the CF doctor to see how much 'wiggle room' we had if we backed away from the battles to some extent, with the ultimate goal to improve Leah's eating. He understood what I was suggesting, told me that the battles were not resulting in eating, and that we should go ahead and try a different way.

Because Leah had potentially serious consequences from her behavior, Maxi was understandably suspicious when I suggested that we make some changes in her behavior for the short run, such as providing Leah with more choices about what to eat, and when to get her treatments. I listened empathically to her concerns, shared the doctor's impressions with her, and helped her devise an emergency plan if this new approach did not work well or Leah showed symptoms of infection. I then explained FT, what it was and how it worked, and why I thought it would help restore Leah's sense of control, and begin to rebuild Maxi's relationship with Leah. As I put it,

> Right now, Leah seems in control of her treatment and that is not going well. I'd like to help her feel in control of something, but not treatment or eating. I'd like her to be in control of something that is acceptable for kids to control—her play!

Maxi understood. I continued,

> I can see how horribly worried you are about her refusals and also how it hurts that she seems to reject you. I think that might actually be more a reflection of her frustrations with what she is going through than it is about her feelings about you. She

doesn't know how to tell you how bad this all feels, so she shows it to you in her unproductive behavior.

After I stopped for questions, I explained,

Filial Therapy is a unique way to approach this problem, but I think it might help Leah feel more in control of some things in her life, help her express her feelings more in her play, and help you show her that you understand. It might seem like a round-about way to get there, but this has worked with children with similar problems, and I'm pretty sure that it will work for Leah, too. My goal is that she will be more willing to eat and take her treatments, but we might have to give her a little space first. Do you think you can do that?

I then reassured her that I would be with her all the way and that we would check in with the doctor frequently. She agreed to move forward with the FT.

The Training Phase of FT

Because time was limited by Leah's physical condition, I suggested that we combine some of the training into two slightly longer sessions. For the first, I did a play session demonstration with Leah while Maxi and her sister watched. Leah was hesitant to engage with me, but I simply empathically listened to what she was doing and feeling, and after 15 minutes, she asked me if we could play dress-up. She dressed herself up as a princess and put the witch's hat on me. She gave me a stethoscope and told me I was the mean old doctor. Taking on the role as it seemed she wanted, I cackled like a witch and said, "I'm the mean old doctorrrrr." Leah laughed, and then gave me a doll to check out. I did so, waiting for a clearer idea of what I was to do. I commented in my 'mean old doctor's voice' that the patient looked sick and I was a smart mean old doctor who could treat her. Again, Leah laughed. She then switched her attention to some other play and did not involve me any further.

Leah left with her aunt, and Maxi and I discussed what had just happened. Maxi was amazed that Leah had turned me into a doctor so quickly, but she was also concerned with the theme of meanness. I listened to her concerns empathically and then suggested that maybe that was how Leah saw the doctors and that she was communicating something important that way. At this, Maxi became quite excited and said she wanted to get started. We then spent the rest of the session going over the play session skills and doing some practice of them together.

The second training session involved two mock play sessions. Maxi had learned quickly in the prior session, so I pretended to be a child and played as Maxi reflected, engaged in imaginary play, or set limits as needed. I coached her along the way to help her be successful, and by the end of it, she had grasped the concepts and simply needed encouragement. I asked how that felt to her and then gave her some skill feedback. She thought it was difficult but was pleased that she was on the right track. After a break, we had a second mock play session in which I again played the child, this time increasing the level of challenge a little bit. I expressed a wider range of emotions, including lots of anger at the doctor puppet, and pretended to break a few more limits. Again,

Maxi learned quickly and seemed to understand the basic skills well. We both thought she was ready to start with Leah during the next session.

First Supervised Filial Play Session

In her first FT play session with her mother, Leah again turned her back and mostly ignored her. As we had practiced before, Maxi kept her distance, and reflected what Leah was doing and seemed to be feeling, "You want to play by yourself. You don't want me to see what you're doing. It's all just for you." Leah glanced at her mother a couple times, seemingly perplexed by this uncharacteristically accepting response. After 15 minutes, Leah turned to face her mother again and announced, "I'm a princess in here and I can do what I want." Maxi reflected, "You're in charge, and you like that idea." Leah smiled faintly. "I'm a princess some of the time, and I'm a mean doctor some of the time. This is my patient (indicating the doll from the session with me)." Maxi, reflected briefly. Leah then put on the witch hat and began to throw the patient around the room, laughing like a witch. She eventually said, "Take that! You are so bad. I'm the mean doctor and you have to LISTEN!" Again, her play changed abruptly after this, and the rest of the session involved more exploratory play.

Maxi and I first discussed her use of the FT skills, which had been excellent. I made a couple of suggestions for improvement, and then we discussed Leah's play. Maxi was both amazed and fearful. She could see that the play was related to strong feelings of anger about the "mean doctor," but she worried that we were unleashing something that could not be contained. I listened and then told her that the play sessions were non directive so that we were not inserting these themes; they were themes that showed us something about Leah's feelings. I complimented Maxi for being so accepting that Leah felt comfortable enough to bring out these strong feelings.

Second Supervised Filial Play Session

In her next session, Maxi became an even meaner doctor, pretending to pinch and hit and claw at the doll patient. Using some of the suggestions we had discussed after her last session, Maxi empathically listened to Leah, touching on some of the deeper feelings below the anger, "That mean doctor is a real witch. The doctor is doing all sorts of mean things to the patient. The patient is helpless and just flying around the room. The doctor is pretty scary and not nice at all." Leah laughed and responded, "That's right! The meanest doctor in the world! Her patients all hate her! She is the meanest of all." Maxi responded beautifully, "She is the queen of mean! No one can rule her. Powe-erful! They must all do what she says, even when they hate it all." Leah laughed heartily and moved closer to her mother. She told Maxi that she needed to be the next patient. Taking her cues from the previous play, Maxi approached the mean doctor with a look of trepidation on her face. Leah began to hit her in the chest, and Maxi set a limit. Leah stepped back for a moment and resumed her mean doctor play. She did not push the limits, but she enacted a scene reminiscent of the airway clearance techniques without touching Maxi. Maxi played the patient throughout, even though I could see that she was uncertain about where this was leading.

At the end of the session, Maxi and I talked again. Maxi had mixed feelings, "I don't know what to think. Those are really strong feelings, but I'm afraid she is getting out of control." We clarified where the boundaries should be if Leah tried to harm her again, and Maxi relaxed. We then discussed the meaning of this play. Leah seemed to be sharing a great deal of intense anger at the doctor, but had placed herself in the most powerful role. I suggested that perhaps this was her way of feeling powerful while helping Maxi see how mad she was. Maxi said, "So this is really working, right?" I agreed.

Subsequent Supervised Filial Play Sessions

When Maxi and Leah arrived for their next session, Maxi asked to speak with me for just a moment before they began. When we were out of earshot, she told me that Leah had relaxed a great deal at home and had agreed to her treatments without fuss for the past few days. She was excited that this had occurred without their usual battles.

In the next few sessions, Leah continued her angry and aggressive play, but she never again broke any limits. Maxi continued to reflect the power and control of the doctor and the helplessness and fear of the patient. Despite the mean doctor theme, Leah seemed to have good emotion regulation, and Maxi could see that. At one point, she again asked Maxi to be the patient, and Maxi took on the role in the way that Leah wanted. At the end of that, Leah told Maxi that now they were both going to be doctors, and they could be nice doctors now. She continued the medical play with far less intensity and expressed pleasant emotions. She moved from this to play in the sand, and she got out the miniature operating room figures and equipment. She asked her mother to help her set up the hospital scene, which Maxi did.

Shift to Home Filial Play Sessions

At this point, Maxi was demonstrating excellent skills in conducting the play sessions, and she seemed to understand when the play was significant and had meaning. She still tended to take some of the play a little personally, but she handled it appropriately when she was with Leah. In everyday life, Leah continued to accept her treatments without resistance. We jointly decided that it was time to begin the home sessions.

Leah was overjoyed that they were going to have play sessions at home in the guest room that had been turned into a FT playroom. During the first home session, she went to the kitchen set and began to cook, making a meal for her guest (Maxi) and herself. She poured water into the cups and bowls, and served them. This transitioned into some restaurant play, where Leah was the server and Maxi was the customer. Leah served the food and whispered to Maxi that she didn't like it. Maxi put on a great show of gagging on the food. Leah then said something surprising, "You need to take smaller bites. They go down easier. I'll cut some of that up for you." Maxi was so surprised that she forgot to respond at all. Leah impatiently said, "Did you hear me? It's all cut up now, so you can eat it! I fixed it so you won't choke."

When she came in to report on this home session, Maxi said that this scenario had struck her like a bolt of lightning. She realized for the first time that maybe some aspects of eating had been physically scary or distressing for Leah. She had realized that the play might convey Leah's fear of choking. As she talked with me, Maxi identified some times when Leah had choked on some food and had appeared momentarily scared, but they had both gone on without discussion.

Maxi decided to take her cues from Leah when cooking, and when she served food that required cutting, she cut it into very tiny pieces. She never said anything to Leah, but she made this adjustment. Leah began eating better. Whether this was because of the smaller food pieces, Maxi's backing off from nagging her to eat, the control needs being met during the play sessions, or some combination of these, the battles around food were greatly decreased. In addition, Leah was beginning to be "her old self," interacting with Maxi in pleasant ways. Maxi said they now had time to have fun together rather than arguing about Leah's CF treatment.

Progress, Generalization of Skills, and Discharge

Maxi continued to have weekly play sessions with Leah, but the most pronounced changes in Leah's real-life behaviors occurred between the fifth and seventh sessions. I met with Maxi to review the home sessions and to generalize the skills to the rest of their lives, and Maxi learned to respond more empathically at home, at doctor appointments, and when Leah was hospitalized. When Leah felt understood, she was less distressed, and no longer needed to show trying to communicate the distress through her resistant behaviors. They had some rough spots from time to time where the resistance resurfaced, but they were short-lived because Maxi understood them and knew how to handle them more effectively. During the discharge phase, Maxi told me that FT had saved their lives. She told me of an epiphany she had while thinking about Leah's play themes. She realized that she, too, had felt angry and helpless. She had been unable to help Leah with her feelings because her own clouded the picture. She had been aware of her fear and frustration, but not the deeper feelings of her own. She attributed this realization to the FT process, the safety she felt in discussing play themes and her own reactions with me, and with her deepening understanding of how Leah's emotions and behaviors were linked.

SUMMARY

FT has been extremely helpful for families of children with chronic medical illnesses. It has helped address the unique needs of all family members while increasing the cohesiveness of the family as a whole. One of my FT groups for families facing medical problems decided to continue meeting after the formal FT sessions were finished, and they continued to do so as a support group for two years. They continued to hold play sessions with their children, discussed them among themselves, and incorporated other forms of fun and support into their process.

FT does require time, but it is a flexible approach, and because it empowers parents to intervene with their own children, the time needed for therapeutic benefit is usually reduced. Children with chronic illnesses, most of all, want their parents to understand them and what they are going through. Healthy siblings want and need the same. Parents want to feel that they can help, that they can do something to alleviate the misery that chronic illness sometimes imposes. FT addresses all of these needs in a comprehensive family intervention.

Interestingly, children often move quickly into playing out their central concerns and worries, usually more quickly than when involved in individual play therapy with the therapist. This is probably due to the fact that they already have an intimate relationship with their parents. While that relationship might be troubled, when children and parents alike begin to understand the dynamics behind the behaviors of concern, they quickly move into deeper levels of communication through the play sessions and in daily life. FT is empowering for every member of the family. The therapist accomplishes this by teaching parents a different way, and then processing the dynamic issues of all family members so that they can be more accepting of each other and themselves. The idea of FT is simple and straightforward, but the actual conduct of it is nuanced and complex. It is, first and foremost, family therapy, but the integrated use of play to build connections and healthier attachments among all family members strengthens families in the face of some of life's most difficult obstacles. When a child has a chronic illness, the whole family has the chronic illness. FT helps them negotiate the challenges together, and most families who have experienced it have commented that it is the most useful thing they have ever done together. Mark Twain said, "Against the assault of laughter nothing can stand." This has particular meaning for families who have participated in FT in the face of chronic illness.

REFERENCES

Bigbee, J.L. (1992). Family stress, hardiness, and illness: A pilot study. *Family Relations, 41*, 212–217.

Bratton, S.C., Ray, D., Rhine, T., & Jones, L. (2005). The efficacy of play therapy with children: A meta-analytic review of treatment outcomes. *Professional Psychology: Research and Practice, 36*(4), 376–390.

Cantrell, M.A., & Kelly, M.M. (2015). Health-related quality of life for chronically ill children. *American Journal of Maternal/Child Nursing, 40*(1), 24–34.

Cleaves, J., Gortmaker, S., & Perrin, J.M. (2010). Dynamics of obesity and chronic health conditions among children and youth. *JAMA, 303*(7), 623–630.

Crenshaw, D.A., Brooks, R., & Goldstein, S. (Eds.). (2015). *Play therapy interventions to enhance resilience*. New York: The Guilford Press.

Donoghue, E.A., & Kraft, C.A. (2009). *Managing chronic health needs in child care and schools*. Elk Grove Village, IL: American Academy of Pediatrics.

Drotar, D. (1997). Relating parent and family functioning to the psychological adjustment of children with chronic health conditions: What have we learned? What do we need to know? *Journal of Pediatric Psychology, 22*(2), 149–165.

Eddy, L.L. (Ed.). (2013). *Caring for children with special healthcare needs and their families: A handbook for healthcare professionals*. Ames, IA: Wiley-Blackwell.

Eisenberg, M.G., Sutkin, L.C., & Jansen, M.A. (Eds.). (1984). *Chronic illness and disability through the life span: Effects on self and family*. New York: Springer.

Glazer-Waldman, H.R., Zimmerman, J.E., Landreth, G.L., & Norton, D. (1992). Filial therapy: An intervention for parents of children with chronic illness. *International Journal of Play Therapy, 1*(1), 31–42.

Graziano, S., Rossi, A., Spano, B., Petrocchi, N., Biondi, G., & Ammaniti, M. (2016). Comparison of psychological functioning in children and their mothers living through a life-threatening and non life-threatening chronic disease: A pilot study. *Journal of Child Health Care, 20*(2), 174–184.

Greening, L., Stoppelbein, L., & Cheek, K. (2016). Racial/ethnic disparities in the risk of post-traumatic stress disorder symptoms among mothers of children diagnosed with cancer and Type-1 diabetes mellitus. *Psychological Trauma: Theory, Research, Practice, and Policy.* Advance online publication. Retrieved December 28, 2016 from: http://dx.doi.org/10.1037/tra0000230

Guerney, B. G., Jr. (1964). Filial therapy: Description and rationale. *Journal of Consulting Psychology, 28*, 303–310.

Guerney, L. F. (1983). Introduction to filial therapy: Training parents as therapists. In P. A. Keller & L. G. Ritt (Eds.), *Innovations in clinical practice: A source book* (Volume 2, pp. 26–39). Sarasota, FL: Professional Resource Exchange.

Guerney, L. F., & Ryan, V. (2013). *Group filial therapy: The complete guide to teaching parents to play therapeutically with their children.* London: Jessica Kingsley.

Hatzmann, J., Peek, N., Heymans, H., Maurice-Stam, H., & Grootenhuis, M. (2014). Consequences of caring for a child with a chronic disease: Employment and leisure time of parents. *Journal of Child Health Care, 18*(4), 346–357.

Hauenstein, E. J. (1990). The experience of distress in parents of chronically ill children: Potential or likely outcome? *Journal of Clinical Child Psychology, 19*(4), 356–364.

Hobbs, N., Perrin, J. M., & Ireys, H. T. (1985). *Chronically ill children and their families.* San Francisco: Jossey-Bass.

Landreth, G. L., & Bratton, S. C. (2015). *Child-parent relationship therapy (CPRT).* New York: Routledge.

Pinquart, M. (2013). Do the parent-child relationship and parenting behaviors differ between families with a child with and without chronic illness? A meta-analysis. *Journal of Pediatric Psychology, 38*(7), 708–721.

Quittner, A. L., Opipari, L. C., Espelage, D. L., Carter, B., & Eid, N. (1998). Role strain in couples with and without a child with a chronic illness: Associations with marital satisfaction, intimacy, and daily mood. *Health Psychology, 17*, 112–124.

Robinson, K. E., Gerhardt, C. A., Vannatta, K., & Noll, R. B. (2007). Parent and family factors associated with child adjustment to pediatric cancer. *Journal of Pediatric Psychology, 32*(4), 400–410.

Rynard, D. W., Chambers, A., Klinck, A. M., & Gray, J. D. (1998). School support programs for chronically ill children: Evaluating the adjustment of children with cancer at school. *Children's Health Care, 27*, 31–46.

Shuman, R. (1996). *The psychology of chronic illness.* New York: Basic Books.

Tew, K., Landreth, G. L., Joiner, K. D., & Solt, M. D. (2002). Filial therapy with parents of chronically ill children. *International Journal of Play Therapy, 11*(1), 79.

Topham, G. L., Wampler, K. S., Titus, G., & Rolling, E. (2011). Predicting parent and child outcomes of a filial therapy program. *International Journal of Play Therapy, 20*(2), 79–93.

VanFleet, R. (1983). *Report on the Filial Therapy skills-training program for parents of pediatric cardiology patients.* Technical report presented to Geisinger Medical Center, Danville, PA.

VanFleet, R. (1985). *Mothers' perceptions of their families' needs when one of their children has diabetes mellitus: A developmental perspective.* Unpublished Doctoral Dissertation, Pennsylvania State University, University Park.

VanFleet, R. (1992). Using filial therapy to strengthen families with chronically ill children. In L. VandeCreek, S. Knapp & T. L. Jackson (Eds.), *Innovations in clinical practice: A source book* (Volume 11, pp. 87–97). Sarasota, FL: Professional Resource Press.

VanFleet, R. (2003). Short-term filial therapy for families with chronic illness. In R. VanFleet & L. Guerney (Eds.), *Casebook of filial therapy* (pp. 65–84). Boiling Springs, PA: Play Therapy Press.

VanFleet, R. (2014). *Filial therapy: Strengthening parent-child relationships through play* (3rd ed.). Sarasota, FL: Professional Resource Press.

VanFleet, R., & Guerney, L. F. (Eds.). (2003). *Casebook of filial therapy*. Boiling Springs, PA: Play Therapy Press.

VanFleet, R., & Mochi, C. (2015). Enhancing resilience through play therapy with child and family survivors of mass trauma. In D. A. Crenshaw, R. Brooks & S. Goldstein (Eds.), *Play therapy interventions to enhance resilience*. New York: The Guilford Press.

VanFleet, R., Ryan, S.D., & Smith, S.K. (2005). Filial therapy: A critical review. In L. Reddy, T. Files-Hall & C.E. Schaefer (Eds.), *Empirically-based play interventions for children* (pp. 241–264). Washington, DC: American Psychological Association.

VanFleet, R., Sywulak, A.E., & Sniscak, C.C. (2010). *Child-centered play therapy*. New York: The Guilford Press.

CHAPTER 15

Play Partners

Incorporating Parents Into Medical Play Practices

Crystal Wilkins

> You make things better . . . even when you are not here.
>
> —Thomas, age 8

The preceding quote is from a patient of mine with whom I worked as a child life specialist. I had been called to his intensive care unit (ICU) bedside "STAT" from the emergency department one night. On the elevator ride up to the ICU, I imagined the worst. A code . . . a death . . . a sibling needing to be prepared to visit their brother or sister for the last time. As I rounded the corner to approach this child's room, I was relieved to find a feisty little boy yelling at his Xbox. My STAT page came because the boy was stressed out his video game didn't work. This little boy also happened to be the child with whom I worked when I was the child life specialist in the Oncology Clinic. I had moved units to give myself the benefit of 12-hour shifts that could also accommodate work I needed to do on off days to obtain training toward becoming a Licensed Counselor and Registered Play Therapist (RPT). This little boy had relapsed about 9 months after I had moved units. I had seen him on and off during his treatment, but it was spotty given my weird hours and my new location of services. My heart broke for his relapse and for my inability to continue the therapeutic relationship we had spent years building in his initial treatment. He loved his new child life specialist, but I knew he missed me too. As we dialogued about the video games and problem solved a solution, I prepared him for my departure to find a new video game cart. As I began to leave, that is when he stated the next words. "Thanks, Crystal, you make things better, even when you are not here." I became teary, thanked the little boy, and walked out on a mission to find another video game cart.

Those words were meaningful to me for many reasons. One, I had it drilled into me from early in my career that my role was to equip, not to enable. I needed to equip children to cope without me. Yes, I advocated being present whenever procedures occurred. Yes, I advocated for children to be able to play with me when I was present. But I also needed to work in such a way that those children and families were equipped to function at 3 a.m. when I was not present. His words articulated an achievement of that goal. His words were meaningful because of the heart behind it. He was stating that even though I left oncology and even though I was not present when he relapsed, the foundation I had set with him and his family had taken root and he was able to cope with the seemingly impossible task of the coping with recurrence of a deadly disease. And third, his words were meaningful because I was in my last 48 hours of working at that hospital before transitioning to a new city, a new hospital, and a new role. These were the kindest words ever spoken to me as a child life specialist, words I will treasure for a lifetime, words that were earned through years of work with this child and his family, through sweat and glitter, blood and paint.

In the pages to follow, I will argue that those words were as meaningful in my work with that child as they were for his family. For that child and for the many others with whom I worked both before and since, it was the inclusion of the parents and family that made my work extend beyond the days, months, or years that I was their child life specialist. In the following pages, you will learn about the vital importance of family to the work of both child life specialists and play therapists, and the ways that I navigated between these two roles in my clinical work with children and their families who struggled with a range of medical challenges. Specifically, you will learn why including parents in medical play is essential to equipping a child to master the health care experiences that threaten and wound, both physically and emotionally.

WHY FAMILIES?

It can be assumed that parents are the most influential people in a child's life (VanFleet, 2005). They provide the genetic makeup and environment that provides incredible influence in a child's physical, spiritual, and emotional development. They nurture their gifts, provide guidance in their mistakes, and support their courage and resiliency in the face of challenges. They are the ones that tuck them in at night, read them bedtime stories, and show up to their recitals and baseball games. They are the child's most important people.

When children are diagnosed with a chronic illness or impacted by a trauma, the whole family system is impacted. According to Tew et al. (2002), families are impacted by illness in a variety of ways including financially, medically, socially, relationally, and in terms of career maintenance and success. Parents, specifically, are faced with the tasks of dealing with their child's illness and coping with the emotional strain that illness causes for them individually, as well as the other members of the family (Tew et al., 2002).

Whether child life specialist or play therapist, there is a responsibility, gift, and challenge of connecting to parents and supporting them in their role when a child is facing an illness of their own or that of a sibling or parent. It is a responsibility because as *kid people*, clinicians may be tempted to marginalize parents out of the desire to focus solely on the child. By doing so, opportunities may be missed to influence the child's life more fully by impacting the people that will guide them forever. Thompson et al. (2009) highlighted that the premise behind family-centered care is the knowledge that families are a constant in a child's life. To make the most impact, a child life specialist and play therapist needs to include the family.

According to Ahmann and Dokken (2012), family-centered care has moved from a growing trend to a *gold standard,* in all levels of health care, but especially in the world of pediatrics. Therefore, it is best practice to equip a family and include them in all levels of care. This enables them to function effectively with or without a child life specialist or RPT on hand. So, when they arrive in the ER, or go through their next challenging experience, they don't need to seek support to function; you've already shown them how. It is a responsibility, because when you connect to the parent, you learn more about the child. You gain a valuable perspective from the people who know the children best, which informs your clinical work and makes you more effective. Strong child life specialists and skilled play therapists know the art of partnering with parents, because it makes their work more effective.

Connecting to caregivers is equally a gift. I have images in my head of parents who have become my heroes. Those parents I fear I learned more from than I contributed to in the face of the crisis they were undergoing. The mother who empowered her 6-year-old to say goodbye to her baby brother based on her instincts, but who needed support out of her fear of the death of her son impacting her daughter's connection to God. The artistic father, who laughed and played as he put ink on his dying sons' feet to create a lasting piece of artwork to remember him after his son died. The mother who appeared to seamlessly grieve the death of her husband and daughter, while attending to the varying developmental and bereavement needs of her surviving children with compassion, wisdom, and her own unique strength. The mother and father whose daughter was in and out of hospice care, seizing daily, who nevertheless found the time to make their backyard an adventure-land for their physically well son, making videos and songs with him to memorize scripture because their first priority as parents was to instill the love of God.

These parents were facing the same crisis as their children. And yet they carry a profound responsibility to themselves, their spouses, and their children to somehow make it through. They are rudderless, and yet expected to have a rudder to guide them through the storm. In your caregiving role, you have the opportunity to be a part of that rudder. It is critical to help steer them through the unforgiving waters, assisting them in making the hardest choices imaginable, and providing support and care for them, as they love their children. To do that effectively, you have to have courage to enter into relationship with them, to have sometimes awkward conversations that you stumble through and attempt to find the 'right words,' and at times let go of the picture in your head of how an intervention should go. It always goes the way it was supposed to—the words always seem to fit, even if they are not yours and even if they are flawed.

Partnering with parents is also a challenge. Parents don't have the same education or experiences as you to guide their parenting. They don't approach things from evidenced based practice or the latest book written by an award-winning neuroscientist. They are parents, who have memories of their own childhood, who have their own strengths and weaknesses, and are doing their best to love their children well during challenging circumstances. As a child life specialist or play therapist, you can help guide them with the wisdom you have gained from your training, but must do so in a way that is approachable, collaborative, and respectful of their autonomy. You must respect a parent's unique wisdom that doesn't come from books or conferences, but from time with their children. And you must validate the insecurity of the parent who inevitably feels like they are screwing up. You can help them be brave, so their children can find their courage, as well.

Partnering with parents, like connecting with children, is a dance. It requires give and take; it inevitably involves stepping on toes or having your toes stepped on, and at times feels like you are going backwards before you get to go forward. But like a dance, there is a beauty and stronger connection once it is complete. So, put on your dancing shoes and enjoy.

Child Life and Play Therapy Practice With Families

Caring for children in the hospital environment is more than taking care of *little adults*. The discipline of Pediatric Health Care must consider how child development has to be taken into consideration when caring for children impacted by illness and injury. According to Dokken, Parent, and Ahmann (2015), patient- and family-centered care initiatives began more than two decades ago. Coyne (2013) defined family-centered care as "a way of caring for children and their families within health services which ensures that care is planned around the whole family, not just the individual child/person, and in which all the family members are recognized as care recipients" (p. 797). In Abraham and Moretz's (2012a, 2012b) two-part article, core concepts of family-centered care were introduced, to include dignity and respect, information sharing, participation, and collaboration. These concepts highlight the importance of prompt information to the family, communication that values the families' perspectives and invites participation at whatever level the family chooses. In summary, these concepts describe a communication process that is informative, respectful, and collaborative in its approach (Abraham & Moretz, 2012a, 2012b).

Child Life and Play Therapy literature both highlight the importance of family involvement. Thompson et al. (2009) highlighted the definition of supportive relationships versus purely clinical or non-clinical. Supportive relationships are defined as those that advocate for psychosocial coping and adjustment, and "promote the interest of or the cause of the individual/family served" (p. 60). Ridge (2015) recognized the value of the child life profession in guiding "not only the patients, but also the parents and siblings" (p. 53). In the Standards of Clinical Practice for Child Life Specialists (2011), education of families and professionals regarding child development and psychosocial care represents a core competency for child life specialists. Furthermore, the Standards indicate that a quality inherent in the provision of Child Life services is the collaborative approach that includes children, families, health professionals, and the community.

From a Play Therapy perspective, the RPT include parents in their initial intake/assessment, as well as their routine parent consults where they monitor progress and evaluate accomplishment of goals. VanFleet (2005) explains that in Filial Therapy, parents are viewed as the primary change agent to assist children in problems that can occur in childhood and to encourage typically developing children as they grow. In Filial

Therapy, parents learn how to connect with their children through play, learning reflective communication skills and play skills that enhance the parent–child relationship (VanFleet, 2005). In further research on Filial Therapy by Ray, Bratton, Rhine, and Jones (2001), the practice of involving parents in the therapy process has been found to have superior results than for children receiving individual play therapy without parent involvement.

As a clinician who has operated in both a child life role and a play therapist role, my inclusion of parents has been important, but different in its application based on the role I am playing. As a child life specialist working in the hospital, I didn't have the benefit of 50-minute sessions with parents. Meeting parents, building a relationship with them, and providing education and support was often done on the fly. It was done in the middle of crowded hallways, during a stressful procedure in between the cries of an anxious child, or through whispers at the child's bedside while they slept. Child life specialists are accustomed to fitting consults, guidance, and techniques into the nooks and crannies of the day because adaptability and flexibility are required in the chaotic environment of the hospital environment.

As an RPT, I set the expectation of doing a formalized parent intake and I set pace with parents of connecting every 3–4 sessions to assess progress and re-assess needs. However, given the chaotic nature of the hospital environment and unpredictability of illness in general, I still had to apply the flexibility that I had learned as a child life specialist to be effective in my work with these families. When working at Dell Children's Medical Center as an RPT, most of my parent intakes and consults were done by phone. Very few parents had the time or ability to make another trip to the hospital for these meetings. Instead, they would share with me when their child typically napped or when they had a window at work where they could visit. I also learned that including parents in my sessions, especially for younger children, was often very valuable to helping parents understand more tangibly the play therapy process, to model the non-directive nature and reflective statements that promote connection through play, and to give the parents a front-row seat into how play allows children to tell their story and to see that story unfold in beautiful ways.

Now that I have transitioned to a community-based setting versus a hospital, I still find that flexibility is the name of the game when working with children impacted by hospitalization. Home visits and hospital visits are sometimes needed when working with children who are dying. When a child's illness progresses to the point of them not being able to walk, or a sibling needs support but parents cannot leave their ill child to get them to your office, you find ways to meet the family where they are. While the process of guiding parents may look different in different roles and different settings, inclusion of parents in the therapeutic process is vital for progress and lasting change to be made.

The remainder of this chapter will highlight a specific intervention called medical play, which is typically utilized by child life specialists and/or hospital-based RPTs. Most of the examples included are from my work as a hospital-based child life specialist, but may be applied to work by RPTs in a variety of settings. Included will be additional information of how clinicians may include parents from the initial introduction of services to the various obstacles that a collaborative relationship may encounter.

MEDICAL PLAY

Medical play is a unique form of play for hospitalized children where they are given an opportunity to explore medical themes with use of medical equipment and other expressive activities. Children often take on the role of a nurse, doctor, or other medical professional and re-enact experiences they have endured, observed, and/or may be fearful of. Medical play may also simply involve a medical theme or include medical equipment in art. Thompson et al. (2009) states "Play is children's most powerful tool. It helps children make sense of their world, develop new concepts, increase social skills, gain emotional support, and take responsibility for their actions through meaningful experiences" (p. 136). Allowing a child who has experienced hospitalization or illness medical-themed toys and activities is as essential as a preschooler being able to play with a toy kitchen or toy tools. Children need the opportunity to explore what is in their environment, and for hospitalized children, syringes, masks, and anesthesia masks are a part of their world.

According to Bolig, Yolton, and Nissen (1991), medical play and psychological preparation are key components in psychosocial programming available in the hospital setting. Kathleen McCue (1988) provided explanation of the specific characteristics that qualify medical play from other forms of play. Characteristics unique to medical play include (1) use of medical equipment or medical themes; (2) initiation by an adult, voluntarily maintained by the child, and not forced, (3) play that can be enjoyable and relaxing, but also intense and aggressive in nature; and (4) occasional use of activities and experiences that are not play-based per se, such as use of medical equipment with the goal of education or preparation for an upcoming procedure (McCue, 1988).

There are a variety of forms of medical play and the role of the clinician is typically on a continuum involving some directive prompts, but all the while allowing the child the control needed to promote mastery (McCue, 1988). For example, when a Certified Child Life Specialist or an RPT offers medical play, they may bring a child a variety of pieces of medical equipment (syringe, anesthesia mask, Band-Aid), with the goal of having them re-enact medical procedures. However, a child may creatively decide the syringe is a rocket ship or the anesthesia mask is a hat. The child can lead and direct the play where they need it to go, and the clinician may have confidence knowing that each time a child explores medical themes, it is a step toward positive coping and resolution of their illness experience. They will get there at their own pace and in their own way.

In medical play, clinicians have an opportunity to educate and empower parents to understand more of the internal landscape of their child's coping and engage with them in a way that supports ongoing emotional expression and mastery of their health care experience. From the initiation of services, clinicians should be providing education about the purposes and goals of medical play. Below are three examples of how a clinician may introduce medical play to a family, and how a clinician may provide education following a structured or unstructured medical play experience.

Introduction of Medical Play to Caregivers

This example shows how a child life specialist or an RPT might introduce medical play for the first time to caregivers in their initial intake or initial assessment. Each situation is different, and the information shared and education provided to families would be individualized to the families' priority needs.

Child life specialist: "Medical play is one thing I do as a child life specialist that helps children cope more positively with being in the hospital and with the procedures that are required. I heard you say that she has had a difficult time with procedures so far. Can you tell me more about that?"

Parent: "Yes, she has had to get poked about 20 times in the past two weeks. We expect her to cry for her procedures because she is 2. But now, when we simply drive near the hospital, she begins to cry. We spend an hour in the waiting room with her crying because she knows what is going to happen next. I tried lying to her so she wouldn't be so anxious, but now she doesn't trust anything I say."

Child life specialist: "I can understand that dilemma of wanting to reduce your child's anxiety and also wanting her to trust you. It can seem impossible to do both at times. With medical play, it allows her to explore the items involved in procedures such as pokes, but in a non-threatening way through play. In play, she gets to be in control; she gets to be the doctor or the nurse or whatever she chooses; and she gets to give a poke versus receiving one to a doll or stuffed animal of her choosing. By doing this, she may learn some things about the purpose behind the pokes, but it also gives her a voice to show us what pokes are like for her, and over time may help reduce her anxiety overall in relationship to the hospital environment."

Parent: "I'm afraid she will see the materials and she will get more nervous. Does that ever happen?"

Child life specialist: "It does. However, I have found that most children, even if nervous initially, benefit from being able to explore items in play. I emphasize that my medical equipment is only for dolls or stuffed animals to alleviate her fear of me doing a procedure on her. I also give children the freedom to refuse. If she becomes so nervous that it does not seem beneficial, I will offer some non-medical play items first to help her build trust with me. And then as she develops more comfort with me, then we can try play with medical equipment again. How does that sound?"

Guided Medical Play

Below is an example of how to introduce a more structured activity for a child to engage with medical themes. The goal for this child is for her to gain knowledge about her illness, but uses play to make exploring that information more comfortable.

Child life specialist: "Hi Alexis! I have an idea for an activity for us to do today while you wait for your procedure. I know you have already been taught all about cancer and chemotherapy from Miss Kelsey. But I have not done this activity before with a child and I wonder if you might tell me if you think it is fun or not, or if you think other kids may learn some important things about their cancer. Would you be willing to try?"

Alexis: "Sure."

Child life specialist: "Okay, so this activity is called blood soup."

Alexis (raising an eyebrow): "That sounds gross."

Child life specialist: "Yes it does. This is a soup that is fun and messy to make, but not one that you eat, because it would be gross. We basically take different kinds of food and make it into a big pile of goop. But each piece of food represents something in our body."

Alexis: "Okay . . . that sounds fun."

Child life specialist: "Okay, so here is what we have . . . marshmallows, red hots and rice. When you learned with Miss Kelsey about cancer, you learned a little bit about different parts of your blood. What parts do you remember?"

Alexis: "Well there are different kinds of cells . . . red ones, white ones, and another one I can't remember."

Child life specialist: "Right! Good memory. The last one tricks me up too . . . it's called a platelet. So the marshmallows, red hots, and rice represent those different parts of the blood. What do you think Marshmallows represent?"

Alexis: "White blood cells."

Child life specialist: "Yep—and what do white blood cells do for the body?"

Alexis: "They are the soldiers."

Child life specialist: "Yes, they are the fighter cells. They are the parts of our body that help fight off infection and keep our bodies healthy and safe."

Alexis: "And the red hots are red blood cells."

Child life specialist: "Yes—and what do they do?"

Alexis: "They help give energy so we can play and learn."

Child life specialist: "Exactly! Red blood cells carry oxygen which is what we breathe. And that oxygen gives our bodies fuel so we have the energy we need to do what we do every day from playing soccer to studying for a big test. Okay, now the hard one . . . what is the platelet?"

Alexis: "Aren't they the Band-Aids?"

Child life specialist: "Yep! Platelets, or the rice here, work like Band-Aids. They help stop bleeding. So when you cut yourself and you see a scab form, that is a bunch of platelets going to that spot to stop that bleeding.

Alexis: "What are the Nerds for?"

Child life specialist: "Great question. So all of these other food we added represent healthy cells that every person has. They help their bodies work the way they are supposed to. But for kids or adults who have cancer, they have cells that are not supposed to be there. They are cells that don't do anything except crowd out the healthy cells from doing their jobs. Those are cancer cells."

Alexis: "Oh I get it."

Child life specialist: "And then we add the corn syrup which is the liquid part of blood called plasma."

Following this interaction, for a family debrief, I may highlight that Alexis seemed to remember quite a bit about the things she had learned from her previous session with another clinician. I could also talk about how parents might refer back to blood soup when discussing symptoms of chemotherapy and the impact chemotherapy has on cancer cells, but also the healthy blood cells that can lead to fatigue, increased risk of infection, and increased bleeding/bruising.

Child-Directed Medical Play

Next is an example of a clinician introducing medical play to a child for the first time and allowing the child open-ended and unstructured medical play. In this situation, a clinician may want to assess the child's comfort level with medical equipment or may want to provide a sense of normalcy through exploration of materials in the child's environment without specific goals or tasks for the child to do in play.

Child life specialist: "Hi Ethan. I wanted to introduce you to Buddy, my doll. He comes to the hospital for the same reason you do. I was wondering if you might be able to help me take care of him. I have a bunch of doctor stuff, and thought you might be the perfect doctor for him."

Ethan: [Quietly begins to explore medical equipment, but looks shy and uncertain.]

Child life specialist: "I bet you've seen a lot of this stuff. I wonder what you would like to try first."

Ethan: [Begins to grab a stethoscope.]

Child life specialist: "It looks like you found something."

Ethan: [Begins to listen to Buddy.]

Child life specialist: "How does he sound, doctor?"

Ethan: "His heart is going bomp bomp, bomp bomp."

Child life specialist: "Is that good?"

Ethan: "Yes, but he is nervous."

Child life specialist: "Ah, I bet lots of kids get nervous coming to the hospital. They aren't sure what will happen."

Ethan: "He is worried about shots."

Child life specialist: "Oh man! My least favorite thing too, Buddy! Does he need a shot, Doctor Ethan?"

Ethan: "Yep, three of them."

Child life specialist: "Oh, wow! That's a lot of shots. I wonder why he needs three?"

Ethan: "Just because."

Child life specialist: "Well, that sounds hard; I wonder how we can help make it easier for Buddy?"

Ethan: "He wants to watch and you should hold his hand. That way he won't stop me."

Child life specialist: "So watching helps him be less nervous, but he needs help not reaching out and trying to stop you. I think we can do those things. All right, you tell me when, and I can help Buddy while you give him the shots."

Family Follow-Up

After engaging a child in a specific activity or medical play session, it may be beneficial to follow up with parents to provide ongoing education about what you assessed from your interaction and what future goals you have for continued work. From the preceding interaction with Ethan, it was clear to me he was shy, but he warmed up quickly and engaged fully in medical play, indicating positive coping. He used play to articulate emotions he may feel, and explored things that are typically threatening related to medical procedures. He communicated different things he may need during procedures. With a family, afterwards, I would ask the parents what parts seemed similar to Ethan's struggles with medical procedures or what parts were different. I would ask the parents if the coping strategies he stated were things they had tried and if they were helpful for him. From that, I might strategize how we could build a coping plan with Ethan through play to help him cope more effectively with his own procedures.

CASE STUDIES

When I began my career as a child life specialist, I was 22 years old, thought I knew everything in all those 22 years of wisdom, and was a perfect combination of cocky and terrified at the exact same time. I was cocky enough to put a medical resident in their place, but tender enough to rock a dying child to sleep. I could share story after story of courage with my colleagues, but didn't tell many that half of the time I walked into the hospital, I had to throw up in the ER bathroom before I started my shift. This work is invigorating and scary as hell. And here I was trying to guide parents in the most critical conversations they will ever have with their children, and my brain was three years from being fully developed. I was a walking oxymoron.

Thirteen years later, with additional training and many letters after my name, I still feel like that oxymoron much of the time. However, I've gained the beauty of perspective that child life specialists at 22 have not had the time to develop yet. And that perspective has come through learning. I've had the privilege of learning from my supervisors and mentors, my colleagues and friends, my students and mentees, my unique experiences, and most importantly, from the mothers, fathers, sisters, brothers, and extended family members I have had the privilege of serving. What follows are a few examples from my work that have changed me as a clinician. Each example will highlight how medical play was influential in supporting coping for these children; in addition, examples of inclusion of parents will be highlighted.

Bobby

Bobby was 3 years old when I met him. He had been diagnosed with lymphoma (a form of cancer) for about one week and had come to the Hematology/Oncology Clinic for the first time to have his port accessed, receive his chemotherapy, and undergo anesthesia for a bone marrow aspiration. Most adults who read this may have to look those words up, but a 3-year-old can't begin processing what that all means, at least not verbally. I was new to the clinic and still trying to figure out my way. An MD jokingly saw me wandering the hallway and stated, "Hey. Do you want to go fix that kid yelling in room 3?" I responded, "Um, sure. How old is he?" And she responded, "5." I was immediately intrigued to meet this feisty child and attempt to "fix" his distress somehow magically. As I rounded the corner, I heard, "I'm not freaking doing it. I'm not getting my port freaking accessed." My child life heart melted by the willfulness that this boy held, which I knew was both an obstacle and strength for the battle he was in.

As I entered the room, I saw this little guy glaring at me, with tears in his eyes, arms crossed and not an ounce of trust. I introduced myself to him and his mother, introduced my role as "helping to make the doctor's visit less scary," and offered him what I knew from my training was the most developmentally supportive method for preparation and eventual mastery, medical play. Mother was on board, stating, "We will try anything." And Bobby just glared. I prepared him for the materials I was bringing in being "only for my doll Buddy," and I gave him the choice of watching how I "get Buddy ready for his medicine by accessing his port," or to help me do it. With materials in hand, I began my medical play and preparation. Bobby chose to watch from his mother's lap, scowl intact, but intently paying attention to the steps that unfolded. My hands were shaking as I accessed Buddy's port; this was my first time to do medical play with an oncology patient, and I was nervous. Mother's eyes were big when she saw my hands shaking, so I had to make a joke to cut the tension. "I know! Look at how my hands are shaking. This is why they only let me do pokes on dolls and not kids. Do not fear. I am not getting you ready for your medicine, Bobby." Awkward laughter followed by me and Bobby's mother. Bobby's scowl did not budge. As I continued with the steps, Bobby became tearful, articulating fear, showing his vulnerability and true emotion. Underneath what many might see on the surface as a surly child was a scared little boy.

Following medical play, Bobby was told that despite his fear and anxiety, we needed to get him ready for his medicine now. The procedure was not pretty. There was fighting, tears, and more "freaking" threats. After the port was accessed, Bobby did what most children do and crumpled into a heap to be scooped up by his mother attempting to provide comfort. This felt like a failure. I quickly judged myself, and by extension, Bobby, in our flawed performances, failing to recognize the baby steps that had just occurred.

The next week, as I wandered the hallway deciding which child to see next, I stumbled upon Bobby also wandering the hallways. This week he was not scowling. Instead, he was wandering the scary land of the clinic, looking for something to do and someone to do it with. "Hey," he said when he saw me. "Hi Bobby. Good to see you," I replied. "You got your doll," he asked. "Uh, yeah, yeah, I do. Should I bring it to your room?" I inquired. "Yep," he stated.

What followed next was a routine of weekly medical play with this young boy who gradually began to do more and more of the port access on doll Buddy independently. He gained confidence week to week in handling the materials that originally seemed so foreign and scary, demonstrating competence, pride in his knowledge, and a swagger as he began to trust himself and his staff more. His procedures continued to look messy, but progress was evident there, as well. He slowly began not to kick or hit the nurses. He then was able to hold still on his own. And then on a magical day, following a port access, he proudly shouted, "I did it without crying!" That was not my goal for him, but it was his goal. Not crying meant he was conquering his fear. And then one day, I walked in late to his procedure, feeling guilty, just in time to see him directing the nurses, stating, "Go . . . go . . . go," with eyes closed as he prepared for the poke. This boy who had been a crumpled ball at the first port access was now directing the whole process with pride, confidence, and ability. I learned the power of medical play and gradual mastery through my young feisty friend, Bobby.

I also learned an important lesson from his mother. Her statement on day one— "We will try anything"—helped me see that parents are looking for help. Where we as professionals may discount what we offer in the face of a distraught child, or where we may say, "what do I know, I don't have kids," a parent is willing to try just about anything to help make their children's experiences more manageable. By working with Bobby's mother, I was able to recognize the strength of what I offered families. Even when it did not work as gracefully as I want it to, or when a child takes months to make the progress we wish could be made in a week, parents want to know they have someone in the fight with them. Jumping into the scary, bringing some humor with my own fear and weaknesses, as well, made me human and fallible, relatable and real. Both Bobby and his mother now had permission to have their hands shake and for them to be imperfect as they navigated the scary world of cancer.

Joseph

As a child life intern, I had the misguided impression that everyone—doctors, nurses, social workers, parents, and children—would happily accept any words of wisdom or techniques I wanted to try because I'm a child life intern and what we do is helpful. I am an optimist to a fault, and quickly learned that sometimes you receive a 'no' when offering services you do out of the goodness of your heart.

Joseph came into the pre-surgery area at 4 years old, and in my assessment with his mother, she indicated he had to have frequent hospitalizations, frequent blood draws, and many, many surgeries. She reported him always struggling with procedures, specifically pokes. I strutted right into problem-solving mode, offering medical play to help normalize and make Joseph more comfortable with the pokes he had to do so frequently. Mother's response took me off-guard when she stated, "No thank you. I want him to be scared of pokes."

I could barely hide the puzzled and somewhat horrified expression of my face when I replied, "Help me understand why you want him to continue to be scared." Her response I will remember and teach forever.

> Crystal, we live in inner-city Baltimore. I work two jobs and will not be around to walk him home from school every day. I live down the street from drug dealers. I don't want Joseph to be so comfortable with pokes that he sees a dirty needle and picks it up to play with it.

My naiveté was soon very apparent, and a much needed dose of humble pie was served. This mother was willing to look at this bright-eyed girl from West Texas and teach me a thing or two about cultural diversity. Growing up in Baltimore, Maryland, was not the same as San Angelo, Texas. Growing up in a middle-class family with a stay-at-home mother was not the norm for all families. My reality was not Joseph's.

As I took my breath, I normalized and validated her concerns. I should have also thanked her for teaching me. I then shared with her an alternative, providing education about how medical play can be supportive, but offering medical play that did not involve actual needles and did include education about why playing with medical equipment was okay ONLY with a supervising adult. Mother was in agreement and allowed to provide him the medical play that could help set up the framework for coping with the medical procedures he would continue to need. Together, we could support his coping needs and his safety needs given the environment in which he was living.

In this situation, the care that I provided required compromise, but it did not compromise the quality of care Joseph received. He was still able to explore medical procedures and medical themes with non-needle items, and could gradually work through his stress with the materials that were still safe to his mother. We could meet Joseph's needs in a way that met the mother where she was in her own coping and within the cultural needs of Joseph's environment. I learned a lot that day about the value of a parent's perspective and how to problem solve, brainstorm, and collaborate with the parents as opposed to telling parents what needed to occur. Together, Joseph's mother and I were able to come up with the best plan for him.

Sophia and Ava

Ava was a 2-year-old girl diagnosed with Wilm's tumor, a form of cancer in the kidney. Her older sister, Sophia, was 7 at the time of her sister's diagnosis. Ava's appointments were a family affair with both sisters, both parents, and often grandparents in tow. The adults in the family all wanted to hear and receive the same information, so they all came together. Two-year-old Ava encountered typical struggles for a toddler facing cancer. She hated the procedures, gave up play at some points of her treatment and, at times, seemed to be about 80-years old in the amount of fatigue she showed.

Sophia, on the other hand, had the typical energy and vitality of a 7-year-old. She was anxious and worried for her sister, but it did not slow her down. She was often shushed to be quiet, told she could not play if her sister did not want to and expected to navigate the scary world of the hospital with a vigorous spirit, but often expected to forfeit that spirit that could be a safe haven for her and for her sister.

In meeting the family, my goal was to help support their entire family. Clearly, they valued the community of family as they brought all family members involved in decision making for Ava. Therefore, my guess was that they would be bought into child life services helping Ava, but also helping Sophia. As I introduced myself to the family, I explained my role in helping both patients and siblings in their coping with hospitalization. I listened as the parents explained what had been hard for Ava, and I offered a variety of ideas that could support the needs they articulated. I also implored how Sophia was doing. They were somewhat dismissive, stating that she was "fine." I provided gentle education indicating that siblings often "seem fine" when their brother or sister is diagnosed with a chronic illness, but often times they are internalizing stress that could be supported. Given Ava's stressors, I stated that initiating my relationship with them through play would be my goal.

We started with normative play, or play materials that she was familiar with. Parents reported that she loved Play-Doh and baby dolls, so those were the items I gathered when we spent time together. Given Ava's lack of initiation with play, I knew that starting with medical play would likely be too much. Instead, I opted to build up to that. There were days that Ava did not engage actively, but she watched her sister through the corner of her eye. Sophia was lively and bright. She was excited to have something to do to fill the long days that clinic typically involved. She was given the opportunity to be herself—the lively 7-year-old she ought to be. We did art, played with dolls, and squeezed Play-Doh. Ava began to engage too. She would ask for materials to play with or hold onto while her sister busily created. She would direct her sister or this specialist to what colors she might like included in a creation. And then, gradually, she began to play herself. Having Sophia play and be herself seemed to revive the spirit in Ava that needed rekindling. As Ava began to play, the parents also began to play. They would join in on art projects and laugh alongside both of their daughters. Clinic appointments became more than just pokes and updates on chemotherapy protocols.

Eventually, I offered the girls the opportunity to engage in "doctor play, or play with medical equipment common in Ava's care" (port-a-cath, port access needle, Tegaderm bandage, tape, cleaning alcohol, etc.). I had shared with the parents that allowing both girls the opportunity to play with medical equipment would give them a way to express what the hospital environment was like for them. I explained to the girls that I would bring in a doll they could "help me take care of." I shared that I would bring in some of the same equipment they've seen in the hospital or things that the doctors sometimes used to help Ava, but emphasized, "But all the things I bring in are just for play and just for my doll."

At first, Ava was hesitant. She did not engage directly or as fully as she had with normative play, and she was offered additional play materials to engage with while Sophia eagerly explored the medical equipment. Again, Ava would watch out of the corner of her eye as Sophia utilized the medical equipment in many of the ways she had seen nurses and doctors care for Ava. Sophia was controlling and bossy, which she often was corrected for by her parents. Because I wanted her to have a venue to be controlling and bossy, I often would interject, "Mother and father, sometimes nurses and doctors can be bossy. I think for our play time, it might be okay for Nurse Sophia to tell me what to do. Is that okay with you?" The parents seemed to understand the cue and gave Sophia a bit more freedom.

Gradually, Ava began to correct Sophia. She would direct Sophia in how things really went during blood draws and port accesses; Sophia would sometimes comply, and other times would refuse. Two sets of materials became a need and both girls worked side by side on their doll patients. In each of their play, different needs and different experiences unfolded. This specialist began sharing with the parents after medical play sessions the themes present in each of their daughters' play that provided gentle explanation of their varying needs in the face of hospitalization. Through play, the children were able to express their unique experiences and perspectives of the hospital, and with coaching, their parents were able to gain insight into how to best support the individual needs of both of their girls.

Working with this particular family was both a challenge and a joy. It was a challenge, as I wasn't sure Ava would ever engage. I knew the power of play, but I was not sure how it would impact this little girl in how sick she was. Seeing her watch her sister's energy and vitality play out and observing the tremendous contagious effect it had on Ava's liveliness was beautiful. At different points in my work with this family, I judged the parents. I grew angry with them at their consistent reprimands of Sophia. I knew she needed an outlet and she also needed their support. But the vehicle for her to express that need was best done gradually and through play. Seeing the insight the parents gained in watching her play spoke volumes louder than my preachiness ever would have. Giving nuggets of wisdom gradually over a slow period of time became a very important teaching tool for me that I continue to use in my work as a child life specialist and as an RPT. Just like children, parents (especially parents who are stressed by illness) need time to understand, retain, and implement what you coach them in. And they will do it imperfectly.

Valerie

Valerie was a 3-year-old Hispanic girl newly diagnosed with leukemia. She was struggling as most 3-year-olds do with procedures surrounding her chemotherapy treatment. I offered medical play, as I routinely did, to help support Valerie's coping development and mastery. Parents were hesitant when I offered medical play, stating, "She gets really nervous anytime medical stuff is brought into the room." I normalized and validated that, offering to bring pretend items in first, and gradually building to the more realistic medical supplies. I shared that often children get upset when nurses bring in supplies because they know their own procedure is about to occur, but that when offered to play with the materials, it can elicit a different response. I also reassured parents that if Valerie chose not to participate, I would accept her refusal. Parents hesitantly agreed. I introduced myself to Valerie as someone who played with lots of children coming to the hospital to help make the hospital "less scary." I told her I would bring in doctor play materials that were just for the doll and other play materials.

As I walked in with my doll Sally, boxes of medical supplies, and some Play-doh as a backup, Valerie's eyes became big and she began to cry and hide and yell in Spanish. I had no idea the actual words she was saying, but I knew "Get out" was the overall message. I tried to hide my huge teaching doll and medical stuff and direct her to Play-Doh, but she was too upset to engage. I then apologized, grabbed my materials and left the room. I returned with several choices of activities Valerie loved to play, without the inclusion of medical equipment. I also extended my apologies to the family and shared a new game plan with the family. I shared with them that children often are too overwhelmed to engage in medical play initially, but that over time, children often will engage. I shared with them my desire to attempt medical play again in a few weeks after Valerie had a chance to view me as a safe person, and was offered normal developmental play consistently. The parents agreed.

Three weeks later, I re-introduced the idea of medical play; the parents were consistent in stating they didn't think Valerie would engage, but were agreeable to another attempt. This second attempt was met with a similar response of fear and refusal. Following the second refusal, I again attempted to normalize and validate medical play as being something that seemed to be too intense for Valerie at her current coping in the clinic environment, but wondered out loud if it might be different at home. The parents reported her having a doctor kit at home, but stated, "She doesn't want to hurt her dolls." I then decided it might be best to try on a stuffed animal that was new and provided by the hospital versus a doll/stuffed animal that Valerie had a special attachment to. The parents agreed to take a stuffed animal and medical play kit home and attempt medical play at home. Upon return to the clinic the next week, the parents laughed, stating, "She loves the stuffed animal. She feeds it and takes it for walks. But she doesn't want to hurt the animal either." At this juncture, I had to laugh too. I was finally seeing that Valerie was communicating her needs quite well. She had no interest in medical play. Despite my experience that most kids enjoy medical play, and can gain mastery through routine medical play, Valerie was not going to fall into that category. I had to adjust my expectations and game plan to fit her individual needs.

Working with this family reminded me how valuable a parent's assessment of their child is. While I do think exploring a parent's hesitation is valuable and coupling that with education on why medical play (or whatever intervention is being offered) is of benefit, at the end of the day, as a child life specialist, sometimes you have to forfeit your agenda and recognize that not every child will benefit from the interventions you lay out. Because this child was continuing to struggle in coping, and medical play and distraction during procedures did not seem to be the best fit, I ended up referring her to play therapy for an alternative mode of support. Valerie thrived in the more nondirective form of support and began to show improvement in her coping that was not feasible through medical play.

FINAL REFLECTIONS: FROM STUDENT TO TEACHER

As a young child life specialist entering the field at 22, I felt ill-equipped to provide parenting guidance. I find now, as a supervisor, a similar trend in the students I train at the practicum and internship level. When I review evaluations with these students, I typically consider involving parents as an 'advanced skill,' but it is something that will only strengthen their work if they are courageous enough to take it on at that stage of their development.

The tricky part of the child life profession is that once you obtain your certification, you may practice as a CCLS with very little observation or coaching. Trends you develop as a new graduate are often the trends that you maintain as a young professional unless you are in the practice of continued mentoring, giving and receiving feedback, and opening yourself up in vulnerability to other child life clinicians who have practiced longer. With support and input from parents specifically, child life specialists have to learn to push themselves if this is a skill set they plan to incorporate more. It is my strong belief that the strongest child life specialists are those who become comfortable with the uncomfortable and become skilled in being vulnerable and learning through their mistakes. Those who do not engage in this practice may become disgruntled and leave the field early.

My experience as a counseling student strengthened my ability to practice vulnerability. The coursework itself was unlike anything I ever experienced in my bachelor's degree. I learned that who I was as a person greatly impacted my work. With that, I had to do my work. I had to go to counseling for the things I was struggling with, and I had to engage in self-care practices that I often sidelined due to 'not enough time.' It was imperative that I do these things. If I could not do this internal work, how could I ever guide a child or a family in the practice of this? If I was going to be a counselor, I *had* to do this. I believe it is imperative for child life specialists too, but I don't think I really learned the importance of this as a priority until graduate school.

For me, I began to be more of a parent coach in Oncology, which happened to also coincide with my training at the University of North Texas to become a counselor. The shift occurred for multiple reasons, I believe. One, I was not ready, nor was I prepared to do it until then. It was also not until then that I encountered families desperate for guidance. Prior to that, I 'told' parents what to do, felt inferior and defensive when they asked me how old I was or asked me if I had children, and spent very little time considering what their experience might be like as a parent of a child with a chronic condition or who had experienced a trauma. I did not care for them. I tolerated them, but I often saw them as an obstacle to doing the work I really wanted to do with their children. As I entered Oncology, not only were they desperate for guidance, I was too. Cancer was this big scary word and this big scary world where I felt ill equipped. In Oncology, I discovered the beauty of the collaborative relationship, much because it was necessary. I was not wise enough to handle it myself. And the parents weren't, either—they needed support. So, I was forced to sit still long enough to listen to the parents—to hear their perspective, to take their perspective to heart, and to guide in what I knew. I learned how to guide from an open-handed place, allowing parents to take the parts that fit for them and to leave the rest. Staying open-handed as a clinician is hard; we believe strongly in what we do. We are passionate, and we want others to see the value in what we do. But, we have to respect a parent's autonomy and insight into their child and to approach their child with what fits them, even when it goes against the grain of what we feel would be best.

I have learned a lot from my work as a CCLS. I have learned the inner workings of the hospital environment. I have seen and served thousands of children impacted by illness, trauma, and grief. I have made awkward mistakes and stumbled through my words to support families. I have fought against parents, and I have gradually learned the art of coming alongside the families in an effort to support their child's coping with medical experiences.

I now consider myself a *baby* RPT as I continue to learn and develop my skills in this new role and new environment. I feel like I am learning something new every day; with each family and each session, I have the unique ability to combine what I have learned from two beautiful professions that have allowed me to learn a ton about myself, have strengthened my gifting and skill sets to serve families and have given me the opportunity to do two roles that are incredibly rewarding. As a CCLS, I gained the experience of doing amazing preventative work with children who were undergoing some of life's hardest challenges. I saw the beauty of play enter into dark spaces and invigorate the spirit of children trying to physically survive an illness, but also emotionally emerge a stronger and more resilient person. I have seen children learn to thrive in circumstances I could not imagine. I have also seen children struggle, and have been thankful for my RPT friends who I could pass the baton to when the child needed something different in addition to the preventative work I continued with them. As an RPT, I am learning what it looks like to support a child in distress. I am learning what it looks like from the pit of despair and helping them find their tools on their way out. There are days I do not feel like I know what I am doing, and I enter in the pit myself. And then there are days where I feel like I climbed a mountain with a child and saw something new and beautiful about the world I am in.

As I reflect, I am thankful for the learning that has occurred over the past 14 years. I am thankful for the families who allowed me to make mistakes with them and their children and trusted me to learn from them—the families who saw my hands and voice shake as I did and said hard things and taught them to do the same, those who saw me as a coach and not an expert, and those who graciously shared their wisdom with me so that we might find the best approach for their child and their family. Not many people get to have their dream jobs or have jobs that make them feel like they are doing what they were put on this earth to do. I am blessed to be one of the few, and I am excited for the opportunity to teach others who have this privilege.

My hope in reading this chapter is that you are inspired to include parents into your work a little more; that you will see the value they bring to the table for you to do your best work. I hope that you will learn both humility and confidence and recognize the continuum those two qualities exist in. I hope that you will be an advocate for children and coach the parents you serve to advocate for their children in beautiful ways that only parents can. I hope that you will see the amazing trickle effect that happens when you show parents the beauty of play and see them begin to play with their child or to see the inner landscape of their child as the playful dance occurs in the play space you create in your relationship with them. This is the magic we are invited into, and I hope you and I both make the most of it.

REFERENCES

Abraham, M., & Moretz, J. (2012a). Implementing patient and family centered care: Part I—understanding the challenges. *Pediatric Nursing, 38*(1), 44–47.

Abraham, M., & Moretz, J. (2012b). Implementing patient and family centered care: Part II—strategies and resources for success. *Pediatric Nursing, 38*(2), 107–109.

Ahmann, E., & Dokken, D. (2012). Strategies for encouraging patient/family member partnerships with the health care team. *Pediatric Nursing, 38*(4), 232–235.

Bolig, R., Yolton, K., & Nissen, H. (1991). Medical play and preparation: Questions and issues. *Children's Health Care, 20*(4), 225–229.

The Child Life Council. (2001). *Chapter 4: Standards of clinical practice.* Retrieved from: www.childlife.org/docs/default-source/the-child-life-profession/standardsofclinicalpractice.pdf

Coyne, I. (2013). Families and health-care professionals perspectives and expectations of family centered care: Hidden expectations and unclear roles. *Health Expectations*, *18*, 796–808.

Dokken, D., Parent, K., & Ahmann, E. (2015). Family presence and participation: Pediatrics leading the way. . . . and still evolving. *Pediatric Nursing*, *41*(4), 204–206.

McCue, K. (1988). Medical Play: An expanded perspective. *Children's Health Care*, *16*(3), 157–161.

Ray, D., Bratton, S., Rhine, T., & Jones, L. (2001). The effectiveness of play therapy: Responding to the critics. *International Journal of Play Therapy*, *10*(1), 85–108.

Ridge, R. (2015). Lessons from a children's hospital. *Nursing Management*, 53–54. https://doi.org/10.1097/01.NUMA.0000470778.25354

Tew, K., Landreth, G., Joiner, K., & Solt, M. (2002). Filial Therapy with parents of chronically ill children. *International Journal of Play Therapy*, *11*(1), 79–100.

Thompson, R.H. et al. (2009). *The handbook of child life: A guide for pediatric psychosocial care*. Springfield, IL: Charles C. Thompson.

VanFleet, R. (2005). *Filial therapy: Strengthening parent-child relationships through play*. Sarasota, FL: Professional Resource Press.

PART VI

Expressive-Creative Research-Driven Practice

CHAPTER 16

Medical Makers

Therapeutic Play Using "Loose Parts"

Jon Luongo and Deborah B. Vilas

> Wonderful ideas are built on other wonderful ideas. In Piaget's terms, you must reach out to the world with your own intellectual tools and grasp it, assimilate it, yourself. All kinds of things are hidden from us—even though they surround us—unless we know how to reach out for them.
>
> —Eleanor Duckworth, from *The Having of Wonderful Ideas*

At a time when free play and recess are disappearing from early childhood homes, classrooms, and school yards across the nation, opportunities for problem-solving and meaning-making through play are on the decline. Children worldwide, in both technologically advanced and developing countries, are learning how to play with technology, sometimes at the expense of other forms of open-ended, hands-on, three-dimensional play. In Cameroon, the youths are called "android generation" or "head tilted down youth" (M. Doh, personal communication, March 15, 2015).

The need for play extends beyond home and school venues into the community at large, and research points to the efficacy of play-based interventions in hospital environments (Koller, 2008). Recent studies examine the neurobiological basis of the necessity for relationship and play as integral components of optimal healing (Gaskill & Perry, 2014). When children face health care issues, the understanding and meaning they bring to the situation influence how they cope and heal. Child life specialists and hospital play specialists play a distinctive role in the provision of open-ended play opportunities that promote development, normalization, understanding, meaning, and coping in hospitalized children. To this end, this chapter will explore the theoretical foundations for such interventions, provide case examples of children making meaning out of their medical experiences, and describe how the role of loose parts and the maker approach serve to deepen play experiences in medical environments.

There are many definitions and functions of play and theories about its role in development and healing across the human life span (Tonkin & Whitaker, 2016). But with so many different types of play, materials, and play approaches, what does good practice look like when it comes to play in hospitals? With this in mind, the authors wish to shine a spotlight on four particular theories, which come together to form a roadmap for play specialists seeking to provide the optimal healing environment. These include the developmental interaction approach, child-centered play, the will to meaning, and loose parts. These four theories, when taken together, form a framework to expand our understanding of and use of play to help children cope with stressful medical experiences. The framework points to ways in which we can deepen and enrich play experiences for children and families in hospitals and community settings.

DEVELOPMENTAL INTERACTION APPROACH

Resting on the shoulders of developmental theorists Piaget and Vygotsky, the developmental interaction approach describes how children's "modes of apprehending, understanding, and responding to the world change and grow as a consequence of their continuing experience of living" (Cuffaro, Nager, & Shapiro, 2000, p. 263). Cognition and emotion are interconnected—how a child feels influences how she thinks and learns. The optimal educational process involves collaborative, interactive engagement with the environment (Cuffaro et al., 2000). In other words, a child learns more fully and effectively when her sleeves are rolled up and she is immersed in three-dimensional materials. Sitting quietly in orderly rows, filling out worksheets, and listening to a teacher lecture produces children who obey, not necessarily children who think . . . or create. Vygotsky also noted that the child's social environment influences her ability to learn. Where Piaget studied what children could do on their own, Vygotsky observed what children might accomplish in the presence of a caring, supportive adult (Vygotsky, 1978). Researchers have examined the disadvantageous effects of adverse childhood experiences (ACEs) on learning and health (Centers for Disease Control and Prevention, 2016). Far from being tabula rasas, children come with their own genetic and environmental histories, some of them traumatic, which then combine influence their ability to learn and to cope.

What does learning have to do with coping in the hospital environment? Cognition is a vital variable in coping with stress. Informed and prepared children who understand what is happening to their bodies cope better with treatment (Koller, 2007). Child life specialists who take the developmental interaction approach with children take this all into consideration. They know that children learn and express themselves through play within a supportive relationship, and that play is the best three-dimensional vehicle to help children understand and cope with their medical experiences.

CHILD-CENTERED PLAY

The child-centered approach grew from Carl Rogers's client-centered therapy (Rogers, 1980) through the work of Virginia Axline, Louise Guerney, and Garry Landreth (Landreth, 2012). It celebrates the healing relationship between therapist and client, acknowledging the locus of healing within the child. Instead of the therapist being the healer or fixer, the child's innate capacity for healing is supported and given a chance to develop in a nurturing playroom setting. Eight principles guide the therapist's relationship and actions with the child:

1. The therapist must develop a warm, friendly relationship with the child, in which good rapport is established as soon as possible.
2. The therapist must accept the child exactly as he is.
3. The therapist establishes a feeling of permissiveness in the relationship so that the child feels free to express his feelings completely.
4. The therapist is alert to recognize the feelings the child is expressing and reflects those feelings back to him in such a manner that he gains insight into his behavior.
5. The therapist maintains a deep respect for the child's ability to solve his own problems if given an opportunity to do so. The responsibility to make choices and to institute change is the child's.
6. The therapist does not attempt to direct the child's actions or conversation in any manner. The child leads the way; the therapist follows.
7. The therapist does not attempt to hurry the therapy along. It is a gradual process and is recognized as such by the therapist.
8. The therapist establishes only those limitations that are necessary to anchor the therapy to the world of reality and to make the child aware of his responsibility in the relationship.

(Axline, 1947, pp. 73–74)

The approach maintains a deep respect for the child's ability to solve her problems and gives the child the opportunity to do so. The responsibility to make choices and to institute change is in the child's hands (Landreth, 2012). Although child life specialists are not conducting play therapy per se, they are able to use child-centered therapeutic techniques to inform their play sessions and a child's play experiences within the hospital. Indeed, these techniques are accessible not only to play specialists, but to parents and teachers as well (Chaloner, 2001; Kraft & Landreth, 1998).

It takes training and skill to truly embrace and implement a child-centered approach, especially in the hectic medical-driven environment. It calls for the child life specialist to give up the notion of themselves as the expert, or the one who can 'fix' the child. It requires specialists to refrain from teaching in a direct sense, and see themselves as more of a 'guide on the side.' Specialists do this by holding back on unnecessary questions; witnessing, tracking, and narrating a child's play; and providing empathic responses that create a holding environment (Winnicott, 1960) for whatever feelings emerge in the child as expressed through their play.

Providing the child with open-ended materials and toys creates the opportunity for children to explore and express a wide range of feelings. Open-ended toys include but are not limited to:

- Toys that encourage nurturing play (dolls, bottles, beds, blankets)
- Toys that encourage aggressive play (bop bags, puppets, and plastic animals with teeth such as sharks, tigers, and lions; handcuffs, plastic and rubber weapons)

- Toys that encourage dramatic play (dolls, costumes, play kitchens, miniatures, puppets, doll houses, vehicles)
- Materials that encourage sensory play (sand, water, Play-Doh, finger paint)
- Toys and equipment that encourage medical play (doctor's kit, IV pole, bed, doll, bandages)
- Toys and materials that encourage building and creating (blocks, LEGO bricks, science kits, cooking materials, fabric)
- Art materials and activities that encourage expression of feelings and allow children and teens to represent their perceptions of illness and identity (paint, drawing tools, blank face masks, collage materials); the Life Line and the Rosebush art activities (Oaklander, 1997; Vilas, 2014).
- Technology that encourages social connection and legacy building (video equipment for filmmaking and capturing medical narratives).

Child life specialists are often called upon to be directive when they are teaching children about their illness and treatment or coaching them through a painful procedure. However, when child-centered language and philosophy are woven into these situations, the specialist supports self-esteem, emotional expression, and internal motivation in children. This empowers children to move at their own pace and find mastery, rather than behaving 'well' in order to obtain an adult's approval.

THE WILL TO MEANING

Victor Frankl sought to understand the psychological and spiritual components of survival in the face of the world's most horrific atrocities, notably that of the Holocaust. He proposed that one's ability to survive trauma and loss, as well as the ability to move beyond mere survival to a meaningful life, requires making meaning out of the traumatic experience. Frankel stated that

> the meaning of life differs from man to man, from day to day and from hour to hour. What matters therefore, is not the meaning of life in general but rather the specific meaning of a person's life at a given moment.
>
> (Frankl, 2006, p. 77)

This piece of the theoretical puzzle resonates as child life specialists empower the child to make her own meaning out of her diagnosis and treatment, as opposed to passively taking on an adult's interpretation of her experience.

Child life specialists provide children and their family members play opportunities to create meaning. Expressive art modalities such as syringe painting, building and exploding model volcanoes, and throwing wet toilet paper at drawings of what frighten or anger them offer outlets for emotional expression. Beads of Courage (2015) give children concrete representations of their medical journey when they string a bead for every poke, scan, treatment, and side effect they encounter throughout their treatment. When a child faces an amputation, casting the body part before it is removed allows the child to build her own legacy and begin to mourn her loss. These are just a handful of ideas. There are countless play opportunities for children and families to make meaning out of their hospital experience.

LOOSE PARTS

The concept of "loose parts," coined by architect Simon Nicholson (1972), provides direction in the provision of play materials that promote mastery and empowerment.

Nicholson believed that "we are all creative, and that 'loose parts' in an environment will empower our creativity" (Belinda, 2009). Unlike prefabricated toys, loose parts are open-ended materials that encourage children to use their imaginations and creativity. They can include anything and everything from masking tape to cardboard boxes and string.

For Nicholson, loose parts include items from the child's natural environment, sand, earth, water, wood, stones, and even fire. Adventure playgrounds proliferated in the United Kingdom in the 1980s. These playgrounds were places where children could use tools to build their own play environments. Play workers took a child-centered approach, overseeing children's activities from a distance, stepping in only when safety issues arose. Access to loose parts materials such as tires, wood, rocks, and rope, and tools such as hammers, saws, nails, and screws, enabled children to create, choose, problem solve, socialize, and implement their imaginations in endless ways. This type of play fosters self-regulation and self-esteem for many children who might struggle to fit into more prescribed and structured social and learning situations. In other words, behavioral problems often disappear when children are given free rein to express themselves and to create (Staempfli, 2009). Recent research shows that loose parts play at lunchtime in school stimulates deeper play and creativity, physical activity, and social skills (Hyndman, Benson, Ullah, & Telford, 2014; Maxwell, Mitchell, & Evans, 2008).

LOOSE PARTS IN THE HOSPITAL SETTING: AN INNOVATIVE TECHNIQUE

The incorporation of loose parts leads our practice away from a prepackaged model of intervention and toward a creative approach that allows children to contribute to the process of making meaning out of their own situations. While loose parts materials have been a hallmark of child life practice for years, theory-driven, intentional application of loose parts in hospitals is a relatively novel idea.

Loose parts in hospitals can extend to medical implements and supplies. A roll of gauze, tubing, paper tape, syringes with the rubber stop removed for safety, and plaster casting material are some examples of materials that can be transformed to create meaning. When I (DBV) found myself in charge of caring for 40 children at a national conference of the Foundation for Ichthyosis and Related Skin Types, I put together my first loose parts activity long before I had the language to describe it. The children in my care were all affected by a congenital skin disorder that caused them physical and emotional suffering. Their daily routines involved lengthy regimens of bathing and lotioning their brittle, dry, and fragile skin. I invited the children to bring in their used and empty lotion bottles, while providing scissors, fabric swatches, pipe cleaners, glue, googly eyes, and paper. The children made dolls out of their bottles, creating a toy out of something that their daily comfort depended on. It was a highly successful activity, giving children a chance to create and play in an emotionally supportive environment with other children just like them.

After a 10-year-old pediatric patient failed a respiratory exam, I (JL) was referred by a pediatric resident physician for child life involvement prior to a second attempt. Until he passed the test, the child could not be discharged from the hospital to home. The physician was concerned the child may have failed the test not due to poor pulmonary function but rather to feeling unnerved when faced with a new piece of medical equipment housed in an unfamiliar area of the hospital, as well as the no-nonsense approach of a technician who seemed impatient with the child. I worked in collaboration with a child life graduate student, with a goal to demystify the medical experience by constructing a toy wind instrument. We brought supplies to the patient's bedside and together fashioned a whimsical "glove-a-phone" out of a cardboard tube from inside a roll of paper towels, a medical glove, a section of clear medical tubing, tape, and a rubber band (RAFT, 2014). When the child blew into the clear tubing, the glove inflated like a bagpipe. The latex, stretched taut across one end of the cardboard tube, vibrated like a drumhead, causing an unexpectedly loud and satisfying HONK. The patient blew into this device with pleasure. He blew it periodically as he sat in his wheelchair for the long trip down the elevator, through the basement, and up a ramp. Along the way he startled several hospital staff people with the noise, who seemed amused, mostly, when they turned and saw the source. The respiratory technician did not seem amused, but the boy showed her the device anyway and blew it hard. Then he passed the exam using the actual medical equipment and was discharged from the hospital within hours. Our session revealed what this child could achieve in the presence of caring, supportive adults as well as what possibilities opened when he could tap into his own (and my) mischievous spirit. Loose parts projects have a way of spreading through the child life community. The child life graduate student who collaborated on the glove-a-phone completed her internship at our small community hospital and went on to take a full-time child life position at a top ranking children's hospital. She recently made a glove-a-phone with a 15-year-old patient awaiting heart transplant (see Figure 16.1). They fashioned it from the cardboard tube inside a roll of exam table paper, so it was extra-large and extra loud (E. Springer, personal communication, December 8, 2016).

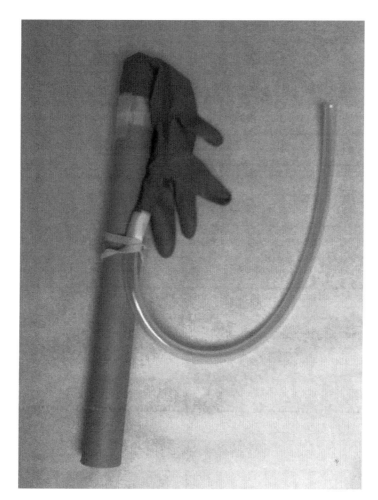

FIGURE 16.1 Glove-a-Phone

DIMENSIONS OF INTERVENTION

The depth of potential healing for hospitalized children rests on a continuum of interventional dimensions (see Table 16.1). The four theoretical concepts described earlier combine to form the cornerstones for best practice. An intervention that includes empathic interaction and play, and incorporates open-ended materials to facilitate creativity and problem-solving, holds the highest potential for healing. In Table 16.1 below, a surgery preparation is deconstructed to illustrate the possible dimensions of intervention.

An example of loose parts in the 6th Dimension is from a colleague who worked with the sibling of a teen who had suffered a brain aneurism and resulting brain damage. The brother, Marco, a 9-year-old boy, shared a room with the teen. He awoke in the middle of the night to frightening gurgling sounds and found his brother unconscious in bed. When his brother was hospitalized, Marco spent many afternoons in the

TABLE 16.1 Dimensions of Intervention (Koch, Passmore, & Vilas, 2014, reprinted with permission)

Dimension	Possible Intervention
−1 (negative one)	The child is lied to about surgery.
0 (zero)	The child is told nothing about the surgery.
1st Dimension	The child life specialist verbally explains the surgery to the child.
2nd Dimension	The child life specialist uses visual aids (books, photos, tablet) to show examples of what the child will see.
3rd Dimension	The child life specialist uses medical equipment and a doll to show the child what he will see, feel, and hear.
4th Dimension	The child is given time and space to play with the materials.
5th Dimension	The child life specialist uses loose parts to customize preparation materials.
6th Dimension	Following a verbal explanation of the diagnosis/procedure, the child life specialist provides the child with loose parts and scaffolding to co-create a 3-D interpretation of the diagnosis/procedure.
7th Dimension	Family members, medical staff, and outside parties are included in using loose parts to build teaching and play materials.

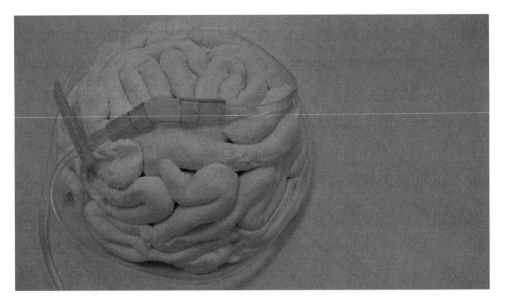

FIGURE 16.2 Three-Dimensional Model of the Brain

hospital playroom, too afraid to visit his brother in the intensive care unit, and unable to express his fears to anyone.

The child life specialist noticed Marco's reticence and somber manner. She approached him and asked if he would like some help understanding what his brother was experiencing. Together, they gathered supplies, as the specialist spoke gently about what had happened to his brother's brain. Together, they created a three-dimensional model of the human brain (see Figure 16.2), using an upside down plastic bowl and modeling clay. Together, they formed an artery out of tubing, replicating the vulnerability in the artery with a piece of rubber glove, and attached it to the brain model. With the help of the specialist, Marco created blood out of red paint and water, filled a syringe with the liquid, and enacted the bursting aneurism by pushing it through the tubing. His affect became excited as he exclaimed, "Now I understand what happened! Can we go show my mom?" The empowerment he felt, along with validation and a new sense of understanding, made a tremendous difference in this boy's ability to process and cope with his family tragedy.

THE 7th DIMENSION: THE MAKER MOVEMENT

There is a movement afoot that plays directly into the 7th Dimension of the Loose Parts Continuum. The maker movement is a tech-influenced DIY community (Moulite, n.d.) that includes tinkerers, craftspeople, frugal design enthusiasts, hobbyists, teachers, computer programmers, mechanical engineers, artists, children, and anyone interested in using tools to make things and solve problems.

Making use of what's at hand to create a clever workaround, or hack, is an age-old pastime. Its current incarnation in the US in the early 21st century is closely tied to recent technologies. For example, 3-D printing now allows everyday people to tweak designs, build prototypes, and generate made-to-order objects. Previously this sort of experimentation was inaccessible to everyday people because of the high cost of manufacturing. Not only are the means of production increasingly accessible, but ideas themselves spread quickly among enthusiasts, thanks to social media, open source hardware, and gatherings called Maker Faires, where people (sometimes in the hundreds of thousands) showcase their work and participate in hands-on activities ("Maker Faire," n.d.). Whereas once the venue for tinkering might have been the workbench, lab, or kitchen table, now places called 'makerspaces' serve as community centers for participants to share tools and ideas. As of 2015 there were an estimated 2,000 makerspaces across the world (Tierney, 2015). Increasingly makerspaces cater to children, a moment in time captured at the first White House Maker Faire, when President Obama stood open-mouthed with an eighth grader as the two of them operated the kid's invention that launched a marshmallow 175 feet across the White House State Dining Room (Kalil & Miller, 2014). Since then, increasing numbers of after-school programs, summer camps, libraries, and pop-up makerspaces across the country promise girls and boys a chance to roll up their sleeves, don safety goggles, learn how to complete electrical circuits, and build robots (Remold, Fusco, Vogt, & Leones, 2016). The maker movement encourages children to approach technology not only as a prepackaged screen experience, but for the deeper level of engagement that comes when they have a problem to solve that has meaning for themselves, and the tools to build a prototype.

A point of entry for the maker movement in health care is the Little Devices Lab at MIT. The researchers there sought health care examples of "lead-user innovation," a term coined by Professor Eric von Hippel to explain what can happen when a person who uses an object regularly designs an improvement, rather than relying upon the traditional flow of innovation from industrial producer to consumer (von Hippel, 2005). Little Devices Lab researcher Anna Young found evidence of such innovators in nurses and other frontline health care workers who improvise affordable solutions to patient care issues. These include tactile call buttons from tongue depressors and tape for patients with low vision, or custom support structures from rolled blankets for patients recovering from surgery (Young, 2015). Through programs such as MakerNurse (http://makernurse.com/) and MakerHealth (www.makerhealth.co/), Young and colleagues sponsor a network of health makerspaces across the country to encourage innovation and improve patient and family experience. In addition, Little Devices Lab sends "MEDIKits" made up of hospital equipment, LEGO bricks, circuitry, and other materials to health care workers in developing countries. Medical teams around the world use these tools to design innovative low-cost solutions to local problems, such as a DIY foot pump nebulizer and a solar-powered autoclave (Gomez-Marquez, 2012).

What opportunities does the maker movement offer for child life specialists to get involved? The first Maker Faire I (JL) attended was sponsored by MakerNurse and located at the hospital where I work. One of the presenters was Victor Ty, a radiation oncology nurse and avid LEGO designer, who demonstrated an impressive array of one-of-a-kind miniature models. He had built a miniature linear accelerator, CT scanner (see Figure 16.3), MRI scanner, and other models, all constructed from LEGO bricks. I told him about how child life specialists can use miniatures

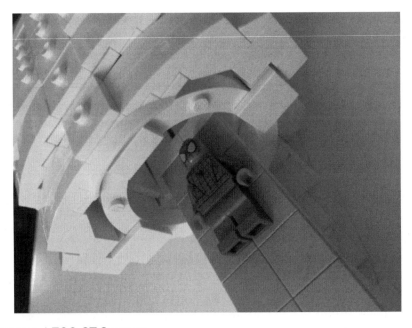

FIGURE 16.3 LEGO CT Scanner

to prepare children as young as 5 or 6 years old to complete MRI scans without anesthesia. In the spirit of collaboration, Ty lent me his model to use. In time the LEGO MRI, alongside child life know-how, became a quality improvement project for the pediatrics and radiology departments. Over the course of 18 months we successfully completed 113 out of 122 studies, meaning that 93% of the young children were able to hold still enough for the MRI to produce diagnostic images. This jump-started a study into how sedation-free pediatric MRIs, completed with preparation by a child life specialist and a miniature MRI model, can save the hospital time and money versus pediatric MRIs completed with anesthesia. Ty and I have gone on to co-present at two World Maker Faires and serve on the advisory board to Health Maker Lab, a new not-for-profit organization based in Brooklyn, NY (www.meetup.com/HCx3DP-NY/). Several 3-D printing enthusiasts on the advisory board are eager to discuss how medicine already uses 3-D printing to image brain tumors, fabricate form fitted cushions for adaptive equipment used by children with disabilities, and produce affordable DIY prosthetic hands that children can customize in playful designs. They seem equally excited to improve patient and family experience in pediatrics by collaborating with the child life community to fabricate new teaching tools and distraction toys (L. Grant, personal communication, August 11, 2016).

When child life specialists teach other health care providers to tinker with loose parts in their interactions with children, we further the collaborative spirit of the maker movement. At the hospital where I (JL) work, pediatric resident physicians complete a developmental rotation with the child life program. I encourage the doctors to tap into their imaginative playfulness to complete what I call the 'tongue depressor challenge.' The task is to co-construct a teaching tool alongside a patient to explain a part of the body, a particular medical condition, or piece of medical hardware. The challenge for doctor and patient is to use at least one tongue depressor in their design; like a single LEGO brick in a set of construction toys, the tongue depressor represents a humble piece of medical paraphernalia with limitless creative building potential. One pediatric resident physician partnered with a 15-year-old patient to construct a medical model of the gastrointestinal tract with ulcerative colitis that located the boy's pain (see Figure 16.4). They used oxygen tubing, a medical glove, clay, tape, a pipe cleaner, and a tongue depressor. Even though the adolescent remained quiet, the doctor didn't talk down or over-explain as they built the model, but rather she used increasingly complex language, such as peristalsis, and the patient appeared very engaged in the explanations. They needed a backdrop to rest the model on and the doctor said, "I'm choosing brown construction paper because you have brown skin like me." The adolescent kept the model on his bedside table for the remainder of his admission and happily showed it to people entering his room. When a child and a caregiver from beyond the child life program work alongside one another to co-construct a loose parts 3-D model, they are engaged not only in optimal cognitive gains for the child but shared meaning-making about the health care experience. In this case, meaning-making included shared cultural identity.

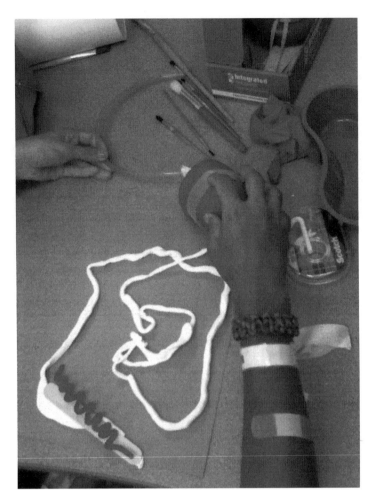

FIGURE 16.4 Loose Parts Model of the GI Tract

LOOKING FORWARD

What's next for the medical maker movement and child life? A trend in US health care delivery is that the patient experience of care is tied to government Medicare and Medicaid reimbursement rates (Centers for Medicare & Medicaid Services, 2016). This makes patient and family experience a key component to the success of hospitals that serve significant populations of patients and families from lower socioeconomic circumstances. A maker approach can improve patient experience by encouraging patients and families—in von Hippel's terms, lead-user innovators (2005)—to engage with issues significant to their wellness. Who knows how to improve the experience of a pediatric hospital stay better than the children and families themselves? They may not know it at the time, but with a creative child life specialist who stands ready to guide them, they become the innovators. One children's hospital initiated a mobile maker cart, staffed by learning scientist and mechanical engineer Gokul Krishnan.

The challenge, for one patient intrigued to use the maker cart, was how to get a good night's sleep. Krishnan gave him a shoebox of loose parts. "I think it was string, wire . . . random stuff, and he told me to make something out of it," remembered the patient. "I wound up making the Nurse Night Light . . . so if the nurses came in at night and opened up the door and flipped the lights on, it wouldn't wake up the child that was asleep" (Nelson, 2015, para. 13). A parent at another hospital needed to figure out a way to prevent her 4-year-old from tangling his IV line in the bedclothes and yanking it out when he turned over. She devised a simple hack by turning over a plastic medicine cup and taping it to the head of the bed at just the right spot to run the IV tubing around it so she could keep track of it. Recently, an adolescent patient, who had experienced multiple admissions for a chronic health condition, shared with the child life team her desire to make a better hospital gown. After many washings, the cloth becomes soft and the flaps that allow access to monitoring wires open immodestly, causing her embarrassment. What opportunities might exist in the future for her to devise a solution? If the patient had the opportunity to participate in a medical makerspace, she might work alongside a textiles engineer to help design a prototype for a hospital gown without flaps, which achieves vital signs monitoring through circuitry integrated into the fabric. "The more we help children to have their wonderful ideas and to feel good about themselves for having them," observed educational theorist Eleanor Duckworth, "The more likely it is that they will someday happen upon wonderful ideas that no one else has happened upon before" (Duckworth, 1996, p. 14).

In health care everything is tightened up, screwed down, shipshape, evidence-based, and code compliant. And that's important! But when we are trying to help children in the hospital to cope, heal, and grow—to make meaning out of their health care experience—we must leave room for loose parts.

REFERENCES

Axline, V. M. (1947). *Play therapy*. New York: Ballantine Books.

Belinda, C. (2009). *Loose parts: What does this mean?* State College: Pennsylvania State University. Retrieved July 13, 2016 from: http://extension.psu.edu/youth/betterkidcare/early-care/our-resources/tips/loose-parts-whatdoes-this-mean

Centers for Disease Control and Prevention. (April 1, 2016). *CDC 24/7: Saving lives, protecting people: Adverse Childhood Experiences (ACEs)*. Retrieved July 12, 2016 from: www.cdc.gov/violenceprevention/acestudy/

Centers for Medicare & Medicaid Services. (November 4, 2016). *Consumer assessment of healthcare providers and systems*. Retrieved December 1, 2016 from: www.cms.gov/Research-Statistics-Data-and-Systems/Research/CAHPS/

Chaloner, W. B. (2001). Play therapy in elementary and preschools: Traditional and new applications for counselor and teacher use. *APT Newsletter, 20*(2), 17–24.

Cuffaro, H. K., Nager, N., & Shapiro, E. K. (2000). The developmental-interaction approach at Bank Street College. In J. L. Roopnarine & J. E. Johnson (Eds.), *Approaches to early childhood education* (3rd ed.). New York: Macmillan.

Duckworth, E. R. (1996). *"The having of wonderful ideas" and other essays on teaching and learning*. New York: Teachers College Press.

Frankl, V. E. (2006). *Man's search for meaning*. Boston: Beacon.

Gaskill, R.L. & Perry, B.D. (2014). The neurobiological power of play using the neurosequential model of therapeutics to guide play in the healing process. In C. A. Malchiodi & D. A. Crenshaw (Eds.), *Creative arts and play therapy for attachment problems*. New York: Guilford Press.

Gomez-Marquez, J. (April 3, 2012). Design for hack in medicine: MacGyver nurses and LEGOs are helping us make MEDIKits for better health care. *Make Magazine*. Retrieved from: http://makezine.com/2012/04/03/design-for-hack-in-medicine/

Hyndman, B.P., Benson, A.C., Ullah, S., & Telford, A. (2014). Evaluating the effects of the Lunchtime Enjoyment Activity and Play (LEAP) school playground intervention on children's quality of life, enjoyment and participation in physical activity. *BMC Public Health*, 14(164). Retrieved from www.londonplay.org.uk/resources/0000/1229/BMC_Public_Health.pdf

Kalil, T., & Miller, J. (February 3, 2014). *Announcing the first White House Maker Faire*. Retrieved November 1, 2016 from: www.whitehouse.gov/blog/2014/02/03/announcing-first-white-house-maker-faire

Koch, C., Passmore, L., & Vilas, D. (2014). Co-creating meaning: Loose parts in the 7th dimension. *Child Life Council Bulletin*, 32(1), 4–5.

Koller, D. (2007). *Evidence-based practice statement: Preparing children and adolescents for medical procedures*. Rockville, MD: Child Life Council.

Koller, D. (2008). *Evidence-based practice statement summary of therapeutic play in pediatric health care: The essence of child life practice*. Rockville, MD: Child Life Council.

Kraft, A., & Landreth, G. (1998). *Parents as therapeutic partners: Listening to your child's play*. Northvale, NJ: Jason Aronson.

Landreth, G. (2012). *Play therapy: The art of relationship*. New York: Routledge.

Maker Faire: A bit of history. (n.d.). Retrieved from: http://makerfaire.com/makerfairehistory/

Maxwell, L.E., Mitchell, M.R., & Evans, G.W. (2008). Effects of play equipment and loose parts on preschool children's outdoor play behavior: An observational study and design intervention. *Children, Youth and Environments*, 18(2), 36–63.

Moulite, M. (n.d.). *The maker movement is the next level in DIY-anything*. Retrieved from: http://socalstories.ascjweb.com/arts-culture/mmoulite/index.html

Nelson, N. (February 4, 2015). A maker space that helps kids create during long hospital stays. *KQED Mindshift*. Retrieved from: https://ww2.kqed.org/mindshift/2015/02/04/a-maker-space-that-helps-kids-learn-during-long-hospital-stays/

Nicholson, S. (1972). Loose parts: An important principle for design methodology. *Studies in Design Education Craft & Technology*, 4(2), 5–14.

Oaklander, V. (1997). The rosebush. In H. G. Kaduson & C. E. Schaefer (Eds.), *101 favorite play techniques*. Lanham, MD: Rowman & Littlefield.

RAFT (Resource Area For Teaching). (2014). *Glove-a-phone: A "note"worthy sound activity*. Retrieved from: www.raftbayarea.org/readpdf?isid=82

Remold, J., Fusco, J., Vogt, K., & Leones, T. (2016). *Communities for maker educators: A study of the communities and resources that connect educators engaged in making*. Menlo Park, CA: SRI International. Retrieved from: www.sri.com/sites/default/files/brochures/maker-educatorcommunities.pdf

Rogers, C. (1980). *A way of being*. New York: Houghton Mifflin Company.

Staempfli, M.B. (2009). Reintroducing adventure into children's outdoor play environments. *Environment and Behavior*, 41(2), 268–280.

Tierney, J. (April 17, 2015). How makerspaces help local economies. *The Atlantic*. Retrieved from: www.theatlantic.com/technology/archive/2015/04/makerspaces-are-remaking-local-economies/390807/

Tonkin, A., & Whitaker, J. (Eds.). (2016). *Play in healthcare for adults: Using play to promote health and wellbeing across the adult lifespan*. London: Routledge.

Vilas, D. (2014). Play maps and life lines: New and borrowed techniques for crossing cultural and generational divides. *Child Life Council Bulletin, 32*(1), 6–7.

von Hippel, E. (2005). *Democratizing innovation.* Cambridge, MA: MIT Press.

Vygotsky, L. (1978). *Mind in society.* Cambridge: Harvard College.

Winnicott, D. W. (1960). The theory of the parent-infant relationship. *International Journal of Psycho-Analysis, 41,* 585–595.

Young, A. (2015). *Anna Young: A maker revolution in health care.* [Video file]. Retrieved from: http://tedmed.com/talks/show?id=527608

CHAPTER 17

With Plush Toys, It Hurts Less

The Effect of a Program to Promote Play to Reduce Children's Postsurgical Pain

Ana M. Ullán and Manuel H. Belver

We must love the child, and encourage his playing.
—J.J. Rousseau, *Emile or Concerning Education*, Book II

INTRODUCTION: PLAY CAN BE A GOOD PAINKILLER

Various non-pharmacological strategies to relieve hospitalized children's pain propose play as a central element. Play is considered an essential resource to improve the negative psychosocial effects of the disease and the hospitalization itself. The goal of the study we wish to present in this chapter was to determine the effect of a program to promote play in the hospital on postsurgical pain in pediatric patients. The research hypothesis was that children will manifest less pain if they are distracted through play during the postsurgical period. We carried out a randomized parallel trial with two groups, an experimental group and a control group. The control group did not receive any specific treatment, only the standard attention contemplated in the hospital. The parents of the children from the experimental group received instructions to play with their children in the postsurgical period, and were given specific play materials with which to play. The results obtained support the research hypothesis. On average, the children from the experimental group scored lower on a pain scale than the children from the control group. This occurred in the three postsurgical measurements of pain. It is concluded that the program to promote play can decrease children's perception of pain.

Relieving children's pain is an essential aspect of pediatric health care. In the past decade, research on children's pain has increased considerably. As a consequence, the knowledge about the assessment and management of pain in these patients has also increased, and there has been a rapid development and expansion of the services that treat pediatric pain (Dowden, McCarthy, & Chalkiadis, 2008). The increasing public sensitivity toward children's rights in the health area has also contributed to this (Brennan-Hunter, 2001; Southall et al., 2000; Ullán & Belver, 2008). Children's right not to suffer unnecessarily is now acknowledged and, consequently, so is the obligation of the health institutions to deal with all the aspects related to children's suffering. Standards and guidelines have been prepared to improve the practices of pain management in a large number of national and international professional settings (American Academy of Pediatrics et al., 2001; Schechter, Berde, & Yaster, 2003; Southall et al., 2000). The key points of these standards are that pediatric pain should be taken seriously, treated aggressively, and managed by multimodal means. This includes non-pharmacological approaches to reduce children's pain, fear, and stress (Finley, 2006; McGrath & Unruh, 1993; Ross & Ross, 1988).

Play Is Part of the Treatment

Various non-pharmacological strategies to relieve hospitalized children's pain and suffering propose play as a central element. Play is a crucial aspect of children's development because it contributes to the cognitive, physical, social, and emotional well-being of children and youth (Ginsburg, Communications & Child Health, 2007). For hospitalized children, play may be a powerful tool to reduce their tension, anger, frustration, conflict, and anxiety (Browmer, 2002; Haiat, Bar-Mor, & Schochat, 2003; Vessey & Mahon, 1990), improve their coping and mastery capacities, their feelings of control, and their cooperation and communication with the clinical staff (Jesse, 1992). Play allows the expression of feelings, exchanging roles, and the control over materials, concepts, and actions. These aspects can reduce the negative impact of hospitalization on children (Bolig, 1990; Hart & Rollins, 2011; William, Cheung, Lopez, & Lee, 2007). Therefore, play is considered an essential resource to improve the negative psychosocial effects of the illness and of the hospitalization itself (Bolig, Yolton, & Nissen, 1991; Huerga, Lade, & Mueller, 2016; Potasz, Varela, Carvalho, Prado, & Prado, 2013).

When children play, they can process emotions and develop a wide range of adaptive skills (Christian, Russ, & Short, 2011). Two aspects of play are especially relevant for pediatric pain: play may distract children and in addition, may improve their mood (Landreth, 2002). When children play, they concentrate on the process of playing and are distracted from other stimuli, both external and internal. There is clear evidence indicating that distraction is clinically effective in the reduction of pain in children (Cramer-Berness, 2007; DeMore & Cohen, 2005; Kleiber & Harper, 1999; Miller, Rodger, Bucolo, Greer, & Kimble, 2010; Vessey, Carlson, & McGill, 1994). Moreover, play offers the children a way to gradually assimilate the anxiety they are experiencing (Gariépy & Howe, 2003; Landreth, 2002). After reviewing the literature on the effect of play in hospitalized children, Rae and Sullivan (2005) concluded that the programs of play for hospitalized children were effective in the reduction of children's hospital-related anxiety and fear, prevention of anxiety, and in the reduction of behaviors that indicate stress.

OVERVIEW OF THE CURRENT STUDY

We conducted a study about the possibilities of using play as a resource to help children's postsurgical pain. The goal of our study (Ullán et al., 2014) was to determine the effect of a program to promote play in the hospital on postsurgical pain in pediatric patients. The research hypothesis was that after recovering from the anesthesia, children will display less pain if they are distracted by play during the postsurgical period. To test this hypothesis, we performed a quantitative study designed to determine the effect on children's postsurgical pain of a program to promote play. A randomized control trial was carried out with two groups, an experimental group and a control group. In this type of design, each participant was randomly assigned to a group, experimental or control, and all participants in the group receive (or do not receive) the intervention. Participants in this study were all the patients between 1 and 7 years of age who underwent surgery in the University Hospital of Salamanca between May and September of 2011. The following exclusion criteria were considered: (1) the children's parents or legal guardians did not give their consent for the child to participate in the study, (2) the child had been admitted in the pediatric intensive care unit after surgery, and (3) the child's operation had been performed in the evening or at night, and not during the normal consulting hours of the hospital, between 8 a.m. and 1 p.m. The study was approved by the Ethics Committee of the University Hospital of Salamanca.

The program to promote play that was used in this study consisted basically of providing the parents with (1) information about the importance of distracting their children through play to relieve their distress, and (2) play material with which to do so. The following procedure was used. Before the children from the experimental group went to the operating theater, a specialist in social education contacted the parents to inform them of the goals of the study and to request their consent for their child to participate. If the parents agreed, the same specialist discussed with them the importance of distracting the children through play to relieve their distress, and she provided them with a brief written summary of the main aspects addressed in the discussion. Figure 17.1 shows the written instructions provided to the parents. In addition to these written instructions, the parents were provided with play material to distract the children after they had undergone surgery. The play material consisted of a plush toy rabbit, dressed as a doctor, with a red cross on its chest. The toy was approximately 50 × 30 cm (Figure 17.2). The plush toy was designed by Ana M. Ullán and Manuel H. Belver especially for use in this study. It was considered appropriate to design a cuddly, soft doll in the shape of a 'rabbit doctor' for two reasons. First, because in the previous pilot studies, we had observed very good acceptance of this type of toy in the hospitalized children, who spontaneously displayed affectionate reactions toward this kind of doll (they hugged them, spoke to them, and refused to be parted from them). Second, we used a 'medical uniform' for the dolls because there is evidence that children who

Playing it hurts less

Play can be a means to help small children overcome episodes of pain. Distracting children with play can contribute to relieving their discomfort and pain. Parents often use these ways to help their children.

The dolls of this hospital are designed to help the parents distract their children while they are in hospital. The doll can be used to play and communicate with the child in many ways, to tell stories, or simply so the child can hug it. Present the doll to the child as just another member of the hospital staff, a very special person who knows how to cure children when they are ill.

Try to develop the child's imagination through play. The doll can help tranquilize and distract the child while he/she is in the hospital. Later on, at home, it is always useful to confide in this kind of "healthcare staff" with experience in curing children when they are ill.

We wish your child a swift recovery and a good stay while in the hospital.

The Pediatric Nursing Team of the University Hospital of Salamanca

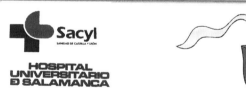

Sacyl
SANIDAD DE CASTILLA Y LEÓN

**HOSPITAL
UNIVERSITARIO
DE SALAMANCA**

Ilustraciones de Clara Hernnández

FIGURE 17.1 Instructions Provided to the Parents of the Experimental Group, Along With the Play Material

play with toys that are symbolically related to medical contents, thoughts, or fantasies about medical procedures may manifest lower levels of anxiety in post-operative situations than children who do not play with these toys (Burstein & Meichenbaum, 1979).

Each one of the children considered eligible for the study was randomly assigned either to the experimental group or the control group. When the children in the study

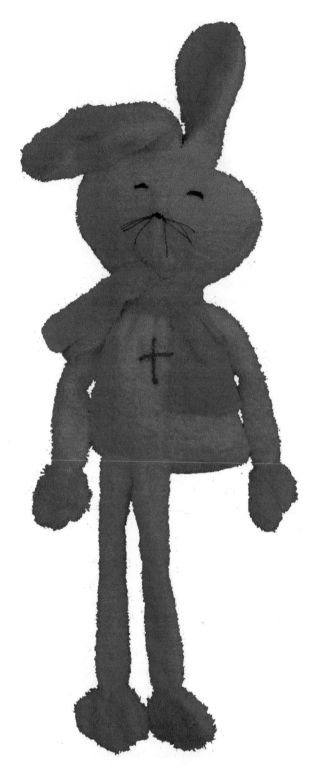

FIGURE 17.2 Play Material Provided to the Children From the Experimental Group

shared a room during their stay in the hospital, we avoided assigning one of them to the control group and the other to the experimental group, and instead, both were randomly assigned to the same group. The children assigned to the experimental group participated in the program of promotion of play described earlier. The children in the control group received the standard care provided by the hospital, and their parents received no special instructions or play material.

How We Assessed the Pain of the Children in Our Study

To assess the children's pain in both groups, we used the FLACC scale (Merkel, Voepel-Lewis, Shayevitz, & Malviya, 1997), which stands for face, legs, activity, cry, and consolability. This observational scale was developed as a simple and consistent tool to identify, describe, and assess small children's (between 2 months and 7 years) pain in clinical settings. It includes five categories of behavior (face, legs, activity, crying, and consolability). Each category is scored on a scale ranging from 0 to 2 points and the total result of the scale ranges between 0 and 10 points. The scale has shown high inter-rater reliability. Its validity was initially proved by the significant decrease observed in the scale scores when analgesics were administered to the children (Merkel et al., 1997). Its validity was also supported by the correlation of its scores with other measures of pain, specifically the scores of the Objective Pain Scale (OPS) and the global scores of pain performed by the nursing staff (Merkel et al., 1997). The FLACC scale is recommended as the first choice to assess postsurgical pain in the hospital as an outcome measure in clinical trials (von Baeyer & Spagrud, 2007).

In this study, three measures of children's pain were taken using the FLACC scale, with a 1-hour interval between them. The first measurement was taken when the children had recovered consciousness after the operation, and the second measurement an hour later. The third measurement was carried out approximately two hours after the first one. If the children were asleep when one of the measurements was supposed to be carried out, we tried to perform the measurement half an hour later, and if they were still asleep, these values were considered missing. All the pain measurements were taken by the same person who had been trained in the use of the scale. In addition to the measures of the children's pain, other variables were registered: sex, age, reason for admittance, and type and quantity of analgesic medication prescribed for each patient. Observations of the children's reactions and the parents' comments were also documented.

Statistical Analysis of the Results

We calculated the descriptive statistics of the three measurements performed for both groups, experimental and control. We conducted an analysis of variance (ANOVA) to determine whether there were significant interactions between the effect of treatment and the children's sex or age. We examined the statistical significance of the differences of means between the measurements of the experimental and the control groups with a t-test. As we wished to verify whether the mean pain score in the experimental group was lower than that of the control group, we used one-tailed tests. Statistical significance was set at alpha value of .10. The sum of the three scores obtained was considered the outcome measurement and was used to compare the effect of the variables sex and age on the children's pain scores. We calculated the descriptive statistics of the sum of the participants' three measures and compared the girls' scores and boys' scores in the younger children (between 1 and 3 years) and in the older children (between 4 and 7 years). We calculated the statistical significance of the differences observed in the mean of the sum of the three measurements of pain between the groups of boys and girls and between the smaller and the older children. We used one-tailed tests and an alpha value of .10. The participants who presented extreme values in the sum of the three measures were considered atypical cases and not included in the analyses. This occurred in three cases: two from the experimental group and one from the control group. The statistical analyses were carried out with the SPSS v.15 (SPSS) and Aabel 3 (Gigawiz) programs.

Figure 17.3 represents the participants' flow chart. Of the 124 eligible patients, 95 participated in the study; their distribution by age and sex are shown in Table 17.1. The mean age was 3.9 years (standard deviation = 1.9); 69% of the participants were boys and 31% were girls. Table 17.2 shows the reason for surgery of the participating patients in this study.

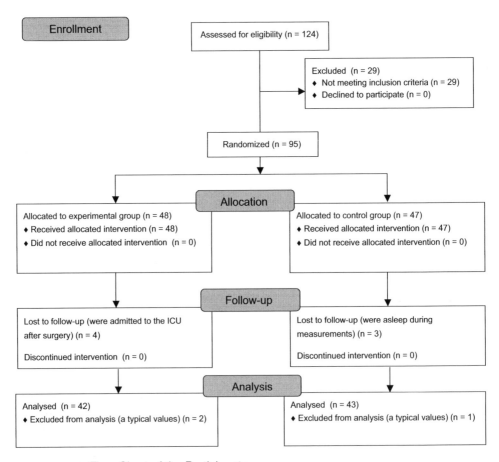

FIGURE 17.3 Flow Chart of the Participants

TABLE 17.1 Distribution of the Number of Subjects of the Sample by Age and Sex

	Group A (experimental, with plush toy)	Group B (control, without plush toy)
Sex		
Boys	32	34
Girls	16	13
Age		
Small (between 1 and 3 years)	24	23
Older (between 4 and 7 years)	24	24

TABLE 17.2 Number of Participants in the Study Who Underwent Each Type of Operation

	Total	Group A (experimental, with plush toy)	Group B (control, without plush toy)
Genital surgery	22	11	11
Ear, nose, and throat	22	12	10
Hernias	19	8	11
Trauma	5	2	3
Ophthalmology	2	0	2
Gastrointestinal surgery	4	3	1
Maxillofacial surgery	3	1	2
Plastic surgery	2	2	0
Other surgery	16	9	7

Our Results: With Plush Toys, It Hurts Less

The goal of this study was to determine the effect on postsurgical pediatric pain of a program to promote play in the hospital. The research hypothesis was that children will display less pain if they are distracted by play during the postsurgical period, after recovering from the anesthesia. The results obtained support the research hypothesis. The children from the experimental group, whose parents had received specific play material and instructions to play with them in the postsurgical period, in general scored lower on the pain scale than the children from the control group, who had only received the standard attention provided by the hospital, and whose parents had not received any specific instructions to play with them or any play material. This occurred in all three postsurgical measurements of pain. In the three measurements of pain carried out, the mean of the experimental group was lower than that of the control group. The statistical significance of these differences observed between the experimental group and the control group are shown in Table 17.3. Table 17.4 represents these means (the error bars represent the mean standard error).

TABLE 17.3 Contrast of Differences of the Means of the Three Measurements of Pain Carried Out in the Experimental Group and the Control Group

	Group									95% CI		Cohen's d
	Experimental			Control								
	n	M	SD	n	M	SD	t	df	p	LL	UL	
First measurement	41	3.7	3.1	42	4.7	3.4	−1.4	81	.08	−2.4	0.4	0.3
Second measurement	42	1.1	1.9	43	1.9	2.8	−1.4	83	.08	−1.8	0.3	0.3
Third measurement	39	0.2	0.6	43	0.8	2.0	−1.7	80	.04	−1.2	0.1	0.4

Note: CI = Confidence interval for the difference of means. LL = lower limit. UL = upper limit.

TABLE 17.4 Contrast of Differences of Means of Boys and Girls in the Sum of the Three Measurements of Pain, in the Experimental and Control Groups

	Boys			Girls						95% CI		Cohen's d
	n	M	SD	n	M	SD	t	df	p	LL	UL	
Experimental group	30	5.8	4.9	12	3.7	3.5	1.3	40	.10	−1.1	5.1	0.4
Control group	31	7.4	5.3	12	5.2	6.2	1.1	41	.13	−1.6	6.0	0.3

Note: CI = Confidence interval for the difference of means. LL = lower limit. UL = upper limit.

TABLE 17.5 Contrast of Differences of Means of Small Children and the Older Children in the Sum of the Three Measurements of Pain, in the Experimental and Control Groups

	Small children			Older children						95% CI		Cohen's d
	n	M	SD	n	M	SD	t	df	p	LL	UL	
Experimental group	21	6.5	4.5	21	3.9	4.4	1.9	40	.03	−0.2	5.3	0.6
Control group	20	8.4	5.2	23	5.4	5.6	1.8	41	.04	−0.3	6.4	0.6

Note: CI = Confidence interval for the difference of means. LL = lower limit. UL = upper limit.

In order to determine the interaction between treatment and the patients' sex, an ANOVA was carried out, which was nonsignificant for all three measurements. The same occurred with the interaction between treatment and patients' age. Considering the mean of the sum of the three measurements of pain in both groups (experimental group and control group), on average, the boys scored higher than the girls. The younger patients (1, 2, and 3 years old) scored higher than the older patients (4, 5, 6, and 7 years old). The statistical significance of these differences is shown in Tables 17.4 and 17.5.

Summary: Why Does It Hurt Less When Playing?

Two relevant mechanisms could explain the results we obtained in our study. The first involves the effect of distraction on the perception of pain (Eldridge & Kennedy, 2010; Quevedo & Coghill, 2007; Wiech, Ploner, & Tracey, 2008). The second is related to the effect of mood on the perception of pain and on the transmission of emotions between the parents and the children in health settings (Goubert, Vervoort, Sullivan, Verhoeven, & Crombez, 2008). Probably, the most frequently studied psychological variable that modifies the experience of pain is the attentional state. Pain is perceived as less intense when people are distracted (Villemure & Bushnell, 2002). Especially in the case of acute pediatric pain produced by immunizations or by upsetting medical procedures, there is evidence that distraction can relieve the children's pain and distress (Cramer-Berness, 2007; DeMore & Cohen, 2005; Kleiber & Harper, 1999; Miller et al., 2010; Vessey et al., 1994). Playing with the plush toy, as proposed herein, may have captured the children's attention during the postsurgical period, which would explain the results obtained, at least partially.

In addition, play could have improved the children's and parents' mood, and the effects of patients' mood and attitudes on their perception of pain have been observed both in clinical and in experimental settings (Villemure & Bushnell, 2002). Play is a useful strategy to help children overcome situations of stress and emotional difficulty (Bratton, Ray, Rhine, & Jones, 2005; Reddy, Files-Hall, & Schaefer, 2005). Moreover, the therapeutic effect of play is more remarkable if the parents participate in the play sessions with the children (Bratton et al., 2005; Leblanc & Ritchie, 2001). The capacity of play to distract children and to improve their mood could explain the lower scores in the pain scales of the children from the experimental group.

Great importance is attributed to play as a resource of well-being in hospitalized children (Bandstra et al., 2008; Ullán & Belver, 2008). Diverse investigations have assessed the efficacy of non-pharmacological techniques, directly or indirectly based on play, to decrease children's acute pain produced by medical procedures such as injections or venipuncture. These assessments have shown the effectiveness of distraction (Blount et al., 1992; Manne, Bakeman, Jacobsen, Gorfinkle, & Redd, 1994), toys (Smith, Barabasz, & Barabasz, 1996; Tüfekci, Çelebioglu, & Küçükoglu, 2009), music (Alegre, 2006), or the presence of the parents (Ross & Ross, 1984; Wolfram & Turner, 1996) to decrease the pain reported by the children. There is less research on non-pharmacological techniques for the management of postsurgical pediatric pain (Pölkki, Pietilä, & Vehviläinen-Julkunen, 2003; Pölkki, Pietilä, Vehviläinen-Julkunen, Laukkala, & Kiviluoma, 2008) but, in general, play is considered a particularly significant element in the care for hospitalized children (Browmer, 2002; Gariépy & Howe, 2003; Haiat et al., 2003; Rae & Sullivan, 2005; Ullán & Belver, 2006). In this sense, this work advances the knowledge about treatment of hospitalized children's pain from non-pharmacological perspectives, underlining two aspects thereof that, in our opinion, are important at a clinical level. The first one involves the ease of the intervention, and the second one is related to the importance of promoting parents' participation in the care of their children in medical settings. Despite the proliferation of standards, guidelines, and services dedicated to the treatment of children' pain, there is extensive evidence that, in practice, pain management in children is far from being optimal (Cummings, Reid, Finley, McGrath, & Ritchie, 1996; Ellis et al., 2002; Wolfe et al., 2000). Moreover, there are discrepancies between the beliefs and knowledge of the health care staff and the clinical practice (Abu-Saad & Hamers, 1997). One of the difficulties faced by pediatric services is how to integrate and deploy the findings of research and the standards in clinical practice. The research design used in this work allows a very simple transfer to clinical practice, which is compatible with the results of previously mentioned investigations, and which matches the mandate of making children's rights effective within health care settings, among them, the right to play and to prevent unnecessary suffering (Parliament European, 1986; Southall et al., 2000). In addition, the proposed intervention shows that, beyond pharmacological treatments of pain in children, there is margin for improvement in relieving pediatric pain, which should be addressed from multimodal perspectives. Lastly, we wish to underline the importance, at a clinical level, of promoting the parents' involvement in the active care of their hospitalized children. Recent research has confirmed parents' desire and expectations to participate in their children's care (Power & Franck, 2008). Parental participation is beneficial to children, parents, and health care facilities, but it depends on the existence of effective routines to facilitate adequate communication among all parties (Kristensson-Hallström, 2000). We believe that the design used in this work can serve to facilitate the establishment of this type of routine that promotes the parents' active involvement in the care of their hospitalized children.

Limitations of Our Study and Looking Forward

In our opinion, our study presents several limitations. One involves the gender bias of the participants; the second revolves around the possible effect of the experimenter's bias; and the third considers not having assessed the extent to which the parents of the experimental group correctly followed the instructions to distract their children through play. With regard to the first limitation, the disproportion observed between boys and girls in the participants reflects the disproportion of hospital admittances in the pediatric surgery service of the hospital, within the age range considered. But, as the proposed play—playing with plush toys—better matches the feminine stereotype of play, we do not think that the greater number of boys than of girls among the participants could reduce the significance of the results obtained. The second limitation seems more important to us. It was inevitable for the person who assessed the children's pain through the observational scale to perceive whether the child had received the play material; that is, whether the child belonged to the experimental group or to the control group. This could have induced a bias in the evaluator's observations in favor of the experimental hypothesis. Given the nature of the intervention, the possibility of performing blind trials is very limited. Another limitation, in our opinion, is that we did not assess the extent to which the parents of the experimental group played with their children differently from the parents of the control group. We can guarantee that they had more information than the parents of the children from the control group about the importance of play and, moreover, they had play material that was not available to the parents or the children from the control group. But this does not necessarily ensure that they followed the instructions.

OUR CONCLUSION

Even taking the preceding limitations into account, our data suggest the need to advance in the systematic assessment of non-pharmacological alternatives to relieve the pain and suffering of children in hospitals. The programs of play in hospitals are a possibility of intervention that, in our opinion, should be seriously considered. Everything indicates that it can contribute to the children's well-being, favoring a multimodal coping with pediatric pain and presenting no adverse side effects.

ACKNOWLEDGMENTS

We wish to express our thanks to Carmen Crego and her team for their work and careful manufacturing of the plush toys used in this investigation. We also want to thank the University Hospital of Salamanca for its support, and very specially, the families who collaborated with us by accepting to participate in the investigation.

REFERENCES

Abu-Saad, H. H., & Hamers, J. P. H. (1997). Decision-making and paediatric pain: A review. *Journal of Advanced Nursing, 26*(5), 946–952. https://doi.org/10.1046/j.1365-2648.1997.00116.x

Alegre, S. (2006). El juego musical como apoyo socioemocional en los niños hospitalizados [Musical play as socio-emotional support in hospitalized children]. In M. H. Belver & A. M. Ullán (Eds.), *La creatividad a través del juego [Creativity through play]* (pp. 275–294). Salamanca: Amarú Ediciones.

American Academy of Pediatrics, Committee on Psychosocial Aspects of Children and Adolescent, & Task Force on Pain in Infant Children and Adolescent. (2001). The assessment and management of acute pain in infants, children, and adolescent. *Pediatrics, 108*, 793–797.

Bandstra, N. F., Skinner, L., LeBlanc, C., Chambers, C. T., Hollon, E. C., Brennan, D., & Beaver, C. (2008). The role of child life in pediatric pain management: A survey of child life specialists. *Journal of Pain, 9*(4), 320–329. https://doi.org/10.1016/j.jpain.2007.11.004

Blount, R. L., Bachanas, P. J., Powers, S. W., Cotter, M. C., Franklin, A., Chaplin, W., . . . Blount, D. D. (1992). Training children to cope and parents to coach them durong routine inmunizations: Effects on child, parents and staff behaviors. *Behavior Therapy, 23*, 689–705.

Bolig, R. (1990). Play in health care settings: A challenge for the 1990s. *Children's Health Care, 19*(4), 229–233. https://doi.org/10.1207/s15326888chc1904_6

Bolig, R., Yolton, K., & Nissen, H. (1991). Medical play and preparation: Questions and issues. *Children's Health Care, 20*(4), 225–229. https://doi.org/10.1207/s15326888chc2004_5

Bratton, S. C., Ray, D., Rhine, T., & Jones, L. (2005). The efficacy of play therapy with children: A meta-analytic review of treatment outcomes. *Professional Psychology: Research and Practice, 36*(4), 376–390. https://doi.org/10.1037/0735-7028.36.4.376

Brennan-Hunter, A. L. (2001). Children's pain: A mandate for change. *Pain Research & Management, 6*(1), 29–39.

Browmer, N. (2002). Therapeutic play and the impact on anxiety in hospitalized children. *Kentucky Nurse, 50*(1), 15.

Burstein, S., & Meichenbaum, D. (1979). The work of worrying in children undergoing surgery. *Journal of Abnormal Child Psychology, 7*(2), 121–132. https://doi.org/10.1007/bf00918893

Christian, K. M., Russ, S., & Short, E. J. (2011). Pretend play processes and anxiety: Considerations for the play therapist. *International Journal of Play Therapy*, 20(4), 179–192. https://doi.org/10.1037/a0025324

Cramer-Berness, L. J. (2007). Developing effective distractions for infant immunizations: The progress and challenges. *Children's Health Care*, 36(3), 203–217. https://doi.org/10.1080/02739610701377855

Cummings, E. A., Reid, G. J., Finley, G. A., McGrath, P. J., & Ritchie, J. A. (1996). Prevalence and source of pain in pediatric inpatients. *Pain*, 68(1), 25–31. https://doi.org/10.1016/s0304-3959(96)03163-6

DeMore, M., & Cohen, L. (2005). Distraction for pediatric immunization pain: A critical review. *Journal of Clinical Psychology in Medical Settings*, 12(4), 281–291. https://doi.org/10.1007/s10880-005-7813-1

Dowden, S., McCarthy, A., & Chalkiadis, G. (2008). Achieving organizational change in pediatric pain management. *Pain Research & Management*, 13(4), 321–326.

Eldridge, C., & Kennedy, R. (2010). Nonpharmacologic techniques for distress reduction during emergency medical care: A review. *Clinical Pediatric Emergency Medicine*, 11(4), 244–250. https://doi.org/10.1016/j.cpem.2010.09.001

Ellis, J. A., O'Connor, B. V., Cappelli, M., Goodman, J. T., Blouin, R., & Reid, C. W. (2002). Pain in hospitalized pediatric patients: How are we doing? *The Clinical Journal of Pain*, 18(4), 262–269.

Finley, G. A. (2006). Pain in children. *Pain Research & Management*, 11(3), 156.

Gariépy, N., & Howe, N. (2003). The therapeutic power of play: Examining the play of young children with leukaemia. *Child: Care, Health & Development*, 29(6), 523–537.

Ginsburg, K. R., Committee on Communications, & Committee on Psychosocial Aspects of Child Family Health. (2007). The importance of play in promoting healthy child development and maintaining strong parent-child bonds. *Pediatrics*, 119(1), 182–191. https://doi.org/10.1542/peds.2006-2697

Goubert, L., Vervoort, T., Sullivan, M.J.L., Verhoeven, K., & Crombez, G. (2008). Parental emotional responses to their child's pain: The role of dispositional empathy and catastrophizing about their child's pain. *Journal of Pain: Official Journal of the American Pain Society*, 9(3), 272–279.

Haiat, H., Bar-Mor, G., & Schochat, M. (2003). The world of the child: A world of play even in the hospital. *Journal of Pediatric Nursing*, 18(3), 209–214.

Hart, R., & Rollins, J. (2011). *Therapeutic activities for children and teens coping with health issues*. Hoboken, NJ: John Wiley & Sons.

Huerga, R. S., Lade, J., & Mueller, F. (2016). *Designing play to support hospitalized children*. Paper presented at the Proceedings of the 2016 Annual Symposium on Computer-Human Interaction in Play.

Jesse, P. O. (1992). Nurses, children and play. *Issues in Comprehensive Pediatric Nursing*, 15(4), 261–269.

Kleiber, C., & Harper, D. C. (1999). Effects of distraction on children's pain and distress during medical procedures: A meta-analysis. *Nursing Research*, 48(1), 44–49.

Kristensson-Hallström, I. (2000). Parental participation in pediatric surgical care. *AORN*, 71(5), 1021–1029. https://doi.org/10.1016/s0001-2092(06)61551-2

Landreth, G. L. (2002). *Play therapy: The art of the relationship* (2nd ed.). New York: Brunner-Routledge.

Leblanc, M., & Ritchie, M. (2001). A meta-analysis of play therapy outcomes. *Counselling Psychology Quarterly*, 14(2), 149–163. https://doi.org/10.1080/09515070110059142

Manne, S.L., Bakeman, R., Jacobsen, P.B., Gorfinkle, K., & Redd, W.H. (1994). An analysis of a behavioral intervention for children undergoing venipuncture. *Health Psychology*, 13, 556–566.

McGrath, J.P., & Unruh, A.M. (1993). Psychological treatment of pain in children and adolescents. In N.L. Schechter, C.B. Berde & M. Yaster (Eds.), *Pain in infants, children and adolescents* (pp. 231–248). Baltimore, MD: Williams and Wilkins.

Merkel, S., Voepel-Lewis, T., Shayevitz, J.R., & Malviya, S. (1997). FLACC behavioral pain assessment scale: A comparison with the child's self-report. *Pediatric Nursing, 23*(3), 293–297.

Miller, K., Rodger, S., Bucolo, S., Greer, R., & Kimble, R.M. (2010). Multi-modal distraction. Using technology to combat pain in young children with burn injuries. *Burns, 36*(5), 647–658. https://doi.org/10.1016/j.burns.2009.06.199

Parliament European. (1986). European Charter for children in hospital (Doc. A 2–25/86). *Official Journal of the European Communities*, C 148/37–38.

Pölkki, T., Pietilä, A.-M., & Vehviläinen-Julkunen, K. (2003). Hospitalized children's descriptions of their experiences with postsurgical pain relieving methods. *International Journal of Nursing Studies, 40*(1), 33–44. https://doi.org/10.1016/s0020-7489(02)00030-5

Pölkki, T., Pietilä, A.-M., Vehviläinen-Julkunen, K., Laukkala, H., & Kiviluoma, K. (2008). Imagery-induced relaxation in children's postoperative pain relief: A randomized pilot study. *Journal of Pediatric Nursing, 23*(3), 217–224. https://doi.org/10.1016/j.pedn.2006.11.001

Potasz, C., Varela, M.J.V.D., Carvalho, L.C.D., Prado, L.F.D., & Prado, G.F.D. (2013). Effect of play activities on hospitalized children's stress: A randomized clinical trial. *Scandinavian Journal of Occupational Therapy, 20*(1), 71–79.

Power, N., & Franck, L. (2008). Parent participation in the care of hospitalized children: A systematic review. *Journal of Advanced Nursing, 62*(6), 622–641. https://doi.org/10.1111/j.1365-2648.2008.04643.x

Quevedo, A.S., & Coghill, R.C. (2007). Attentional modulation of spatial integration of pain: Evidence for dynamic spatial tuning. *Journal of Neuroscience, 27*(43), 11635–11640. https://doi.org/10.1523/jneurosci.3356-07.2007

Rae, W., & Sullivan, J. (2005). A review of play interventions for hospitalized children. In L. Reddy, T. Files-Hall & C. Schaeffer (Eds.), *Empirically based play interventions for children* (pp. 123–142). Washington, DC: American Psychological Association Press.

Reddy, L., Files Hall, T., & Schaefer, C. (2005). *Empirically based play interventions for children*. Washington, DC: American Psychological Association.

Ross, D.M., & Ross, S.A. (1984). Childhood pain: The school-aged child's viewpoint. *Pain, 20*(2), 179–191.

Ross, D.M., & Ross, S.A. (1988). *Childhood pain: Current issues, research and management*. Baltimore, MD: Urban & Schwarzenberg.

Schechter, N., Berde, C., & Yaster, M. (2003). Pain in infants, children and adolescents: An overview. In N. Schechter, C. Berde & M. Yaster (Eds.), *Pain in infants, children and adolescents* (2nd ed., p. 3). Philadelphia: Lippincott Williams & Wilkins.

Smith, J., Barabasz, A., & Barabasz, M. (1996). Comparison of hypnosis and distraction in severely ill children undergoing painful medical procedures. *Journal of Counseling Psychology, 43*, 187–195.

Southall, D.P., Burr, S., Smith, R.D., Bull, D.N., Radford, A., Williams, A., & Nicholson, S. (2000). The child-friendly initiative (CFHI): Healthcare provision in accordance with the UN Convention on the Rights of the Child. *Pediatrics, 106*(5), 1054–1064.

Tüfekci, T.G., Çelebioglu, A., & Küçükoglu, S. (2009). Turkish children loved distraction: Using kaleidoscope to reduce perceived pain during venipuncture. *Journal of Clinical Nursing, 18*, 2180–2186.

Ullán, A.M., & Belver, M.H. (2006). Jugar para estar mejor: El juego de los niños en los hospitales [Playing to feel better: Hospitalized children's play]. In M.H. Belver & A.M. Ullán (Eds.), *La creatividad a través del juego [Creativity through play]* (pp. 249–272). Salamanca: Amarú Ediciones.

Ullán, A.M., & Belver, M.H. (2008). *Cuando los pacientes son niños: Humanización y calidad en la hospitalización pediátrica pediátrica [When the patients are children: Humanization and quality in pediatric hospitalization]*. Madrid: Eneida.

Ullán, A.M., Belver, M.H., Fernández, E., Lorente, F., Badía, M., & Fernández, B. (2014). The effect of a program to promote play to reduce children's post-surgical pain: With plush toys, it hurts less. *Pain Management Nursing, 15*(1), 273–282.

Vessey, J.A., Carlson, K.L., & McGill, J. (1994). Use of distraction with children during an acute pain experience. *Nursing Research*, 43(6), 369–372.

Vessey, J.A., & Mahon, M.M. (1990). Therapeutic play and hospitalized children. *Pediatric Nursing*, 5(5), 328–333.

Villemure, C., & Bushnell, M.C. (2002). Cognitive modulation of pain: How do attention and emotion influence pain processing? *Pain*, 95(3), 195–199. https://doi.org/10.1016/s0304-3959(02)00007-6

von Baeyer, C.L., & Spagrud, L.J. (2007). Systematic review of observational (behavioral) measures of pain for children and adolescents aged 3 to 18 years. *Pain*, 127(1), 140–150.

Wiech, K., Ploner, M., & Tracey, I. (2008). Neurocognitive aspects of pain perception. *Trends in Cognitive Sciences*, 12(8), 306–313. https://doi.org/10.1016/j.tics.2008.05.005

William, L., Cheung, H., Lopez, V., & Lee, T.L.I. (2007). Effects of preoperative therapeutic play on outcomes of school age children undergoing day surgery. *Research in Nursing & Health*, 30(3), 320–332.

Wolfe, J., Grier, H.E., Klar, N., Levin, S.B., Ellenbogen, J.M., Salem-Schatz, S., . . . Weeks, J.C. (2000). Symptoms and suffering at the end of life in children with cancer. *New England Journal of Medicine*, 342(5), 326–333. https://doi.org/10.1056/NEJM200002033420506

Wolfram, R.W., & Turner, E.D. (1996). Effects of parental presence during children venipuncture. *Academic Emergency Medicine*, 3(1), 58–64.

CHAPTER 18

Playing With Biofeedback

A Practical, Playful Approach to Using Biofeedback in Pediatric Health

Jason L. Steadman and Michael E. Feeney

A game is an opportunity to focus our energy, with relentless optimism, at something we're good at (or getting better at) and enjoy. In other words, gameplay is the direct emotional opposite of depression.
—Jane McGonigal, *Reality Is Broken: Why Games Make Us Better and How They Can Change the World*

The human body is a wondrous engine driven by a complex mixture of corporeal physiology and transcendental psychology. Although theorists define the human engine differently—some reduce almost all human function to physiological mechanisms, others focus exclusively on psychology—science repeatedly reveals close interactions between humanity's non-physical and physical selves. This principal of cooperation and coordination between psychology and physiology is a driving force that has informed mental health practice now for decades. Overwhelming evidence supports that most treatments (for both medical and psychiatric problems) must address physical AND psychological realms to be most effective (Masters, France, & Thorn, 2009).

Play-based approaches to treatment are no exception to these principles. When humans play, both psychology and physiology respond to that play. It is essential that clinicians and researchers begin to more purposefully take advantage of play to invigorate the human engine toward healthier functioning on both physical and non-physical realms. In this chapter, we review some of the techniques developed through decades of research to better understand connections between the mind and body. Specifically, we present research on biofeedback training as a means to teach humans to monitor and then psychologically alter their physiological state for therapeutic purposes. We then review more recently developed techniques we have used in our own clinical and research practice that specifically incorporate play into biofeedback training. In this manner, we seek to capitalize on play to teach children psychological control over their physiology.

In this chapter, we define play broadly to include traditional, 'old-fashioned' play (defined here as any play that is not digital) as well as modern, digital play. Before the close of the chapter, we will discuss at least one old-fashioned, completely non-digital means to teach play-based biofeedback to children. However, the clear majority of biofeedback play is based in a digital world. Hence, most of our discussion highlights modern advances in video game–based play that uses biofeedback as a key component of gameplay.

BIOFEEDBACK: A PRACTICAL APPROACH FOR THE NON-PSYCHOPHYSIOLOGIST

Biofeedback training (BFT) is an evidence-based therapeutic intervention that can be used to enhance learning in a number of behavioral treatments. There is a long, empirical history of successfully using biofeedback for generalized stress and anxiety management (Lehrer, Woolfolk, & Sime, 2007), applicable to a number of psychiatric disorders. In addition, biofeedback training has also grown increasingly popular in recent years as an effective treatment for health-related complaints, as described in more detail in this chapter. However, despite the evidence base surrounding BFT, many clinicians may be reluctant to use it due to challenges with accessibility, cost, and discomfort related to a perceived lack of sufficient educational background to use the equipment. As result, its utility is often believed to be limited to specialty clinics and/or research labs. Additionally, many clinicians may be hesitant to use biofeedback training, particularly if they do not feel they have the appropriate training in psychophysiology needed to properly interpret results.

Nevertheless, recent technological innovations have allowed biofeedback training to be more accessible to the general public and requires little to no specialized training in interpretation. In the interest of making clinical recommendations for practitioners who may not be trained in advanced applied psychophysiology, we focus the majority of this chapter on a practical approach to biofeedback training that can be implemented by the average clinician and with the average youth client. Researchers and developers have created a number of games that greatly simplify biofeedback interpretation. These games respond directly to the physiology of the player and change the game in some way as a means to inform the player about his or her internal physiological state. In this way, biofeedback no longer requires a trained specialist, but *anyone*, even a child, can play a biofeedback game to monitor changes in his or her own physiology. In this chapter, we review some empirical literature investigating such interventions with children and will present a number of play-based means to teach children essential stress management and relaxation skills through biofeedback training. Guidelines for practical implementation of biofeedback training in clinical practice will also be offered, based on the authors' own clinical experiences and on empirical literature. By the end of the chapter, readers should be prepared to institute biofeedback training (once appropriately trained) in their own clinical practice, using basic principles of play and other creative/expressive therapies in various pediatric applications.

History of Biofeedback

One of the earliest descriptions of BFT can be found in a 1938 publication by Edmund Jacobson. Jacobson had begun researching the effects of 'progressive relaxation' on tension and other ailments at Harvard in the early 1900s. Progressive muscle relaxation involves a purposeful process of tensing and then relaxing muscles across several different muscle groups. Although this technique is not unique to Jacobsen, he was among the first to make an effort to actually measure the level of tension present in given muscle groups during the progressive relaxation process. He did this by using electromyography (EMG), described further later. Over the next 30 years, interdisciplinary researchers continued to develop the science of biofeedback, following similar models as that described earlier. Research flourished, and in 1969 the Biofeedback Research Society was formed. This event is generally judged to be the official birth of biofeedback training as a profession.

Since its formal introduction into the medical field and literature, biofeedback researchers and practitioners have capitalized on our understanding of psychophysiology to treat various presentations of pathology—many in the general domain of stress. As we came to understand more about the links between stress and neurophysiology, BFT grew into a logical means to teach humans the capacity to regain control over their physiology, and thereby conquer some of the effects of stress. In the general setup for administering BFT as a therapeutic intervention, there are always at least three components: the patient, the sensor(s), and the processor, which feeds the information back to the participant. A biofeedback loop is then created, where the patient learns to self-monitor the information given by the processor and then practices skills that generate changes in the output. The changes in the output tell the patient which techniques are successful, which are neutral, and which are countertherapeutic. The therapeutic effect comes from the participant gaining increased control over the feedback loop.

Therapeutically, biofeedback is most often paired with techniques common to mindfulness-based stress reduction (MBSR). Mindfulness involves cognitive training to refocus the mind only on present occurrences and learning to receive these occurrences without judgement. Patients in therapy typically receive some form of coaching in mindfulness and then they are instructed to practice mindfulness at least daily, which serves generally to help reduce distress and other negative affect over time.

There is an abundance of research on using MBSR to treat both adult and pediatric medical and psychiatric problems. In the medical field, MBSR has been used as a psychosocial intervention for pediatric cancer patients (Jones et al., 2013; Kanitz, Camus, & Seifert, 2013), to promote positive disease management in youth infected with HIV (MacDonell, Naar-King, Huszti, & Belzer, 2013), to support other weight loss interventions for obesity (Koithan, 2010; O'Reilly, Cook, Spruijt-Metz, & Black, 2014), and to improve pediatric sleep problems (Bei et al., 2013). Within psychiatry, MBSR has been shown to be an effective treatment for children with post-traumatic stress disorder (PTSD) (Catani et al., 2009), as a means to improve parent management of attention deficit hyperactive disorder (ADHD) symptoms (van der Oord, Bögels, & Peijnenburg, 2012), and for generalized stress in school-aged children

(White, 2012). Given that adding biofeedback to traditional MBSR is most often associated with reinforced effects of treatment, the potential applications of bio-feedback gaming in the aforementioned areas would be expected to achieve similar results.

The Nervous System in Biofeedback

In order to truly appreciate and understand biofeedback mechanisms, it is useful to first review some key components of the nervous system as they relate to BFT. All biofeedback mechanisms are designed to measure physiological changes that occur in the body as a direct result of neural input (hence, the term '*psycho*physiology'). Other biological mechanisms (e.g., blood glucose level) are *not* a target in biofeedback. The nervous system is divided into two major components: the central nervous system (CNS) and the peripheral nervous system (PNS). Although a full description of the functions of each is beyond the scope of this chapter, a simplified means of differentiating the two is that the CNS consists of the brain and the spinal cord while the PNS contains everything else. The PNS has additional divisions, including the somatic and autonomic nervous systems. The somatic system consists of nerve fibers that send sensory information to the CNS. It also contains motor nerve fibers that project to skeletal muscle. The autonomic nervous system (ANS) has three additional subdivisions: the parasympathetic, sympathetic, and enteric nervous systems. The parasympathetic branch is primarily responsible for maintaining a homeostatic state when the body is at rest, and is often summarized as having the 'rest and digest' or 'feed and breed' functions, because it controls sexual arousal, salivation, lacrimation, urination, digestion, and defecation. The sympathetic branch, on the other hand, responds primarily to perceived threats and controls the 'fight or flight' response. In other words, the sympathetic branch forms the main circuitry for the body's automatic and immediate stress response. The enteric nervous system is the final branch, and controls the function of the gastrointestinal system.

The preceding discussion is important to remember because different mechanisms of biofeedback measure neural functioning in different systems. However, very few neural systems communicate in isolation. Activity in one system can both directly and indirectly impact activity in another system. These interactive effects are important to consider in BFT (see Gevirtz, 2007, for more details). An inexperienced BFT user may believe that a spike, for example, in heart rate means they are 'stressed,' as heart rate can increase as a result of sympathetic activity. However, heart rate can also increase slightly during active sexual arousal, during digestion, or as a result of other parasympathetic activities. Therefore, as we discuss various methods for BFT later, it is important to remember that several can be 'contaminated' by neural activity that is not the target of the specific BFT implementation model being used.

At the same time, these previously described interactive effects can also be used to the advantage of the patient in BFT. Because the systems interact, therapeutic intervention in one system is likely to also lead the therapeutic benefit in other systems. For example, as the sympathetic nervous system functions in a healthier manner, so will the parasympathetic system. Likewise, the CNS may also be changed. Thus, although interactive effects make assessment difficult, they provide a grand benefit to therapy and intervention. This interactive benefit is especially useful in medical applications of BFT, in that therapy can theoretically target medical needs (e.g., improved digestion, healthier cardiac function) in addition to psychological needs.

Electromyography

One of the most common forms of biofeedback in a clinical setting is electromyography (EMG). EMG uses small electrodes placed on specified muscle groups to measure the electrical potential of motor ganglia (neurons) in that particular area. When muscles in the specified group receive neural stimulation, the muscles become tense. EMG also receives that input. Thus, EMG informs participants about the amount of energy being sent to a muscle area, indicating the amount of tension in that muscle.

One of the best logical applications of EMG is its usage in progressive muscle relaxation (PMR). PMR is a very commonly applied intervention in the management of stress and anxiety reduction (see Manzoni, Pagnini, Castelnuovo, & Molinari, 2008; McGuigan & Lehrer, 2007). In PMR, individuals are instructed to gradually tighten, hold tight, and then relax muscle groups in a progressive fashion until the whole body has been covered. As patients tighten and relax their muscles in PMR, EMG gives direct, immediate feedback to the patient about this process. EMG is particularly useful in patients who have poor conscious control of muscle tone. Several research studies have demonstrated EMG guided PMR to be quite effective in patients with incontinence and elimination problems (Agnihotri, Paul, & Sandhu, 2008; Chiarioni & Whitehead, 2008; Cox et al., 1994; Dedeepya, Nuvvula, Kamatham, & Nirmala, 2014; Woodward, Norton, & Chiarelli, 2014). Additionally, at least one study supports the effectiveness of biofeedback on relieving pediatric headaches (Bussone, Grazzi, D'Amico, Leone, & Andrasik, 1998).

EMG has also been applied to pediatric neuromuscular and pain disorders and has shown positive effects on debilitating physical and developmental conditions. One study observed a reduction in pain and improved muscle strength in a sample of juvenile patients with rheumatoid arthritis (Eid, Aly, & El-Shamy, 2016). Additionally, EMG-assisted biofeedback has been shown to have a greater efficacy compared to traditional rehabilitation techniques in improving the gait of children with cerebral palsy (Dursun, Dursun, & Alican, 2004). Other studies have similarly applied EMG for a variety of neuromuscular rehab needs for adults and children, such as improving head control, balance, and use of upper extremities (Bolek, 2006; Middaugh, 2007).

Incorporating electromyography into one's practice may present some challenges. Like many forms of biofeedback, EMG often requires a wired connection between sensor and processor. This wired connection can restrict mobility, which may impact some applications of therapy. Technological innovations have been developed that do allow full mobility. Mobile options tend to be costlier, but they have several added benefits of feeling more natural to patients and thereby reducing procedural anxiety common to children, who may display some fear of being connected to large machines. Another drawback is that EMG only measures tension in the muscle groups on which sensors are placed. In practice, this means that the amount of muscles being targeted at any given time is limited by the number of sensors available. A full body scan (commonly used in PMR), then, would require numerous sensors placed all over the body. Some patients (and practitioners) may consider this placement process to be time-consuming and aversive, which can decrease effects. For these reasons, we do not recommend EMG for standard biofeedback practice with every patient. However, as described earlier, there are several specific applications (e.g., neuromuscular disorders, localized pain) where EMG is a wonderful treatment option, and by incorporating play (see later examples), clinicians may find numerous children are quite receptive to EMG in BFT.

Electrodermal Activity

Electrodermal activity (EDA) is an umbrella term used for describing a myriad of psychophysiological changes in the electrical properties of the skin. For the purposes of our discussion, EDA can be used interchangeably with skin conductance, although technically skin conductance is only one type of EDA. Skin conductance includes both the baseline skin conductance level (SCL) and the rapid changes that occur in response to various stimuli (skin conductance responses, SCRs). It is measured by sending a harmless electrical impulse across two electrodes, both of which are attached to the skin. EDA measures the electrical flow between these two electrodes, using skin as an electrical conductor.

An important quality of EDA is that it is unique among other methods of biofeedback in that it is the only measure that is controlled solely by sympathetic activity. In fact, EDA is often considered to be the most useful index of psychological and emotional stress because it is the only psychophysiological marker that is not also tainted by parasympathetic functioning (Boucsein, 2012; Braithwaite, Watson, Jones, & Rowe, 2013). Because of this property, changes in EDA can be predicted to very likely result from an immediate stress response, rather than from longer term homeostatic mechanisms.

Electrodermal activity has a robust empirical history as an effective measure to be used in BFT for a breadth of conditions (Boucsein, 2012). In one study (Pop-Jordanova, 2009), EDA-assisted BFT was found to be a successful, brief treatment for non-organic somatic complaints (i.e., somatic symptom disorder, illness anxiety disorder, conversion disorder) in a sample of 220 children who presented in medical settings. Given that somatic complaints are a common referral for behavioral health clinicians in integrated medical practices (see Hoffses et al., 2017), it is important for clinicians to consider ways to implement EDA-BFT in practice. In another study, Teufel and colleagues (2013) utilized EDA-assisted BFT to train obese patients to reduce arousal in the presence of food, which reduced food cravings and improved food-related self-control in the sample. These findings suggest that practitioners of BFT may be able to use techniques to reduce potential problematic food-related behaviors in patients, which may serve as a useful guide toward generalized healthy functioning overall.

In addition to being a relatively 'pure' measure of sympathetic activity, EDA has numerous other advantages that allow it to lend itself well to BFT. EDA requires only two sensors that can be attached on any area of skin. The two sensors most often are placed in proximity either on two fingers or, occasionally, on the wrist. Because EDA can be measured on the wrist, there are now several wearable devices that can monitor and record EDA accurately over long periods of time (see Poh, Swenson, & Picard, 2010). In fact, although they are not currently routinely marketed or used, some commercial fitness watches (e.g., Microsoft Band, Jawbone UP3) contain technology capable of measuring long-term EDA. Recently (late 2016), developers have begun to release and market wristwatches for 'emotional fitness,' which measure EDA over time and report direct feedback to wearers about their relative stress levels over time. The Feel wristband is one example. The Feel interacts with smartphone or computer apps to show daily levels of stress. Users can learn when their most common times of physiological arousal occur and can then schedule relaxation activities around that time to reduce overall distress. Another example is the Embrace watch from the company Empatica (www.empatica. com), which is based on technology and research developed at the Massachusetts Institute of Technology (MIT). Embrace uses long-term EDA and other measurements to be able to predict onset of epileptic seizures. A clinical trial is currently being conducted to test its effectiveness in reducing overall risk and improving everyday life for people with epilepsy. The fact that people can wear these monitors long term in an unobtrusive manner is perhaps the most significant benefit of EDA over other measures of human physiology. We expect that soon this technology will initiate a plethora of potential clinical applications relevant to pediatric behavioral and mental health practice.

Heart Rate Variability

Another form of biofeedback involves measuring the time between heart beats that changes with inhaling and exhaling, termed heart rate variability (HRV). The most accurate way to measure HRV is with an electrocardiogram (EKG), but simpler (and less expensive) devices use heart rate and blood pressure sensors that can attach to fingertips, earlobes, or wrap around one's wrist (most fitness watches described earlier also measure HRV). HRV is an indicator of cardiovascular status. Decreased HRV is associated with numerous cardiovascular diseases, including hypertension, sudden cardiac death, ventricular arrhythmia, ischemic heart disease, and other related diseases (see Lehrer & Gevirtz, 2014; Hillebrand et al., 2013; Wheat & Larkin, 2010). It is also associated with increased risk for anxiety, panic attacks, depression (Angelink, Boz, Ullrich, & Andrich, 2002; Gorman & Sloan, 2000; Kemp et al., 2010; Kemp, Quintana, Felmingham, Matthews, & Jelinek, 2012), and asthma (Kazuma, Otsuka, Matsuoka, & Murata, 1997). Thus, it is clear that decreased HRV is a major risk factor for serious illness, representative more broadly as a general vulnerability to stress. Thus, a goal of some biofeedback training is to increase HRV, which then improves one's overall physiological adaptability to stressors. HRV-mediated BFT is most often accomplished using simple breathing training. Lehrer (2013) presents a manualized model that has been researched predominantly with adults. However, the method can be easily adapted to children.

In the method described by Lehrer and colleagues (2013), HRV-mediated BFT is a complex process that requires a trained clinician to interpret biofeedback. A full protocol is described in detail (session by session) within the original article. In short, the protocol begins by orienting the participant to the equipment (sensors) and explaining the output, which will usually involve at least heart and respiratory rates. Next, baseline data is gathered, assessing the patient's natural HRV. Then, participants undergo a series of breathing exercises, alternating breathing rhythms (different rates of respirations) until an optimal (maximal) HRV is achieved. This is the point at which an expert is needed to assist with monitoring output to find the optimal HRV. Target breathing rate generally varies between 4.5 to 6.5 breaths per minute. Once an optimal rate is observed, patients are instructed to repeat it and encouraged to practice at this optimal rate in between sessions at home (even if the HRV monitoring equipment is not available there). This method has been used to treat pain, asthma, anxiety, depression, chronic obstructive pulmonary disease, food cravings, and hypertension (see Lehrer et al., 2013). As an intervention for youth, breathing training is very simple and can be implemented by a wide range of practitioners and clients. Also, HRV can be measured easily and non-invasively, making it a very friendly model to be used in BFT with young clients.

Electroencephalography and Neurofeedback

Another form of biofeedback (often called neurofeedback, in this case) utilizes information gathered from electroencephalography (EEG). EEG is among the more complex and time-intensive mechanisms of biofeedback, typically requiring advanced neurological training in the interpretation of EEG and also requiring extensive, precise setup of electrodes around the head. Once placed correctly, electrodes display active brain waves, which can indicate behavior or other mental states. EEG and neurofeedback have been used clinically to treat seizure disorders, ADHD, and various presentations of anxiety (for in depth reviews, see Hammond, 2005; La Vaque et al., 2002; Simkin, Thatcher, & Lubar, 2014; Sterman, 2000a; Sterman, 2000b; Tan et al., 2009). However, due to the complexity of EEG and the specialized equipment necessary to use it (e.g., contact gel), we do not recommend it for routine clinical practice of BFT with children, as other, less involved methods appear to provide the same benefits for most patients.

INCORPORATING BIOFEEDBACK TRAINING INTO PLAY THERAPY

Having reviewed BFT as a general approach, we can now move toward describing play-based biofeedback. In response to common limitations of BFT described earlier (required technical knowledge), researchers have developed processors that convert biofeedback results into a more readily interpretable format. Most often, these are task-oriented, inviting the patient to work to accomplish some goal in a game, which can only be accomplished by maintaining adequate control over his or her own physiology. In the subsequent sections, we review some of these recent innovations that have arisen within the literature, with particular attention paid to techniques the first author (JLS) has used in his own practice and research.

Biofeedback Game Design

In the coming sections, we will be discussing two forms of biofeedback gaming, split generally into 'high tech' and 'low tech' options. We will begin by reviewing video game–based biofeedback (high tech), which will compose the majority of our review. Then, we will explore a technique that we have found successful in traditional play therapy and that requires little to no advanced technological equipment.

Video Game–Based Biofeedback Training

Before we progress to describing specific games that use biofeedback, it is first important to understand the work game designers have conducted that inform biofeedback game design. In a wonderfully informative review article, Nacke, Kalyn, Lough, and Mandryk (2011) described several innovations used by game designers to evaluate (1) how players respond when physiological sensors are used during gameplay, and (2) which types of sensors work best for which in-game tasks. Physiological game sensors are divided into two categories: direct-input and indirect-input. Direct-input sensors are those that are more easily controlled without specific training and include EMG through muscle flexion and sensors that measure breathing rate and temperature change (achieved through blowing hot air). Indirect-input sensors are those that require specialized training (i.e., through mindfulness and relaxation) to control and include HR and EDA.

Biofeedback gaming has been around for decades, beginning in the late 1970s and early 1980s. One of the first examples was an EDA sensor placed in a computer mouse, which was used to control a racing game called CalmPrix, released in 1984. Nintendo also released an electrocardiographic biosensor that interacted with Tetris 64 (released in 1998). In this version of Tetris (released primarily in Japan), the sensor measured heartrate and the speed of falling pieces changed accordingly. Similarly, the Nintendo Wii Vitality sensor is a pulse oximeter connected to the Wii remote that can be used in select games, usually relaxation-based games. However, the market for these innovations proved to be relatively small at the time, and as a result, widespread release never occurred. Some early efforts at biofeedback gaming were judged to be tedious and/or uncomfortable for users. For example, one early game for the Atari system used forehead EMG sensors for game control, but users complained of headaches resulting from repetitive forehead muscle contraction (shrugging eyebrows).

Another important consideration is to understand what kinds of game-related changes are possible to achieve through biofeedback input. Nacke and colleagues (2011) describe numerous approaches they have explored in their research using a first-person shooter game they designed for the Xbox 360 (a first person shooter is any game where a player views their environment from the perspective of a protagonist and attempts to conquer enemies through gun-based combat). In one example, the size of enemy targets was altered depending on arousal, where increased calmness would increase size of targets (making them easier to shoot). In another example, game designers introduced variable lengths of flame that shoot out of a flamethrower weapon depending on relative arousal. Additional examples included altering character speed and jump height, the rate of snowfall in the environment (with heavier snow fall impairing vision), and modifying difficulty level of bosses. These changes were controlled either through HR, EDA, temperature (again, through blowing hot air), or through breathing rate. These are just a few examples of the potential game-design features that can be implemented through biofeedback gaming.

Another finding from game designers who have researched user reactions to biofeedback gaming is that many players do report enhanced and more enjoyable gaming experiences when well-designed biofeedback is used (Nacke et al., 2011). However, many users do seem to report increased fatigue associated with difficulty using some of the sensors. From an entertainment perspective, this perceived difficulty may be seen as less desirable; however, from a clinical perspective, it suggests that players may benefit from training in how to use the sensors. We know from decades of BFT research that bio-control can be improved with practice, and that this practice leads to numerous beneficial clinical outcomes (see above). Therefore, biofeedback gaming has a tremendous potential to teach youth (and adults, too) increased physiological control in an entertaining, palatable environment. With regard to clinical work, this enhanced enjoyment has several implications for play therapy practice. Importantly, by increasing palatability of psychotherapy, overall adherence, tolerance, and maintenance of psychotherapeutic gains are expected to also improve.

Review of Specific Sensors and Games

In the next section, we review several sensors and games that have either been subjected to initial clinical research or that the first author (JLS) has used in clinical practice. Readers should be aware, however, that clinical research specifically for biofeedback gaming is still in its infancy and that most research findings reviewed are preliminary and still require replication. Also, in the spirit of this volume, which is intended to be a practical handbook for clinicians to use play therapy principles in practice, we limit our discussion to relatively low-cost, easy-to-learn techniques, which are well-suited to young players. There is far greater research, for example, in virtual reality (VR) therapy, but a full VR setup can be extremely expensive and require very specialized space. Instead, in our review, we focus only on systems and techniques that can be completed with one or two low-cost sensors and a standard, gaming-capable computer, tablet, or console. In this way, patients can potentially obtain and utilize these technologies in their own homes to allow out-of-clinic practice, which is an essential component of long-term maintenance of therapeutic gains (Kazdin, 2007).

The Pip (www.thepip.com; see Figure 18.1) is a small, lightweight (16 g), inexpensive handheld device that functions as an EDA reader (see Figure 18.1). It interacts with several smart apps, compatible with smartphones and tablets, to assist with BFT. Patients hold the Pip between their thumb and forefinger (placed on gold plates on each side of the Pip) while interacting with one of several apps, 1) *Clarity*, 2) *Four Steps to*

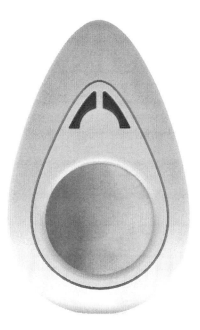

FIGURE 18.1 Pip

Mindfulness, 3) *The Loom*, 4) *Relax & Race*, and 5) *Stress Tracker*. Each app contains different functionality to provide various options for users. In our pediatric practice, patients have generally expressed a preference for *Relax & Race* and *The Loom*.

Relax & Race

Relax & Race challenges players with the task of using relaxation skills to make a character (either a dragon, hot air balloon, or fish, in the current version of the app) race toward a finish line. In all versions, the more relaxed a player is, the higher and faster their character flies/swims. Peaceful music plays in the background during the race. *Relax & Race* can be played by two players (using two pips) or by one single player, who races against his or her own previous time. In clinical intervention, it is usually recommended that children race against themselves, and not each other. Individual baseline differences in EDA make competitive trials unfair. However, sometimes there can be some therapeutic benefit to allowing the child and therapist to race each other (e.g., to build rapport, to demonstrate relaxation skills, as a reward for completion of a successful session).

Each race is generally short-lived, with most people being able to finish the race within 1–3 minutes. This allows the activity to be repeated numerous times over the course of a single session. In the screenshot in Figure 18.2, one can see that two dragons are pictured, but one is so far behind in this case that it cannot be seen on the main screen (and is instead captioned in the bottom left corner). This design gives children direct feedback about their relaxation skills. In this case, they know that whatever they are doing to relax now is working much better than their previous attempt (the dragon in the bottom left, which is far behind). Through repetition of this process numerous times, children learn individualized skills that work best for them.

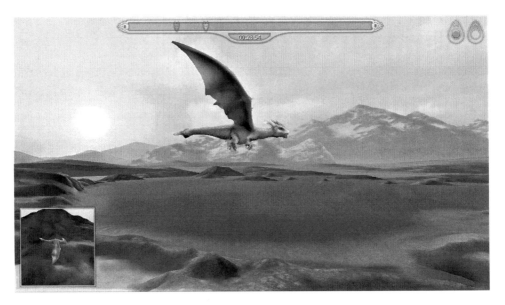

FIGURE 18.2 Dragon

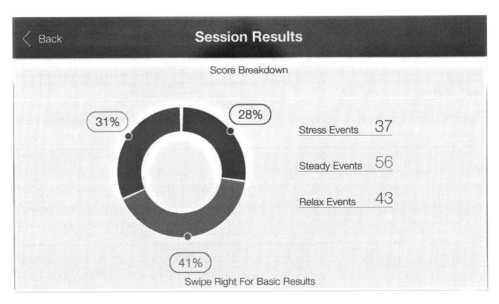

FIGURE 18.3 Session Results

At the end of each race, participants are given data on their performance (pictured in Figure 18.3). These data report in a very user-friendly manner. Rather than showing a graph of their EDA in micro Siemens (the traditional output), the graph displays an easily interpretable summary of 'stress events' (in red), 'steady events' (in orange), and 'relax events' (in green). These data are then saved in a cloud-based server containing all of that person's previous scores called "My Pip," which patients and providers can use to monitor progress over time.

Another app that interacts with the Pip is called *The Loom*. In *The Loom*, patients view a scene and then use relaxation skills to move the scene toward resolution. The screenshots in Figures 18.4 and 18.5 show the "New Life" scene, in which participants

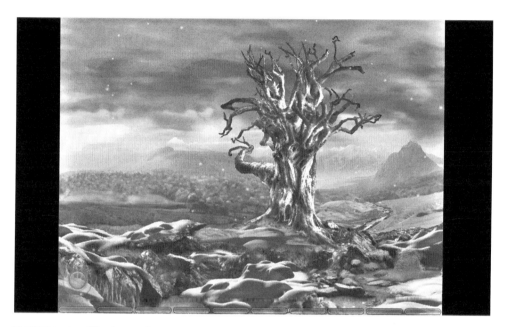

FIGURE 18.4 The Loom I

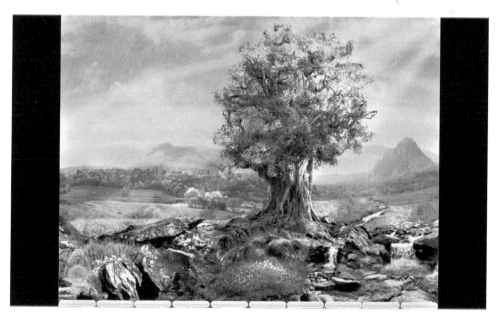

FIGURE 18.5 The Loom II

attempt to change a wintry scene into spring. There also two other scenes from which to choose. *The Loom* takes slightly longer, on average (3–5 minutes), than *Relax & Race*, and thus has a benefit of allowing a longer practice period in which to build relaxation skills. Like *Relax & Race, The Loom* also plays peaceful music in the background. With both apps, if patients do not like the music, it can be silenced without loss of functionality. Also like *Relax & Race, The Loom* displays session data at the end of each session that is saved to the My Pip cloud.

Research Support for the Pip and Related Apps

A game nearly identical to the Pip's *Relax & Race* interface called *Relax to Win* has been previously shown to be effective in clinical research for helping children with anxiety (Sharry, McDermott, & Condron, 2003). The Pip itself has only been explored so far in a young adult population (ages 18–35). In a recent study, researchers completed a randomized-controlled trial comparing the Pip to a non-biofeedback game in 50 participants (Dillon, Kelly, Robertson, & Robertson, 2016). Participants in each condition of the study played games for one 30-minute session, and their anxiety and self-reported stress levels were measured before and after. Results showed a significant decrease in stress and heart rate for the Pip compared to control. The Pip reduced rated stress by 50% compared to 18% in the control group, while it reduced heart rate by 8% compared to 2% in the control group. These findings provide some initial support for the Pip, and the previous findings from similar games support its use in youth.

Additional Special Considerations in Using the Pip

My Pip is a cloud-based platform, and thus, some clinicians may have concern with using the app, due to the possibility that it may publish protected health information to the server. However, My Pip was developed with awareness of HIPAA laws and other legal protections of health care information in mind, and it meets minimal HIPAA standards. Nonetheless, if clinicians or clients are still uncomfortable with cloud-based data management, identifying information can easily be removed from My Pip by using anonymized identifiers. In our research, we enter a seven-digit patient identifier, a uniform and impossible date of birth (1/1/1900), and a unique, anonymized email address.

Some additional procedures are also useful in preparing clients to use the Pip. We generally ask clients to wash their hands prior to use, to remove any lotions, excess dirt, or other contaminants that may impair EDA readings. In clinical practice, we have anecdotally found that clients across the age span (as long as they are old enough to hold the device) accept the intervention, and no adverse experiences have arisen in our clinical practice. We use it most frequently with pediatric anxiety, sleep, pain, and gastrointestinal disorders, in the same manner as described below, as an adjunct to other evidence-based treatment. In all cases, the goal is to provide generalized stress relief, which then translates to improved functioning in other areas. We typically conduct the intervention in 15- to 30-minute increments over the course of several sessions.

Initially, we start with general psychoeducation about mind–body connections, which we perform in a playful manner. To help illustrate concepts for children, we engage them in a collaborative physiological arousal and relaxation activity at the beginning of each session. First, baseline arousal levels are collected with the Pip. Next, children are instructed to start by "doing something to get our bodies excited," which they are told is meant to mimic what happens in our bodies when stressed. Children are able to choose their activity, and they may run in place, do push-ups, perform jumping jacks, or dance. This lasts only briefly (about 1–2 minutes) to prevent children from getting so engaged in the exercise that they get overaroused, but long enough to allow their physiology to respond. Following this activity, we measure physiology again with the Pip over another brief period. Initially, during psychoeducation, this period lasts only 2–3 minutes to illustrate the arousal that has occurred. In later sessions, after relaxation skills have been learned, the resting period also includes relaxation practice, so that children can practice calming their physiology and seeing the output through biofeedback. Occasionally, older youth catch on to the artificiality of the activity—that they are aroused due to exercise, not due to stress. If this occurs, youth are praised for their astute observation but then told that the artificiality is done purposefully to encourage practice when not stressed, so that they can use it better when they really need it. Eventually, youth can be instructed to simulate psychological stress (e.g., thinking about a stressful math test) and seeing the output in biofeedback; however, doing so does not always result in noticeable changes in the output. The changes (or lack thereof) depend on individual variations in general electrodermal reactivity. Some people only exhibit very subtle changes, which are only notable over extended practice periods. Therefore, clinicians are cautioned to warn youth that some people won't notice changes in game performance right away on the Pip, but that over time, their *average* performance typically does get better.

Nevermind

In an ongoing study, we have recently begun investigating a biofeedback-based game called *Nevermind* (www.nevermindgame.com). *Nevermind* is a PC game that began development in 2012 and was released in September 2015 by a small company called Flying Mollusk, LLC. *Nevermind* is unique among modern commercial games in that it uses several forms of biofeedback technology in its interface, including HRV, facial expression–based emotional biofeedback (a webcam reads facial expressions), and eye tracking (with compatible hardware, sold separately). The game itself is an adventure game in which the player must explore a world, deciphering puzzles to solve a mystery. In this case, the player is a 'Neuroprober'—a physician who can enter the minds of patients with traumatic backgrounds and for whom traditional treatment has been ineffective. The Neuroprober is then tasked with entering the subconscious minds of several trauma victims and walking through the traumas to help bring them toward resolution. Thus, the game itself has at its core a design that is already based heavily in psychological science.

The game is designed to be a horror game, and has been assigned a rating of "Mature" by the ESRB due to themes of "Violence, Blood, Sexual Themes, Partial Nudity, Strong Language, and Use of Drugs." Given the Mature rating, this game is likely not suitable for all youth. However, some youth, at their guardians' discretion, may still benefit from it. *Nevermind* uses biofeedback in several unique and interesting ways. The more stressed players become, the harder and scarier the game gets. The screenshot below depicts this process. The image on the right demonstrates how a room that is fully visible when the player is calm floods with water when the player is stressed (see Figure 18.6). If the player does not gain control over his or stress in time, he or she would be at risk of 'dying' in the game. In this way, players are forced to monitor and master their own physiological and emotional states in order to progress through the game.

As noted, we are currently testing *Nevermind* in a small, randomized clinical trial, seeking to explore its utility in a sample of mildly (but clinically) anxious adults. Once we understand more about its therapeutic potential in adults, we hope to expand our research on *Nevermind* to youth as well. Due to the mature themes in *Nevermind*, however, we recommend caution in using it with children.

Technologically, *Nevermind* can function with inexpensive biotechnology. The game is compatible with an array of commercial heartrate monitors commonly used for exercise tracking. We use (and recommend) a chest strap HR monitor (which can be purchased for around $40–$60), as chest strap monitors are generally more reliable and accurate than wristwatch monitors for heartrate. Facial recognition can be accomplished with nearly any web camera. Recently (October 2016) a VR version of *Nevermind* was released for the Oculus Rift, which is a VR mask/interface similar to other consumer-grade VR devices that have recently entered the market. Obviously, this version enables even more advanced technological capabilities. However, VR devices require extra expense. For the clinician or consumer on a budget, the game does work well with only an HR monitor and/or webcam.

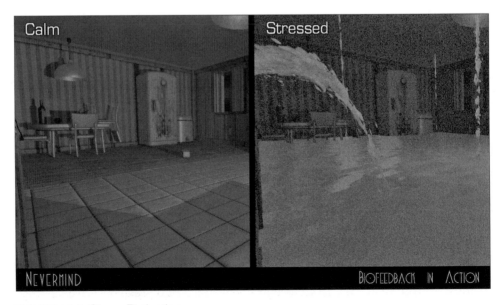

FIGURE 18.6 Stress Reduction

Nevermind has had limited research so far, but studies across several research labs are underway. In one example, a team of researchers including some from the team that developed the game presented a poster at a recent conference based on a study that sought to determine whether an ability to downregulate (decrease arousal) during the game corresponded to real-world emotion regulation strategies (Lobel et al., 2015). Testing a sample of 47 young, emerging adults (aged 18–24), Lobel and colleagues found that players who needed more time to return to a calm state after a negative arousal were also less likely to use the cognitive strategy of reappraisal as a skill for coping with anxiety in the real world ($r = -.330$, $p = .046$). Although these are only preliminary findings and more research is needed, these results at least suggest that physiological observations made during gameplay can translate to real-world implications.

Wild Divine

Wild Divine (www.wilddivine.com) is another popular commercial product (purchase price ranges from about $120 to $350, depending on the package purchased) that was developed in collaboration with numerous leading researchers and practitioners in biofeedback-based therapy. With an interface very similar to that described above in the Pip, *Wild Divine* uses a device that attaches to three fingers to simultaneously measure HRV and EDA. *Wild Divine* is marketed as an entertaining meditation trainer, rather than a 'game' per se, but the principles are similar to that described in previous examples. *Wild Divine* can be played on PC or a tablet, and the devices connect via Bluetooth or USB.

RAGE-Control

RAGE-Control is a game system that was developed by a team of researchers and clinicians from Boston Children's Hospital and Harvard Medical School (Kahn, Ducharme, Rotenberg, & Gonzalez-Heydrich, 2013). The game incorporates heart rate–based biofeedback (as measured by a pulse oximeter) into a video game based loosely on the arcade game *Space Invaders*. Players must maintain heart rate below their resting heart rate threshold to be effective at the game. In preliminary studies, clinical researchers have shown promising results suggesting that *RAGE-control*, in addition to cognitive behavior therapy, may be an effective way to teach youth improved emotional control to which children respond better than treatment as usual (Ducharme et al., 2012; Kahn et al., 2013). Over the course of several sessions, children learn several relaxation and cognitive restructuring techniques that help them achieve better emotional control, which they can practice inside a safe gaming environment.

Biofeedback in Traditional (Non-Digital) Play

In our clinical practice, we have also found success incorporating some biofeedback into traditional play therapy. In a procedure nearly identical to that described with the Pip, we regularly engage children in a physiological hyperarousal and relaxation activity during our play therapy sessions. However, instead of using the Pip or another high-tech sensor, we simply have children measure heartrate in beats per minute (BPM) using a stethoscope or by feeling their pulse with their figures. They measure their pulse at baseline, after arousal, and then again after relaxation. For the relaxation intervention, we use a number of therapeutic skills, including storytelling (telling a 'story about relaxing'), interactive play, progressive muscle relaxation (in the form of an interactive game or dance), or art-based approaches. The point of the activity is that children learn to monitor their own physiology as a means to also monitor relative distress and then they learn to respond in an adaptive manner to maladaptive increases in arousal. Although not as sophisticated as EMG, EDA, HRV, or EEG, the simple act of counting heartrate in BPM can be an effective means to teach children about mind-body physiological connections.

The first author (JLS) has conducted some mixed quantitative and qualitative research on children's and parents' reactions to this biofeedback play in a manualized approach to play therapy described elsewhere (Steadman, 2014), and children and parents have both reliably described this biofeedback portion as being the "most helpful" aspect of therapy targeting pathological anxiety. More research is needed to confirm these pilot findings, but these preliminary results suggest that patients find great value in adding a biofeedback component to traditional play therapy. Although some of the digital forms of BFT described in previous sections offer unique advantages in a modern format, low-tech biofeedback play can be used with a wide array of children and a wide array of settings and without requiring access to equipment. This makes BFT applicable to even the most impoverished clients and clinicians.

SUMMARY AND PERSONAL REFLECTIONS

In the modern world, where nearly all youth play at least some form of video game on a regular basis, play therapists must begin to harness the potential for video games to be used in psychotherapy with youth (Steadman, Boska, Lee, Lim, & Nichols, 2014). Biofeedback gaming is an ideal means to accomplish this feat, as it allows users a means to practice a specific, evidence-based therapeutic skill (MBSR and relaxation training) while simultaneously doing something fun—playing a game. However, as we've seen, biofeedback gaming need not only be limited to the digital world, but children can be taught and encouraged to monitor and augment their own physiology through nearly any play-based format. It is also a relatively brief intervention that can be taught and practiced in short chunks (e.g., 10 minutes at a time). These features make biofeedback gaming an excellent adjunct to any psychotherapy.

Based on our own experiences, we find that biofeedback gaming can be learned and implemented by novice and experienced therapists and does not require an advanced technical background. However, before pursuing biofeedback gaming in practice, we do still advise a consultation with a technical team to ensure your equipment does meet proper technical specifications. We particularly advise this consultation for computer requirements. It is wise to ensure not only that your computer has the processing power to manage games and sensors, but also that any data saved and any network or other connections used are compliant with HIPAA standards. Remember that saved data may constitute protected health information (PHI). It is important to consult with a local

HIPAA-compliance officer to ensure any PHI meets all minimum security standards. With all of the techniques and software we reviewed in this chapter, we have found that secure data management is possible. Still, clinicians implementing these techniques in their own practices should exercise due diligence to ensure their own data is also secure.

Lastly, it should be noted that many forms of commercially available biofeedback gaming are still considered investigational products. In our own research, for example, using *Nevermind* and the Pip, we have had to label our devices as 'investigational' devices under FDA standards, meaning they should not be understood by users as being designed or established to evaluate or treat any clinical illness. This labeling is done to avoid any confusion among patients that these commercial devices should be considered 'medicinal.' They simply are commercial devices being used in the practice of psychotherapy, similar to the way a notebook may be used in therapy that uses journaling or that toys may be used in traditional play therapy. Although most patients intuitively understand that a notebook or a toy are not 'medicinal' in and of themselves, this knowledge may be less intuitive for high-tech biofeedback devices. Therefore, we recommend an extended informed consent process with patients where it is possible to more thoroughly discuss the nature of these products and their use in therapy.

We hope the preceding discussion and examples were an informative introduction to biofeedback training as a clinical intervention for a wide variety of pediatric medical and psychological issues. We believe that biofeedback gaming not only has a bright future in the entertainment industry, especially with the recent movement toward VR gaming; it also will play an important role in making biofeedback-based clinical therapy a readily accessible, relatively user friendly means to improve clinical prognosis for a significant number of clients.

REFERENCES

Agnihotri, H., Paul, M., & Sandhu, J. (2008). The comparative efficacy of two biofeedback techniques in the treatment of generalized anxiety disorder. *Pakistan Journal of Social and Clinical Psychology, 6,* 35–46.

Angelink, M. W., Boz, C., Ullrich, H., & Andrich, J. (2002). Relationship between major depression and heart rate variability: Clinical consequences and implications for antidepressive treatment. *Psychiatry Research, 113*(1), 139–149.

Bei, B., Byrne, M. L., Ivens, C., Waloszek, J., Woods, M. J., Dudgeon, P., . . . Allen, N. B. (2013). Pilot study of a mindfulness-based, multi-component, in-school group sleep intervention in adolescent girls. *Early Intervention in Psychiatry, 7,* 213–220.

Bolek, J. E. (2006). Use of multiple-site performance-contingent SEMG reward programming in pediatric rehabilitation: A retrospective review. *Applied Psychophysiology and Biofeedback, 31*(3), 263–272.

Boucsein, W. (2012). *Electrodermal activity.* New York: Springer.

Braithwaite, J. J., Watson, D. G., Jones, R., & Rowe, M. (2013). A guide for analyzing Electrodermal Activity (EDA) & Skin Conductance Responses (SCRs) for psychological experiments. *Psychophysiology, 49,* 1017–1034.

Bussone, G., Grazzi, L., D'Amico, D., Leone, M., & Andrasik, F. (1998). Biofeedback-assisted relaxation training for young adolescents with tension-type headache: A controlled study. *Cephalalgia, 18,* 463–467.

Catani, C., Kohiladevy, M., Ruf, M., Schauer, E., Elbert, T., & Neuner, F. (2009). Treating children traumatized by war and Tsunami: A comparison between exposure therapy and meditation-relaxation in North-East Sri Lanka. *BMC Psychiatry, 9*(22), 1–11. https://doi. org/10.1186/1471-244X-9-22

Chiarioni, G., & Whitehead, W. E. (2008). The role of biofeedback in the treatment of gastrointestinal disorders. *Nature Clinical Practice Gastroenterology & Hepatology, 5*(7), 371–382.

Cox, D. J., Sutphen, J., Borowitz, S., Dickens, M. N., Singles, J., & Whitehead, W. E. (1994). Simple electromyographic biofeedback treatment for chronic pediatric constipation/encopresis: Preliminary report. *Biofeedback and Self-Regulation, 19*(1), 41–50.

Dedeepya, P., Nuvvula, S., Kamatham, R., & Nirmala, S. V. S. G. (2014). Behavioural and physiological outcomes of biofeedback therapy on dental anxiety of children undergoing restorations: A randomized controlled trial. *European Archives of Pediatric Dentistry, 15*(2), 97–103.

Dillon, A., Kelly, M., Robertson, I. H., & Robertson, D. A. (2016). Smartphone applications utilizing biofeedback can aid stress reduction. *Frontiers in Psychology, 7*(832), 1–7. https:// doi.org/10.3389/fpsyg.2016.00832

Ducharme, P., Wharff, E., Hutchinson, E., Kahn, J., Logan, G., & Gonzalez-Heydrich, J. (2012). Videogame-assisted emotional regulation training: An ACT with RAGE-Control case illustration. *Clinical Social Work Journal, 40*, 75–84.

Dursun, E., Dursun, N., & Alican, D. (2004). Effects of biofeedback treatment on gait in children with cerebral palsy. *Disability and Rehabilitation, 26*(2), 116–120.

Eid, M. A., Aly, S. M., & El-Shamy, S. M. (2016). Effect of electromyographic biofeedback training on pain, quadriceps muscle strength, and functional ability in juvenile rheumatoid arthritis. *American Journal of Physical Medicine & Rehabilitation/Association of Academic Physiatrists, 95*(12), 921–930.

Gevirtz, R. (2007). Psychophysiological perspectives on stress-related and anxiety disorders. *Principles and Practice of Stress Management*, 209–226.

Gorman, J. M., & Sloan, R. P. (2000). Heart rate variability in depressive and anxiety disorders. *American Heart Journal, 140*, S77–83.

Hammond, D. C. (2005). Neurofeedback with anxiety and affective disorders. *Child and Adolescent Psychiatric Clinics of North America, 14*(1), 105–123.

Hillebrand, S., Gast, K. B., de Mutsert, R., Swenne, C. A., Jukema, J. W., Middeldorp, S., . . . Dekkers, O. M. (2013). Heart rate variability and first cardiovascular event in populations without known cardiovascular disease: Meta-analysis and dose—Response meta-regression. *Europace, 15*(5), 742–749.

Hoffses, K. W., Riley, A. R., Menousek, K., Schellinger, K., Grennan, A., Cammarata, C., & Steadman, J. L. (2017). Professional practices, training, and funding mechanisms: A survey of pediatric primary care psychologists. *Clinical Practice in Pediatric Psychology, 5*(1), 39–49.

Jacobson, E. (1938). *Progressive relaxation*. Chicago: University of Chicago Press.

Jones, P., Blunda, M., Biegel, G., Carlson, L. E., Biel, M., & Wiener, L. (2013). Can mindfulness-based interventions help adolescents with cancer? *Psychooncology, 22*(9), 2148–2151. https://doi.org/10.1002/pon.3251

Kahn, J., Ducharme, P., Rotenberg, A., & Gonzalez-Heydrich, J. (2013). 'RAGE-Control': A game to build emotional strength. *Games for Health Journal, 2*(1), 53–57.

Kanitz, J. L., Camus, M. E. M., & Seifert, G. (2013). Keeping the balance—An overview of mind-body therapies in pediatric oncology. *Complementary Therapies in Medicine, 215*, S20–S25.

Kazdin, A. E. (2007). Mediators and mechanisms of change in psychotherapy research. *Annual Review of Clinical Psychology, 3*(1), 1–27.

Kazuma, N., Otsuka, K., Matsuoka, I., & Murata, M. (1997). Heart rate variability during 24 hours in asthmatic children. *Chronobiology International, 14*, 597–606. https://doi. org/10.3109/07420529709001450

Kemp, A. H., Quintana, D. S., Felmingham, K. L., Matthews, S., & Jelinek, H. F. (2012). Depression, comorbid anxiety disorders, and heart rate variability in physically healthy, unmedicated patients: Implications for cardiovascular risk. *PLoS ONE*, 7(2), e30777.

Kemp, A. H., Quintana, D. S., Gray, M. A., Felmingham, K. L., Brown, K., & Gatt, J. M. (2010). Impact of depression and antidepressant treatment on heart rate variability: A review and meta-analysis. *Biological Psychiatry*, 67(11), 1067–1074.

Koithan, M. (2010). Mind-body solutions for obesity. *Journal for Nurse Practitioners*, 5(7), 536–537.

La Vaque, T. J., Hammond, D. C., Trudeau, D., Monastra, V., Perry, J., & Lehrer, P. (2002). Template for developing guidelines for the evaluation of the clinical efficacy of psychophysiological interventions. *Journal of Neurotherapy*, 6(4), 11–23.

Lehrer, P. (2013). How does heart rate variability biofeedback work? Resonance, the baroreflex, and other mechanisms. *Biofeedback*, 41(1), 26–31.

Lehrer, P. M., & Gevirtz, R. (2014). Heart rate variability biofeedback: how and why does it work? *Frontiers in Psychology*, 5, 1–9.

Lehrer, P. M., Vaschillo, B., Zucker, T., Graves, J., Katsamanis, M., Aviles, M., & Wamboldt, F. (2013). Protocol for heart rate variability biofeedback training. *Biofeedback*, 41(3), 98–109.

Lehrer, P. M., Woolfolk, W. L., & Sime, W. E. (Eds.). (2007). *Principles and practice of stress management*. New York: Guilford Press.

Lobel, A., Gotsis, M., Reynolds, E., Annetta, M., Engles, R., & Granic, I. (May 2015). *Nevermind: Emotion regulation in a biofeedback game*. Presented at the Experiential Technology Conference and Expo, San Francisco.

MacDonell, K., Naar-King, S., Huszti, H., & Belzer, M. (2013). Barriers to medication adherence in behaviorally and perinatally infected youth living with HIV. *AIDS and Behavior*, 17(1), 86–93.

Manzoni, G. M., Pagnini, F., Castelnuovo, G., & Molinari, E. (2008). Relaxation training for anxiety: A ten-years systematic review with meta-analysis. *BMC Psychiatry*, 8(1), 1.

Masters, K. S., France, C. R., & Thorn, B. E. (2009). Enhancing preparation among entry-level clinical health psychologists: Recommendations for 'best practices' from the first meeting of the Council of Clinical Health Psychology Training Programs (CCHPTP). *Training and Education in Professional Psychology*, 3(4), 193–201.

McGuigan, F. J., & Lehrer, P. M. (2007). Progressive relaxation. *Stress Management*, 57.

Middaugh, S. J. (2007). Electromyographic feedback for evaluation and neuromuscular re-education in Cerebral Palsy. *Biofeedback*, 35(1), 27–32.

Nacke, L. E., Kalyn, M., Lough, C., & Mandryk, R. L. (May 2011). *Biofeedback game design: Using direct and indirect physiological control to enhance game interaction*. Paper presented at the Conference on Human Factors in Computing Systems, Vancouver, BC, Canada.

O'Reilly, G. A., Cook, L., Spruijt-Metz, D., & Black, D. S. (2014). Mindfulness-based interventions for obesity-related eating behaviors: A literature review. *Obesity Reviews*, 15(6), 453–461.

Poh, M. Z., Swenson, N. C., & Picard, R. W. (2010). A wearable sensor for unobtrusive, long-term assessment of electrodermal activity. *IEEE Transactions on Biomedical Engineering*, 57(5), 1243–1252.

Pop-Jordanova, N. (2009). Biofeedback application for somatoform disorders and Attention Deficit Hyperactivity Disorder (ADHD) in children. *International Journal of Medicine and Medical Sciences*, 1(2), 17–22.

Sharry, J., McDermott, M., & Condron, J. (2003). Relax to win: Treating children with anxiety problems with a biofeedback video game. *Eisteach*, 2(25), 22–26.

Simkin, D. R., Thatcher, R. W., & Lubar, J. (2014). Quantitative EEG and neurofeedback in children and adolescents: Anxiety disorders, depressive disorders, comorbid addiction and attention-deficit/hyperactivity disorder, and brain injury. *Child and Adolescent Psychiatric Clinics of North America*, 23(3), 427–464.

Steadman, J.L. (2014). *Fantasy-Exposure Life-Narrative Therapy (FELT) for anxious children: A pilot and feasibility study.* Unpublished Doctoral Dissertation, Baylor University, Waco, TX.

Steadman, J.L., Boska, C., Lee, C., Lim, X.S., & Nichols, N. (2014). Using popular commercial video games in therapy with children and adolescents. *Journal of Technology in Human Services*, 32(3), 201–219.

Sterman, M.B. (2000a). Basic concepts and clinical findings in the treatment of seizure disorders with EEG operant conditioning. *Clinical EEG and Neuroscience*, 31(1), 45–55.

Sterman, M.B. (2000b). EEG markers for attention deficit disorder: Pharmacological and neurofeedback applications. *Child Study Journal*, 30(1), 1–1.

Tan, G., Thornby, J., Hammond, D.C., Strehl, U., Canady, B., Arnemann, K., & Kaiser, D.A. (2009). Meta-analysis of EEG biofeedback in treating epilepsy. *Clinical EEG and Neuroscience*, 40(3), 173–179.

Teufel, M., Stephan, K., Kowalski, A., Käsberger, S., Enck, P., Zipfel, S., & Giel, K.E. (2013). Impact of biofeedback on self-efficacy and stress reduction in obesity: A randomized controlled pilot study. *Applied Psychophysiology and Biofeedback*, 38(3), 177–184.

van der Oord, S., Bögels, S.M., & Peijnenburg, D. (2012). The effectiveness of mindfulness training for children with ADHD and mindful parenting for their parents. *Journal of Child and Family Studies*, 21(1), 139–147.

Wheat, A.L., & Larkin, K.T. (2010). Biofeedback of heart rate variability and related physiology: A critical review. *Applied Psychophysiology and Biofeedback*, 35(3), 229–242.

White, L.S. (2012). Reducing stress in school-age girls through mindful Yoga. *Journal of Pediatric Health Care*, 26(1), 45–56.

Woodward, S., Norton, C., & Chiarelli, P. (2014). Biofeedback for treatment of chronic idiopathic constipation in adults. *The Cochrane* Database, Issue 3.

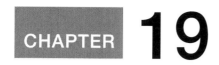

CHAPTER 19

The Future Is Now

Using Humanoid Robots in Child Life Practice

*Jacqueline Reynolds Pearson
and Tanya Nathalie Beran*

> And above all, watch with glittering eyes the whole world around you because the greatest secrets are always hidden in the most unlikely of places.
>
> —Roald Dahl, *The Minpins*

In the spirit of searching for hidden treasures, the most recent issue of the Association of Child Life Professionals Bulletin encourages readers in the endless pursuit of finding something not yet known (Bennett, 2017). This chapter presents an endeavor to do just that, as we describe the process of our MEDi robot 'coming into being' and gaining its own unique position within the comprehensive health care team. We begin with a description of our early research on children's reactions to an unsophisticated robot, then outline the various applications of many types of robots in hospitals, and with children in other settings. Given children's enthusiasm for robots and knowing how medical experiences can be challenging and overwhelming for them, we describe the next stage of our research—introducing a robot to help children during needle procedures. Its impact is described next, followed by a full explanation of how humanoid robots were then integrated into a Child Life program and their specific uses by child life specialists as enhancements to their therapeutic interventions with children and families. We then focus on MEDi's role during specific interventions currently employed by child life specialists (Goldberger, Mohl, & Thompson, 2009; Humphreys & LeBlanc, 2016). These include play, procedural support, conscious choice of alternate focus (historically referred to as 'distraction'), preparation, medical play, and empowering children and parents through learning coping strategies. We explain each construct and provide examples of MEDi's involvement including vignettes covering a range of areas within the hospital. We end the chapter by presenting a list of what we have learned about implementing a robot in a hospital.

OUR EARLY RESEARCH ON CHILDREN AND ROBOTS

The idea of introducing robots to children began in 2010. Having been inspired by research showing that children express social behaviors toward a robotic dog (Melson, Kahn, Beck, & Friedman, 2009), we were curious to learn how children ages 5 to 16 years would interact with other types of robots. We used a small industrial electric robot arm with five degrees of freedom and with pre-programmed bio-inspired control mechanisms (for full description, see Beran & Ramirez-Serrano, 2011). To make it appealing to children, we decorated it in craft materials to give the appearance of eyes, ears, and a mouth (see Figure 19.1).

We programmed the robot to stack blocks, and enhanced its autonomous characteristics by also programming it to release the last block, as if it were accidentally dropped. The robot arm then swept from side to side in the area to 'look' for the dropped block. We watched children's reactions under several experimental conditions. To our surprise, the majority of children (70%) attempted to help the robot stack the last block (Beran, Ramirez-Serrano, Kuzyk, Nugent, & Fior, 2011). They expressed considerable emotion, moreover, in their attempts to help: shouting ("It's right here!"), encouraging ("You can find it!"), and crying out ("The robot needs help!"). Children tried a variety of strategies to help the robot, including putting the block in front of its eyes to better 'see' it, into its mouth to help hold it, and on the tower of blocks to complete the task for the robot. These helping behaviors were particularly surprising given that they were spontaneous: children were not asked to help the robot.

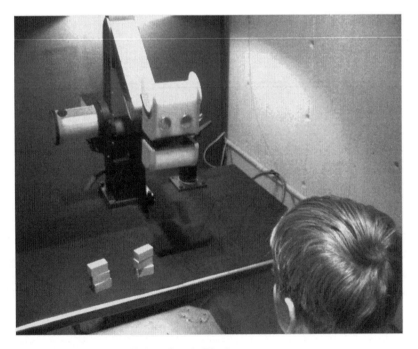

FIGURE 19.1 Child Watching Robot Stack Blocks

In addition to providing this form of support to the robot, we were curious to learn how children regarded the robot; would they see it as alive in its ability to think, feel, and behave? We were shocked to find that children thought the robot had abilities that clearly it did not have (Beran, Ramirez-Serrano, Kuzyk, Fior, & Nugent, 2011). In terms of their beliefs about the robot's cognitive capacity, more than half thought the robot could remember them, and almost a third thought it knew their feelings. Children also attributed affective characteristics to the robot, with more than half stating that they thought the robot liked them, and that the robot would feel rejected if not played with. Finally, more than a third of children thought it could see the blocks and many stated that the robot could play with them in a variety of ways, such as playing soccer (even though the robot had no legs).

If children believed the robot possessed these human characteristics, perhaps they would enter into a friendship with one. So, we asked children if they thought the robot liked them, could be their friend, could cheer them up, and if they would talk to the robot and share secrets with it. We were amazed to discover that the majority of children endorsed a positive response to these questions (Fior, Nugent, Beran, Ramirez-Serrano, & Kuzyk, 2010). These results were in response to a robot arm (no torso, legs, or arms) with craft materials (wood, foam). If this level of enthusiasm was demonstrated toward an unsophisticated robot, perhaps it underestimated the extent of endorsement children would show toward a humanoid robot, capable of a variety of human behaviors such as talking and walking.

Through this series of studies, it became apparent that children entered into magical thinking about the robot (Beran & Ramirez-Serrano, 2010). With it programmed to act in autonomous ways, children seemed to believe that its actions were deliberate and purposeful—which are properties of animism—or the characteristic of life. Indeed, they believed that the robot had human capabilities that it did not have. Perhaps they were projecting their own human experiences of thoughts, feelings, and behaviors onto the robot. Upon seeing a robot's animated actions to appear as if it is intentionally looking for a dropped block with the goal of completing the tower stacking task, children's own empathy may have been triggered. This experience seemed to activate an emotional reaction toward the robot.

Given this enchanting child–robot connection, we wondered if there could be some sort of beneficial application. At the time, research to address the significant pain and distress experienced by children receiving immunizations was well underway (Chambers, Taddio, Uman, McMurtry, & HELPnKIDS, 2009; Uman, Chambers, McGrath, & Kisely, 2008). These reviews indicated that psychological strategies could be helpful in managing pain associated with needles but were not always incorporated into the medical experience. We continue to need to find ways to better help children having trouble coping with painful medical procedures, especially needles. If children express such an affinity toward a simple robot arm, perhaps a more endearing robot could be used to help them manage medical procedures?

This argument becomes plausible when we consider children's propensity for technologically enhanced devices such as computers and cell phones. In fact, according to the Kaiser Family Foundation (2006), U.S. children in grades 7 to 12 are exposed to 6.38 to 12.49 hours of media (TV, computers) per day. With television programs now available on cell phones, it is likely that these numbers are even higher today. This engagement with technology suggests that children would also be enthusiastic about a robot, and because robots are now being used in schools for a variety of education purposes, perhaps children would enjoy them in a health care setting as well.

ROBOTS IN HEALTH CARE

In 2011, we launched the first study, to our knowledge, of the use of a humanoid robot for pediatric pain management. At that time, robots were not new to health care. Robotic applications for surgery were explored in the late 1980s (Kwoh, Hou, Jonckheere, & Hayall, 1988) and systematically tested in hospitals in the early 2000s (Melvin, Needleman, Krause, & Ellison, 2003; Talamini, Chapman, Horgan, & Melvin, 2003). Then in 2013, the Food and Drug Administration (FDA) approved the first robot (RP-VITA) that navigates through the hospital environment and allows a doctor to communicate with a patient through a tablet (U.S. Food and Drug Administration, 2012). Robots are also used to dispense medication in hospitals (e.g., ScriptPro) and deliver food and supplies (e.g., AZO Robotics).

For application with children specifically, robots have been used to help children with autism to develop social skills. For an overview of the various robots used, see Kozima, Michalowski, and Nakagawa (2009). In general, they are shown to encourage dyadic (robot and child) and triadic (robot, child, caregiver) interactions. That is, children exhibit social behaviors such as touching and approaching the robot, smiling at it, initiating behaviors to gain a reaction from it, imitating it, and expressing protective and gentle behaviors toward it. They also turn to their caregiver during engagement with the robot. Robots may be appropriate for a wide range of ages. Research shows that even children as young as 7 months of age will use a joystick to drive themselves on a robot chair (Galloway, Ryu, & Agrawal, 2008).

In terms of pediatric pain management, the application of robotics had not been previously explored. Other strategies for reducing children's pain and anxiety such as blowing bubbles, listening to music, and watching cartoons do not consistently show a significant benefit (Cassidy et al., 2002; Megel, Houser, & Gleaves, 1998). Perhaps stronger and more stimulating interventions are needed when children encounter needles and other painful procedures. Indeed, counterconditioning suggests that a positive response such as laughter to a positive stimulus such as a dancing robot can replace an undesirable response, such as crying, to a negative stimulus such as a needle.

We believed that a child-friendly humanoid robot, with the ability to talk, move, and play sounds, could serve as a highly engaging positive stimulus. There were two primary factors to consider in formulating such an intervention: the robot's appearance and actions. The most endearing and intelligent robot available at a reasonable cost is the NAO robot produced by Softbank Robotics. Weighing 11 pounds and standing 2 feet tall, with LED lights for eyes that change color and shape to express emotions, 14 motors to move head and limbs, and moving fingers that can hold objects, it seemed that this robot would be attractive to a wide age range of children. In regard to its actions, we programmed the robot with cognitive behavioral strategies such as role modeling deep breathing, embedded in the form of play (such as helping to blow off dust from a rubber duck). These strategies significantly reduce pain and anxiety, but when we teach them to children they tend to forget to use them, and they are rarely taught to parents. Once they are programmed into a robot, they are delivered just the way they were designed every time they are played.

THE EMERGENCE OF MEDi IN OUR RESEARCH

To examine the implementation of the NAO robot in a medical setting, and with it programmed to be medically and socially appropriate, we gave it the name MEDi— Medicine and Engineering Designing Intelligence. In collaboration with an engineer at the University of Calgary, and clinician-scientists at the Alberta Children's Hospital (ACH), we designed a randomized control trial to test MEDi during flu vaccination. We randomly assigned children to nurse-administered vaccination under standard care (minimal distraction sometimes used such as "Look at the dinosaur on the wall") or nurse-administered vaccination while interacting with MEDi. We programmed the robot to play music, share personal experiences, play popular and familiar sounds, and invite children to blow together. Full details of the study have been published (Beran, Ramirez-Serrano, Vanderkooi, & Kuhn, 2013). We found a significant reduction in children's pain and anxiety. In addition, children and parents smiled significantly longer with MEDi than in the control group (Beran, Ramirez-Serrano, Vanderkooi, & Kuhn, 2015). Unexpectedly, there were several children in the control group who could not be vaccinated because they were kicking and attempting to bite their caregiver. In those situations, the nurses said they were unable to vaccinate. All of those children agreed to be calmly vaccinated with MEDi. Then a snowball effect occurred whereby families told others about the robot at the hospital and families contacted the hospital and drove from out of town to have their children vaccinated with MEDi. Perhaps most surprising, however, was the number of unsolicited emails our research assistants received in which they shared stories of what their children were saying and telling others about the robot. We then received requests from parents to have MEDi present during other longer procedures, such as blood tests.

Our second randomized control trial was, therefore, using MEDi during blood tests (see Beran, Manesh, Greenberg, & Sharlin, 2015). This time, the robot engaged children in interactive games involving questions and answers, hand games, storytelling, and friendship behaviors. In this study, parents reported significantly lower pain for children with MEDi compared to children without MEDi. Considerable validation for the effectiveness of this study came from patients who spontaneously shared their stories. One family notified our research team that after her daughter completed her blood test with MEDi, she spoke with her oncologist for the very first time. Perhaps MEDi's support comforted her and gave her courage to face other medical challenges.

FIRST PATIENT STORIES

Parents and children shared a variety of reactions to MEDi during and after our research. Some children felt empowered and encouraged from being with MEDi:

> My 8-year-old daughter usually goes "ballistic" when knowing she has to take the vaccine. Last year she was terrified and tried bolting out of the room but none of that happened this time [with the robot]. I didn't even have to hold her. I'd say there was 90 percent improvement.
>
> (Beran et al., 2015)

More neutral reactions included some but not major changes in the child's experience during the medical procedure:

> My 10-year-old son had a nose bleed last year but didn't this year because of the robot. It was different this time. At one point he was really engaged with the robot and was smiling. Then he remembered the needle and became anxious again. If I had a choice, I'd pick the robot again.
>
> (Beran et al., 2015)

Positive feedback included, "My 5 year-old son wants to have the robot for every needle until he's a grown-up" (Beran et al., 2015). These comments suggest that for some children the robot had a greater effect than for others, which seems to be a realistic response to a painful and frightening medical experience.

These patient stories, in combination with the statistical evidence of effectiveness in reducing children's pain and anxiety, opened our eyes to the possibility that pediatric patients could gain and benefit from support from a little robot. In Roald Dahl's words, we found a hidden secret in an unlikely place. This possibility gave us further impetus for continuing our research as well as beginning implementation in hospital. Given that the role of Child Life is to reduce anxiety and create positive health care experiences for children, working with these professionals was a logical next step.

INTEGRATING MEDi INTO CHILD LIFE AT THE ALBERTA CHILDREN'S HOSPITAL

The Alberta Children's Hospital (ACH) is a tertiary care teaching and research hospital located in a major urban center in Western Canada. It is closely affiliated with the University of Calgary and is an integral part of Alberta Health Services, which includes many other hospitals and health centers throughout the province. ACH serves infants, children, and adolescents, and is Southern Alberta's major treatment facility for complex pediatric medical problems and also provides mental health services.

Within ACH, Child Life and Therapeutic Arts (art, horticultural, and music therapy) form a team and work collaboratively with other health professionals throughout the facility. Historically, child life specialists concentrated primarily on the inpatient units; however, in recent years they have broadened their focus to the emergency department and several ambulatory clinics. Currently, there are 12 child life specialist positions. In congruence with the Association of Child Life Professionals' Mission Statement (www. childlife.org), child life specialists at ACH focus on supporting patients and families through therapeutic play, preparation, and education regarding pain management and coping strategies. Primary goals include building resiliency, promoting empowerment, and facilitating confidence for future health care experiences.

A major theme within the culture of this health care center is a concerted commitment to helping children and their families understand and cope with pain. Various innovative pain management strategies and coping techniques have recently been integrated into the care provided throughout the hospital and by a wide range of health care professionals. The use of humanoid robots is one of several contemporary enhancements provided by a unique donor funded program aimed at further advancing the quality of patient care.

In response to Dr. Tanya Beran's work on the development of MEDi, ACH purchased four robots under the Vi Riddell Pain and Rehabilitation Centre for integration into clinical programming. ACH also agreed to be the official test site for the robots and became the first hospital in the world to work with humanoid robots in this way. When the robots arrived in 2015, the hospital's leadership team had some evidence of 'why' but had not yet established the specifics of 'where' or 'how' the robots would be used in the day-to-day provision of health care.

Building on the studies of MEDi's role during vaccinations and blood tests (Beran et al., 2013; Beran et al., 2015), it was initially thought the robots would be used primarily as supports for children ages 4 to 12 years who were experiencing potentially painful medical procedures while staying on certain units within the inpatient area of the hospital. A quality improvement study was designed to monitor any changes in these units. At the start, nurses were asked which procedures were most painful for children. Intravenous (IV) placements, tube insertions/removals (such as nasogastric, catheter, chest tubes, and drains), and dressing changes were identified as the top three categories. A series of behaviors to align with the steps and types of psychological support typically beneficial to children were designed and programmed for the robots.

During the planning phase of the study, the practical side of implementing the robots began to emerge. Many questions arose, including "Where will the robots stay when not in use?" "How will their batteries be charged?" "Which staff will have access to them?" "How can we ensure their security and cleanliness?" "Who learns to operate them and how?" "Who is responsible for technical issues?" As we worked through the answers to these questions, we realized that a home for the robots within the Child Life program was a natural fit given that a primary component of the child life specialist's role is providing procedural support, which is what the robots were also initially programmed to do. It was also established that a project leader was key to help on this journey of learning, and as a long-time Certified Child Life Specialist with expertise in technological applications to child life, Jacqueline Reynolds Pearson was assigned in June 2015. The quality improvement study began with the assistance of an undergraduate student on a summer scholarship and was completed by the team of child life specialists learning how to use the robots and operating them during the procedural support interventions designated by the quality improvement study. The results of this study are being prepared for publication.

A referral system for ongoing implementation of MEDi was developed. Through educational sessions and contact with health professionals as requests arose, staff and physicians were encouraged to submit a referral to child life for support. Once referrals are received, they are triaged, and individual child life specialists then assess and determine whether MEDi will be used during their intervention. Type of procedure, location, timing, the child's developmental level, prior health care experiences, coping skills, and preferences are all factors for consideration. Most referrals are discussed with other health care professionals and within the child life team so as to implement MEDi in the best possible way for each child.

Along with the excitement of hearing about the robots through media stories and in-service trainings, came requests from health care professionals and families. This enthusiasm provided the impetus for child life specialists to begin creatively exploring the potential use of the robots to help patients with a much broader range of needs and treatment regimens than those initially defined in the quality improvement study. These ideas of integration of the robots into child life specialists' therapeutic interventions are described next.

PLAY

It has been said that play is an "essential component of a child life program and the child life professional's role" (American Academy of Pediatrics, 2014, p. e1473) and that therapeutic play is the "essence of child life practice" (Koller, 2008, p. 2). Therapeutic play centers around specialized activities that are supportive of normal development while also facilitating the emotional well-being of children in difficult situations such as medical experiences (Koller, 2008). Developmental, expressive, and health care/medical play are examples of types of therapeutic play interventions commonly used by child life specialists (Humphreys & LeBlanc, 2016). In fact, in their recent summary of the interventions frequently used by child life specialists, the definition of almost every one of them includes the word 'play.'

The value of play rests on our knowledge that it provides children opportunities for control and mastery, decision making, practice of developmental and social skills, and is usually perceived as enjoyable (Humphreys & LeBlanc, 2016). Based on the work of Erikson in the 1940s, we also believe that play provides a means for children to work through stressful circumstances (American Academy of Pediatrics, 2014).

There are many ways to set up therapeutic play opportunities for children in the hospital, but a very popular option now is to involve technology in some way. Electronic toys and devices such as iPads and other tablets have, in the last decade, become common additions to the child life specialist's toolbox. Are humanoid robots the next natural step?

It is through the use of play that child life specialists often take the first step toward building a relationship with a child in the hospital. It did not take long for ACH (Alberta Children's Hospital) child life specialists to notice the potential for involving MEDi in this process. Upon receiving the robots, child life specialists immediately began to realize just how captivating they are. During the first MEDi training session, child life specialists noticed that almost every child who walked by stopped, came closer, and wanted to engage with MEDi. It was fun to see how quickly he would catch their attention.

The first item on the mind of a child life specialist when meeting a new patient is how to begin to build rapport. Between MEDi's small stature, cute childlike features, pre-programmed playful behaviors, and the novelty of encountering a humanoid robot in a health care environment, it is hard for children and adults alike to not be intrigued (see Figure 19.2).

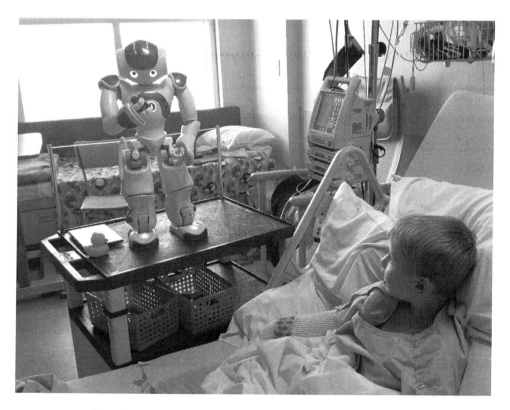

FIGURE 19.2 Child Captivated by MEDi

One of the first things I (JRP) noticed about MEDi upon introduction was that the robot said my name: "Hello, Jackie. It's a pleasure to meet you!" It felt like eye contact was genuinely made, and the robot's arm was extended as if to shake my hand. I remember I was smiling and experienced a warm feeling in response to the fact that MEDi actually said my name. Dr. Beran reassured me that it was okay to shake its hand, and just tap the red sensor as I did it. "I'm so lucky I get to meet friendly people like you!" said MEDi enthusiastically. I get to relive this feeling almost every time I introduce MEDi to a new patient, sibling, parent, or staff member. The reactions are almost always similar with big smiles, expressions of delight, and a lively, playful interaction often following. Sometimes this response occurs at the bedside, or in the playroom, art studio, hallway, or even the elevator, and it is almost always incredible to see how easily the ice is broken and rapport effortlessly begins.

A child life intern provided the following testimonial as to MEDi's initial effect on a child. "I introduced MEDi to a little boy with Down Syndrome during preparation for surgery. He was so excited when MEDi said his name, he jumped up with excitement and fell over from laughter."

There are many parallels between play therapy and the value child life specialists place on relationship building. Landreth (1991) explains,

> The development of the relationship with a child, which we refer to as play therapy, is facilitated by the therapist's subtle use of self in responding to the child's communication of self in the process of play and is dependent on the therapist's understanding of the dynamics of the child's world, as well as the child's emotional expression communicated in the relationship. Only when the child begins to feel safe with the therapist, will he/she begin to express and explore the emotionally meaningful and sometimes frightening experiences which have been experienced.
>
> (p. 180)

According to Landreth (1991), therapeutic relationships begin with the adult conveying sensitivity for the child's world. Weaving MEDi into an introduction can be a positive first step toward demonstrating awareness of a child's interests—elements of their world. The following thank-you note from a mother of an 8-year-old with significant needle fears who attended the Child Life Needle Coping Clinic illustrates this dynamic:

> I cannot thank you enough. Today was amazing for my son. To walk in the room and see [the same] robot from his special book was amazing for him. He couldn't believe it! The activities helped him and I look forward to seeing how he goes forward with needles now. The first thing he did when we got home that night was grab his *National Geographic* book. Such an excited boy because he has dreamed of one day seeing this robot from his book. THANK YOU!

Given children's magical thinking and projection of human qualities onto MEDi, it appears that a friendship bond of sorts is often formed between the child and the robot. This playful connection can bridge the gap between the child and child life specialist and facilitate trust, which then can help the child life specialist make the procedure or event more manageable.

Vignette of a Play Invitation

We have observed MEDi encourage children to comply with requests from health care staff to do something challenging, particularly in the area of physiotherapy. Non-adherence to movement and exercises are common problems, especially among children in pain. One of our favorite stories involving MEDi to date came early on in our integration of the robots into child life practice. Child life specialists were asked to collaborate with nurses and physiotherapists to motivate a 5-year-old to get out of bed after several days of rest following treatment of pneumonia, including surgery for chest tubes. There were many physical, medical, practical, developmental, and psychosocial reasons why it was important and beneficial for this young patient to begin to move around, but she was so afraid that she would not budge an inch. Her sheets had not been changed in days and she was beginning to develop bedsores. Physiotherapists, nurses, and her parents tried everything they could to convince her to move, but she only refused. A child life specialist decided to introduce MEDi as a play partner. She set the little robot up on the floor like another child, then had MEDi invite her to play. To everyone's surprise, she agreed, and allowed the nurses to lift her to MEDi's side and join in a game of Simon Says, moving her entire body in concert with MEDi while exclaiming enthusiastically to everyone who came by "Look at my friend, MEDi the robot!"

From an educational perspective, the timing could not have been better. The chief resident happened to enter the room with a group of junior residents as the interaction unfolded and noticing the patient, her mom, MEDi, the physiotherapist, and the child life specialist all sitting on the floor, instructed the residents to do the same. Surely, they will always remember the value of getting down to a child's level and interacting through play.

PROCEDURAL SUPPORT

The manner in which MEDi interacted with patients during the vaccination and blood test studies is similar to what is known in the child life literature as procedural support. This construct refers to the process of providing specific strategies aimed at assisting children in coping with medical tests or procedures while the child is undergoing the test or procedure (Humphreys & LeBlanc, 2016). When MEDi is involved, the robot guides the child through the steps of a medical procedure, reframing medical language in a child-friendly way and providing alternative focus by telling jokes or doing a dance at key times. Deep breathing is a coping technique that is well supported by the literature and has often been integrated into MEDi's procedural support script. Additional cognitive behavioral strategies are also embedded in the procedural support MEDi delivers, including affirmation, encouragement, guided imagery, humor, positive reinforcement, preparation, role modeling, and therapeutic storytelling.

Building on the approach to providing support to children during vaccinations and blood tests, additional applications (apps) were added to MEDi's repertoire, including intravenous (IV) insertion, catheter removal, nasogastric tube insertion, port access, dressing change, and electroencephalogram (EEG). At the time of writing, apps to support children during more than a dozen different medical tests or procedures have been programmed for MEDi. For each of these, the second author (TNB) observed the medical test or procedure in action, worked collaboratively with child life specialists, and created a script and program for MEDi's words and movements. In some apps, the approach is linear, guiding the child step by step through a specific test or procedure whereby MEDi describes what the child is to do or what the health care practitioner will do next (see video at www.rxrobots.com/hospital.html).

In other apps, the format is more abstract and may integrate therapeutic storytelling as a cognitive strategy employing the benefits of metaphorical content (Goldberger et al., 2009). For example, in the IV insertion app, MEDi tells the story of *The Little Engine That Could*. While the nurse is preparing the child's hand or arm for IV placement, MEDi talks about the train preparing for its journey. Throughout the steps of the IV insertion procedure, MEDi conveys different parts of the story, leading up to a request from MEDi to blow on the fire in the train's engine. This part is delivered during the potentially most bothersome part of the procedure, when the child would benefit most from blowing.

There are two main challenges in using MEDi during procedures. It can be difficult to synchronize MEDi with the dynamic nature of many tests and procedures and each individual health professional's pace and manner. Also, the theme, language, and types of interactive activities embedded might not be inclusive of the ages, developmental levels, and individual interests of every child.

This challenge creates an opportunity where the child life specialist can greatly enhance the outcome. Knowing a child's interests, and what is involved in each medical procedure, the child life specialist may choose an app that can be accommodated to a different test than for which it was originally designed. For example, *The Little Engine That Could* IV insertion app can be effectively used with preschool or early school-age children undergoing just about any test or procedure because the train theme is popular with this age group. The script does not involve explaining the steps of a particular medical procedure and the child life specialist can align the blowing part to occur during the most opportune time. The language used is encouraging and the theme is centered on perseverance. The story captivates the child's attention, the blowing engages the child in focusing on something other than the procedure and helps to relax the child's body, and the positive language models a resilient outlook. ACH child life specialists have used the IV insertion app effectively with children receiving Xolair injections for asthma treatment.

Certain parts of each procedural support app, particularly alternative focus activities, are also available on MEDi's tablet so that child life specialists can choose specific behaviors to fit each unique situation. Sometimes this selection is as simple as selecting a lively dance like "Gangnam Style" or "Mister Funk" for MEDi to perform to divert the child's attention during a tense moment, or using the calming music and fluid movements of tai chi in an attempt to de-intensify the situation.

Vignette of MEDi in Minor Surgery Clinic

Child Life was asked to become involved in the Minor Surgery Clinic by a surgeon/urologist who was looking for some support during a specific urological procedure. Because all of the surgeries are done using only local anesthetic and focus on the penis, boys can be both uncomfortable and anxious. The doctor was finding that many of the boys became upset during the procedure and wondered if MEDi could help by providing a distraction. He had heard about the robot and thought it might captivate the interest of this age group of boys.

It turned out that MEDi helped do much more than distract the boys. The surgeon developed a flow for the clinic that included him going out to the waiting area to meet the family, briefly letting them know what to expect, telling them about child life and enticing them by alluding to a surprise or to a robot. Adding a child life specialist to the team allowed the nurse to focus on her charting, paperwork, and calculations, the surgeon to focus on his procedure, and leave the role of talking with the families to the child life specialist. This collaboration allowed for a "One Voice" approach, which was appreciated by all the staff.

The boys usually entered the operating room suite with one or two parents. This room is sterile, bright, and can be intimidating. MEDi and the child life specialist became a focus for everyone immediately. The families were curious about the robot so were easily encouraged to take their places in the room beside the robot as the medical staff continued to prepare for the procedure.

In this clinic, it is necessary for the boys to come into the room so a topical numbing cream can be applied, leave for a short time, then return for the procedure. On the first visit to the room, the child life specialist introduced MEDi, asked if the boys would like to see how he works, read a little story about him (Bell-Graham, Gregson, & Pearson, 2016), and found out if they were interested in seeing him in action when they returned to the room. Most boys were keen and returned to the room eager to see what the robot could do. If they were not interested in the robot, the child life specialist offered a choice of an alternative focus activity. Some of the older boys chose to engage in an activity on their own tablet instead.

During the procedure, a parent took the role of supporting through use of physical touch and positioning, holding hands and stroking the boy's head. The child life specialist encouraged the boys to focus on the robot, which was positioned near their head. This position allowed the nurse and doctor to concentrate on the surgical procedure. The child life specialist could easily control MEDi, turn him off and move on to another app as needed, and be available to reassure and encourage the family.

Overall, MEDi is perceived as a good tool in the Minor Surgery Clinic. Not only was anxiety reduced for the young patients and parents, staff in the room appeared more relaxed than usual, singing and dancing along with MEDi when appropriate. Another staff member even came out of her office to find out what the laughter was all about, as in the past she had never heard that sound from that particular clinic. A humanoid robot presents a unique and somewhat interactive alternative focus activity that does not disrupt the flow of the procedure or increase the time it takes to complete it. The surgical team remains supportive and agree that MEDi is a fun and helpful tool in this setting. The challenge may be ensuring that staff members do not become too overwhelmed with the repetitive programs.

MEDi helped open the door for child life specialists to find a valuable place in the Minor Surgery Clinic. There are many ways child life specialists can help support families in this stressful environment, and MEDi introduces a unique approach and enables this multidisciplinary team to focus on reducing anxiety for everyone.

CONSCIOUS CHOICE OF ALTERNATE FOCUS

'Conscious choice of alternate focus' is described by Goldberger et al. (2009) as a cognitive strategy for coping with painful procedures. Utilizing cognitive processes to shift attention away from a medical test or procedure, it is similar to the concept commonly referred to as distraction, but different in that the former implies active choice on the part of the child/family of an activity that they believe will help them to cope. Cognitive tasks such as counting, reciting the alphabet or spelling words, listening to or telling jokes, looking at something intriguing like an electronic device, or participating in a virtual reality experience (also combines behavioral and sensory strategies) are all examples of activities to divert focus away from a potentially painful procedure. Using Melzack and Wall's Gate Control Theory of Pain (Helms & Barone, 2008), health professionals often talk about "keeping the brain busy" to close the metaphorical gate to processing of painful stimuli. The ideal approach involves the child life specialist preparing the child for the procedure, including selection of planned alternative focus activities based on the individual interests of the child. In this approach, the child (and sometimes the parents, too) are actively involved in customizing the coping plan, including selection of activities that they believe will focus the child's attention away from the test or procedure.

Recently, we began to trial a Child Life Needle Coping Clinic. ACH patients are invited to attend a group program centered on teaching strategies for coping with needles to children and their parents. A variety of learning activities are offered, including medical play with real needles, an art activity involving creation of a 'find it tube,' an expressive art activity involving drawing then squirting away fears with a water-filled syringe, and an interactive station with MEDi in the role as educator, teaching the specifics of how to deep breathe. During the clinic, families develop an individualized coping plan including their own selection of conscious alternate focus activities. Some families have taken videos of MEDi in action to keep as reminders of how to deep breathe or as alternate focus activities for use during upcoming needle procedures.

Vignette of MEDi's Role in a Cystic Fibrosis Clinic

At ACH, child life specialists are integrating MEDi into their approach to facilitating children's selection of alternate focus activities. A longtime child life specialist who works with patients in the Cystic Fibrosis (CF) clinic often includes the robot in her practice in this way. Children with CF typically have one to two examinations per year, which regularly require blood testing. Based on the cumulative effect of negative experiences with this test over the years, fear levels can be high when these children come in for their checkups. Many have heard about MEDi through their online support communities and ask to meet the robot. The child life specialist often meets these patients outside of the laboratory, introduces MEDi, demonstrates its capabilities including dances, interactive games, and stories, and asks each how they would like to involve MEDi as a support during their procedure. Some choose a particular dance for MEDi to perform, then watch eagerly while completing their bloodwork. Others practice the strategy of deep breathing with MEDi in advance, then during their blood test use the strategy on its own or in combination with another cognitive behavioral strategy (like blowing on a pinwheel as demonstrated by the robot). Others are so aware of their own reactions that they know that playing with MEDi during the wait time (also conscious use of alternate focus) will be enough to regulate their anticipatory anxiety and make the procedure manageable without the robot even entering the laboratory.

PREPARATION AND MEDICAL PLAY

When surveyed about their role in pain management, child life specialists report that they perceive providing information/preparation as being the most effective strategy for reducing pain (Bandstra et al., 2008). Preparation is a core child life intervention and is considered an evidence based technique for pain management (Uman et al., 2008). Play is often the modality through which child life specialists convey information about medical experiences.

MEDi has been programmed with a medical play app that provides information in a playful manner about the sensations and experiences associated with surgery and other procedures, including demonstrations of how real medical equipment is used. Children may follow MEDi's lead when the robot demonstrates how medical equipment is used. Child life specialists have used this approach as an enhancement to traditional individual or small group preparation for children who appear to need extra enticement to participate in preparation or are particularly interested in robots.

Health care or medical play involve engaging children in play about health concepts or using materials related to the hospital environment to help children express their worries, ask questions, gain knowledge and mastery, clear up misunderstandings, practice coping strategies, and work through feelings (Humphreys & LeBlanc, 2016). Early on in MEDi's integration, we introduced the robot in our Child Life Clinic—a group program offering a medical play component. A surprising discovery during these sessions was that children immediately wanted to carry out medical procedures on MEDi in the same way they had been performed on themselves. In other words, children used MEDi in these play sessions in a similar manner to how they would use a doll or stuffed animal, with the exception that the robot can talk to them (see Figure 19.3). Upon learning of this unique opportunity for role play, we programmed MEDi and created an app whereby child life specialists could type text for the robot to speak and demonstrate friendly human qualities. For example, when

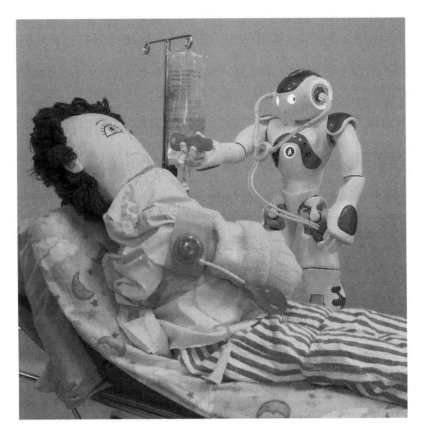

FIGURE 19.3 Role Play With MEDi

a child puts a bandage on MEDi's arm, MEDi can say that the child is taking good care in being gentle. This suggestion can help children develop positive perceptions of their health care providers. The child life specialist can also use this opportunity to reinforce behaviors or attitudes, correct misconceptions, and answer questions through MEDi. Overall, this type of medical play session can help children to gain mastery of treatment processes and coping strategies and play out feelings.

Vignette of Medical Play and Preparation for EEG Testing

In this next example, neurological testing was anticipated for 2- and 3-year-old boys. The child life specialist assigned to their care invited them for a preparation and play session to assess their understanding of what they would soon experience, and provide them with experiential learning activities to alleviate anxiety about both the hospital environment and the tests to come. In addition to sensory materials related to EEG testing, the child life specialist also organized MEDi for involvement. She set up MEDi with wire sensors and gauze to model what the children would wear for their EEG tests. The child life specialist then invited the children into the clinic area and introduced MEDi already prepared for his pretend EEG and showed the children a few of MEDi's interactive behaviors. The children easily engaged with the robot in a playful way. Next, she explained to the children that MEDi was ready for his EEG and she would show them on a doll how he was prepared. She demonstrated the steps of applying the wire sensors and gauze, then offered the children an opportunity to get ready too, just like MEDi. Both were very keen to do so and cooperated beautifully as she gently applied the materials. As a wrap-up to the session, the children played in the vicinity of MEDi with toys of their selection to confirm for them that the EEG 'hat' was comfortable. Both boys appeared to enjoy the experience and did not express any signs of discomfort or fear of putting on and continuing to wear the sensors and gauze wrap for an extended period of time.

Magnetic resonance imaging (MRI) testing may also be required for each of the boys. Given their affinity for MEDi, a future plan is for MEDi to attend the MRI preparation and 'watch' them practice in the Mock MRI Scanner so that they can show the robot what they have learned. The child life specialist anticipates that the boys will be motivated to come back to the hospital and be very cooperative if MEDi is part of this preparation intervention.

EMPOWERMENT THROUGH COPING

Empowerment involves the process of becoming strong and confident, especially in controlling one's life. Child life specialists can help in facilitating children's and parent's development of empowerment through educational initiatives and increased involvement in planning of their care.

Recent research in the field of pain memory suggests that children's pain experiences are influenced by their parents' own memories of childhood pain and feelings of self-efficacy regarding managing pain (Noel, Palmero, Chambers, Taddio, & Hermann, 2015; Simons & Sieberg, 2015). Educational interventions to increase parents' and children's understanding of pain management and coping strategies may be one avenue to increasing feelings of empowerment and positively affecting pain memories for both generations.

Given the efficacy of deep or belly breathing for coping with pain and fear associated with injections (Chambers et al., 2009), extra work has gone into creating apps for MEDi that emphasize the specifics of how to use this technique. MEDi has been programmed to explain the concept of deep or belly breathing to children and their parents and encourage them in a fun way to practice this strategy. We have observed that children are receptive to the robot's instruction and have seen some use of the strategy taught by the robot even when MEDi was not there during the subsequent procedure. As mentioned, we also teach parents this strategy so that they have a skill for reducing pain and fear for their children and can practice and encourage their children to use it during medical tests or procedures. It is our hope that by facilitating learning of this skill through MEDi's programming and delivery, parents will feel effective in managing their children's pain and fear, thereby helping to build positive pain memories. Moreover, MEDi facilitates this opportunity by inviting the parent to participate with their child so both can develop mastery in dealing with painful procedures.

We are currently investigating, through a randomized controlled trial, the effects of MEDi's delivery of an educational intervention regarding deep breathing to children and parents in advance of an IV placement for induction for surgery. At the time of writing, we were nearing the end of the data collection phase and anticipate sharing our findings in the next year.

Helping families feel connected to their care can also promote feelings of increased empowerment. Throughout the process of developing MEDi, we continually invite children and families to share their ideas and contribute feedback involving them in the ongoing process of the expansion of MEDi's role. Children and parents appear to appreciate this opportunity and often go out of their way to provide suggestions and praise (e.g., bringing a list of child-friendly jokes). It also becomes a means for families to share their learning from health care experiences with others, which appears to have a positive effect for all.

Vignette of MEDi in Mental Health

Coping strategies are not just for pain and medical procedures. They are also applicable to other stressful circumstances. Children and adolescents who enter the Day Treatment and Acute Care Emergency Services programs at ACH often feel stress associated with their lack of familiarity with the hospital environment and separation from their families, friends, schools, and regular daily activities. The child life specialist's role in this program concentrates on supporting children by normalizing the experience, and teaching social and emotional self-regulation skills through group activities. Group counseling programs can provide individuals with the kinds of experiences that help them learn to function effectively, to develop tolerance for stress and anxiety, and to find satisfaction in working and living with others (Corey & Corey, 2006; Gazda, Ginter, & Horne, 2001).

The child life specialist in this area has used MEDi to change the process for a brief time, from a typical group about the children's own problems to a group about helping others. In 2016, the second author (TNB) also joined the group to assist in facilitating a discussion of ways in which MEDi could be potentially helpful to other children who are just like them. They came up with the idea of developing an app for MEDi to help others with bullying—a common experience for them. The group, ages 8–13 years, who identified as being bullied or bullying others, were invited to give input on what MEDi should say or do. The result was a script and set of behaviors for MEDi to talk about feeling hurt by peers and consider various ways to respond to this situation. The children named it the "Feeling Left Out" app.

MEDi and this app are used to help group facilitators generate discussion about bullying. The timing of the facilitator in managing MEDi's responses is essential to create the 'magic' associated with a robot being part of a group. When MEDi conveys a story about being rejected and encourages empathy, children begin to identify, share, and regulate their own feelings to help them develop the skills for improved peer and family relations and adaptation to the school environment.

The group provided feedback and suggestions for modification of the app a few times. Based on the group's recommendations, the ending of the app was changed to include an empowering song about being brave. After each session, the children were presented with an 'app developer certificate' to acknowledge the time spent using communication skills, sharing creative ideas, and, most importantly, using their experience to 'teach' MEDi how to talk to other children about bullying. The purpose of the group meetings is to improve children's self-esteem; this goal was achieved through their sharing of insights about bullying to teach MEDi how to help others. This teaching role seemed to empower them to stand up to a bully and use the communication and coping skills they were learning in the group sessions. Thus, MEDi had the primary effect of helping children develop mastery around coping with bullying, and the secondary effect of empowering them in the role of leadership to help other children.

WHAT WE HAVE LEARNED ABOUT ROBOTS IN HOSPITALS

Our work has shown us that the robot is a multipurpose tool. In addition to all the areas described earlier, robots can be used to share standard information about medical procedures to prepare families in advance. In addition to acting as a pain coach, it can be used to encourage children to swallow pills (MEDi role modeling and making sounds of drinking), used a walker (race MEDi down the hallway to see who is faster), as a means in teaching children to be still for diagnostic tests (playing the statue game to see who can be still the longest), and so on. Other applications include fundraising, such as radiothons (telling jokes, sharing stories), golf tournaments (MEDi can putt a golf ball), and special events (speeches) to attract donations and media attention. MEDi has also been used as an ambassador to the hospital—to introduce families to different areas of the hospital through media such as books, websites, and videos. As the robot can be given any name, hospitals can also name it in honor of one of their financial donors. In addition to all the insights we gained in the aforementioned areas, we learned how to manage its day-to-day operation.

- The robot can be sanitized between patient visits by first turning off devices and then cleaning the robot with hospital grade disinfectant wipes.
- Transportation, storage, and battery charging must be considered. Wheeling the robot on a cart while secured to a harness prevents breakage while allowing the robot to perform its actions while on the cart. The power management system designed for the cart allows the robot and devices to be plugged in with one cord. Charging is recommended whenever the robot is not in use.
- Child life specialists, nurses, volunteers, parents, and children are able to use a tablet to operate the robot.
- Pre-programmed behaviors like those described earlier are useful for a variety of medical procedures, and the use of a tablet to operate the robot allows the user to type messages for the robot to stay in the moment to ensure it is responsive.
- With the robot able to speak more than one language, it can communicate with a variety of patients.
- Some children may be initially apprehensive of visiting with a robot. Some of these children may warm up to one, particularly when introduced in a friendly way.

CONCLUSION

As robotic arms in manufacturing have replaced some assembly line jobs, we are some-times asked if a robot will replace the role of a child life specialist. Although we may have an imagination for such a possibility due to 'live' robots featured in movies, the most advanced technology does not have this capability. In fact, our observations are that children spent the most interactive time with MEDi when child life specialists used it purposefully to achieve therapeutic goals. Just as we found in our earliest research that children were most likely to help the robot when the experimenter presented the robot in a positive way, so can patients gain the most support from the robot when Child Life uses the robot as a therapeutic tool. All the many ways in which MEDi touches the lives of our patients have been discovered only through the close col-laboration between our child life specialists and researchers who are actively watching for and discovering hidden secrets little MEDi has to offer our families. Our team is excited to continue the exploration of things not yet known.

The second author (TNB) wishes to disclose a conflict of interest. At the time of writ-ing this chapter, she was involved in MEDi's commercial use with other hospitals and dental offices.

ACKNOWLEDGMENTS

The authors would like to thank Alberta Health Services, Alberta Children's Hospi-tal, and the Vi Riddell Pain and Rehabilitation Pain and Rehabilitation Centre for the support and encouragement to explore and share new ways of helping children and families. We also offer a special acknowledgment for the creativity, risk-taking, and collaborative effort contributed by the Child Life and Therapeutic Arts Team. The authors wish to also thank the research support from Alex Ramirez-Serrano, Sue Kuhn, Otto Vanderkooi, Ehud Sharlin, Saul Greenberg, Setareh Manesh, Sarah Nugent, Meghann Fior, and Roman Kuzyk—and thank you to Brad Uphill for his help with the photos. We especially thank the patients and families for their participation.

REFERENCES

American Academy of Pediatrics, Committee on Hospital Care Child Life Council. (2014). Child life services. *Pediatrics, 133*(5), e1471–e1478. https://doi.org/10.1542/peds.2014-0556

Bandstra, N. F., Skinner, L., LeBlanc, C., Chambers, C. T., Hollon, E. C., Brennan, D., & Beaver, C. (2008). The role of child life in pediatric pain management: A survey of child life special-ists. *Journal of Pain, 9*(4), 320–329.

Bell-Graham, L., Gregson, B., & Pearson, J. (2016). *What will you see? At the Alberta Children's Hospital*. Calgary, Alberta: Blurb.

Bennett, K. L. (2017). You tend to find what you're looking for. *Association of Child Life Profes-sionals, 35*(2), 1.

Beran, T. N., & Ramirez-Serrano, A. (Jun 2010). *Can children have a relationship with a robot?* Paper presented at the International Conference on Human-Robot Personal Relationships, the Netherlands.

Beran, T. N., & Ramirez-Serrano, A. (2011). Robot arm–child interactions: A novel application using bio-inspired motion control. In S. Goto (Ed.), *Robot arms* (pp. 241–262). Croatia: InTech.

Beran, T. N., Ramirez-Serrano, A., Kuzyk, R., Fior, M., & Nugent, S. (2011). Understanding how children understand robots: Animism in the 21st century. *International Journal of Human-Computer Studies, 69,* 539–550.

Beran, T. N., Ramirez-Serrano, A., Kuzyk, R., Nugent, S., & Fior, M. (2011). Would children help a robot in need? *International Journal of Social Robotics, 3*(1), 83–92.

Beran, T. N., Ramirez-Serrano, A., Vanderkooi, O., & Kuhn, S. (2013). Reducing children's distress towards flu vaccinations: A novel and effective use of humanoid robotics. *Vaccine, 31*(25), 2772–2777.

Beran, T. N., Ramirez-Serrano, A., Vanderkooi, O., & Kuhn, S. (2015). Humanoid robotics in health care: An exploration of children's and parents' emotional reactions. *Journal of Health Psychology, 20*(7), 984–989. https://doi.org/10.1177/135910531350479

Beran, T. N., Manesh, S., Greenberg, S., & Sharlin, S. (May–June 2015). *Discovering how humanoid robotics can be used for pediatric procedural pain.* 10th International Symposium on Pediatric Pain, Seattle.

Cassidy, K.-L., Reid, G. J., McGrath, P. J., Finley, G. A., Smith, D. J., Morley, C., . . . Morton, B. (2002). Watch needle, watch TV: Audiovisual distraction in preschool immunization. *Pain Medicine, 3*(2), 108–118.

Chambers, C. T., Taddio, A., Uman, L. S., & McMurtry, C. M., for the HELPnKIDS Team. (2009). Psychological interventions for reducing pain and distress during routine childhood immunizations: A systematic review. *Clinical Therapeutics, 31B,* S77–S103.

Corey, M. S., & Corey, G. (2006). *Groups: Process and practice* (7th ed.). Belmont, CA: Thompson Higher Education.

Fior, M., Nugent, S., Beran, T. N., Ramirez-Serrano, A., & Kuzyk, R. (2010). Children's relationships with robots: Robot is child's new friend. *Journal of Physical Agents, 4*(3), 9–17.

Galloway, J. C., Ryu, J. C., & Agrawal, S. K. (2008). Babies driving robots: Self-generated mobility in very young infants. *Intelligence Service Robotics, 1,* 123. https://doi.org/10.1007/s11370-007-0011-2

Gazda, G., Ginter, E., & Horne, A. (2001). *Group counseling and group psychotherapy: Theory and application.* Boston: Allyn & Bacon.

Goldberger, J., Mohl, A., & Thompson, R. (2009). Psychological preparation and coping. In R. Thompson (Ed.), *The handbook of child life: A guide for pediatric psychosocial care* (pp. 160–198). Springfield, IL: Charles C. Thomas.

Helms, J. E., & Barone, C. P. (2008). Physiology and treatment of pain. *Critical Care Nurse, 28*(6), 38–49.

Humphreys, C., & LeBlanc, C. K. (2016). Promoting resilience in paediatric health care: The role of the child life specialist. In C. DeMichelis & M. Ferrari (Eds.), *Child and adolescent resilience within medical contexts* (pp. 153–173). Switzerland: Springer International.

Kaiser Family Foundation. Media multitasking among American youth: Prevalence, predictors and pairings—Key findings. (2006). Retrieved April 20, 2017 from: www.kff.org/entmedia/7593.cfm

Koller, D. (2008). *Child life council evidence-based practice statement: Preparing children and adolescents for medical procedures.* Rockville, MD: Child Life Council.

Kozima, H., Michalowski, M. P., & Nakagawa, C. (2009). Keepon: A playful robot for research, therapy, and entertainment. *International Journal of Social Robotics, 1,* 3–18.

Kwoh, Y. S., Hou, J., Jonckheere, E. A., & Hayall, S. (February 1988). A robot with improved absolute positioning accuracy for CT guided stereotactic brain surgery. *IEEE Transactions on Biomedical Engineering, 35*(2), 153–161.

Landreth, G.L. (1991). *Play therapy: The art of the relationship.* Muncie, IN: Accelerated Development.

Megel, M.E., Houser, C.W., & Gleaves, K.S. (1998). Children's responses to immunizations: Lullabies as a distraction. *Issues in Comprehensive Pediatric Nursing, 21,* 129–145.

Melson, G.F., Kahn, P.H., Beck, A., & Friedman, B. (2009). Robotic pets in human lives: Implications for the human—animal bond and for human relationships with personified technologies. *Journal of Social Issues, 65*(3), 545–567.

Melvin, W.S., Needleman, B.J., Krause, K.R., & Ellison, E.C. (February 2003). Robotic resection of pancreatic neuroendocrine tumor. *Journal of Laparoendoscopic & Advanced Surgical Techniques, 13*(1), 33–36.

Noel, M., Palmero, T.M., Chambers, C.T., Taddio, A., & Hermann, C. (2015). Remembering the pain of childhood: Applying a developmental perspective to the study of pain memories. *Pain, 156*(1), 31–34.

Simons, S.E., & Sieberg, C.B. (2015). Parents-to help or hinder pain memories in children. *Pain, 156*(5), 761–762.

Talamini, M.A., Chapman, S., Horgan, S., & Melvin, W.S. (October 2003). A prospective analysis of 211 robotic-assisted surgical procedures. *Surgical Endoscopy, 17*(10), 1521–1524.

Uman, L.S., Chambers, C.T., McGrath, P.J., & Kisely, S. (2008). A systematic review of randomized controlled trails examining psychological interventions for needle related procedural pain and distress in children and adolescents: An abbreviated Cochrane review. *Journal of Pediatric Psychology, 33*(8), 842–854.

U.S. Food and Drug Administration. (October 11, 2012). *Remote Presence System, Model RP-VTATM 870.2910 regulation number.* Retrieved April 20, 2017 from: www.accessdata.fda.gov/cdrh_docs/pdf12/k123229.pdf

Appendix

Taking Your Child to the Doctor or the Hospital: Helpful Suggestions and Practical Tips to Make Your Child's Visit More Comfortable

Patricia Weiner

Prepare yourself for your child's visit. If you feel at ease, your child can sense that and react in the same way. Prepare a written list of questions that you want to ask the doctor. It is important to include details of your child's symptoms and any concerns you might have. A great way for toddlers and preschoolers to prepare for going to the doctor is to play doctor. Let your child use a toy doctor's kit and give her a doll or stuffed toy so she can give her doll a checkup. She can check her doll's heart, reflexes, ears, and eyes, weigh her, reassure her, and feel her tummy. Toy doctor's kits come with a play stethoscope, otoscope, reflex hammer, and a pretend syringe for shots/injections. You can use materials found in your house: Band-Aids, alcohol (to show how cold an alcohol wipe is), and gauze pads. It's fun and educational for your child to 'play doctor'! Speak to your child's physician about types of pain relief before your first visit. You might want to discuss pain medicine for immunizations, injections, or other painful medical procedures. Sometimes local anesthetics that you can apply at home prior to or following a procedure are recommended. Some pediatricians use other methods for pain relief. Stay with your infant or young child during the doctor's office visit whenever possible. Separation is one of the most difficult experiences for a young child. A parent's presence is comforting and healing. It's important to use comforting positions for your infant or child. Holding infants or having them sit on your lap gives them a sense of security, control, and comfort. Take a familiar toy, teddy, or blanket to the doctor's office. It may help comfort your infant or child.

HELPING YOUR BABY TO BE SOOTHED AND COMFORTED

- Babies and young children love to be held or sit in a comforting position on their mom's or dad's lap.
- As the children get older, they may want one of their parents to hold their hand.
- Babies love to suck and it is soothing to them—whether breast- or bottle-fed, help them find their fingers or pacifier.
- Infants love movement, it soothes them. Hold, walk, sway, or rock with your baby.
- Stroke your infant's face—infants love gentle touch.
- Sing or hum softly to your baby. Infants enjoy music and familiar voices.
- Bottle or breast-feed after appointment or procedure is completed.
- Bring your child's favorite snack and offer it to her after the appointment or procedure.

FOR CHILDREN

Children find comfort in routine and discipline.

- Do something fun when the visit is done.
- Use simple, concrete language.
- Be honest. Give information to your child that will help prepare her for a visit to the doctor, hospital, or for a specific procedure. What will she see, hear, smell and have to do (i.e., weight, height, hold still, answer doctor's questions)?
- Help your child express her feelings and/or fears and prepare her through play. Playing doctor is one way of helping your toddler or preschooler prior to your visit.
- Reading some of the books listed in the 'Suggested Readings' page to your child before you go to the doctor or hospital will help prepare her for health care experiences.
- Call your local library or contact the hospital's Child Life Department for additional age-appropriate books and toys for your child.
- Reassure your child. Make sure your child knows going to the doctor or hospital is not a punishment and is not necessarily a place where she will feel pain. Sometimes your child will need immunizations or medicines given by injection or a blood test to find out how her body is working. Reassure your child that her body keeps making more blood all the time.
- Give your child choices when possible. Choices give your child a sense of control. Your child can choose which arm to use for an injection, or whether or not to watch a procedure. She can pick out her favorite Band-Aid or sticker! Having choices will help her to get through the procedure. Try not to make promises you can't keep.
- Listen to your child's concern. It is OK to ask questions, to want to watch the procedure, cry, and talk about her feelings. Crying is a release for tension, anger, and hurt.
- Use comforting positions and other coping techniques familiar to your relationship with the child. Use photographs for distraction or guided imagery. Bring bubbles, rattles, or other distraction toys that your child likes.

- Bring crayons for drawing. Exam table paper makes a great canvas.
- Bring your child's favorite music and earphones with you, or sing a familiar song to your child. Music is a wonderful way to support and soothe your child.
- Praise your child and bring small rewards with you for positive reinforcement.
- Encourage her during the procedure.

TECHNIQUES

1. Preparation and Medical Play
2. Comforting Positions
3. Positive Reinforcement
4. Distraction
5. Deep Breathing
6. Guided Imagery
7. Positive Self-Talk
8. Relaxation.

1. Preparation and Medical Play (15 Months Through All Ages)

Children benefit by being prepared briefly for visits to the doctor or hospital. Consider preparing toddlers and preschoolers one day ahead of their visit or on the way to the doctor. School-age children sometimes are best prepared 1 day prior to their visit. Adolescents should be informed sooner, especially if they are going to the hospital. Parents are the best judge of when to tell their children about doctor or hospital visits. If your child is going to the hospital, more preparation is usually needed. Call the director of the Child Life Program at the hospital and ask about any 'pre-admission' or 'pre-operative' programs.

The following are some suggestions to help prepare your child:

- Prepare yourself first. Ask your child's doctor for more specific information about the procedure.
- You know your child best of all. Help your child get ready by talking with her.
- Choose a quiet time to talk to your child. Using a calm and comforting voice will help your child to be relaxed.
- Explain the reason for the visit or procedure.
- Offer your child honest, sensitive, and developmentally appropriate information that she can understand.
- Prepare your child for what will happen. Use 'hands-on materials' for young children.
- Ask your child what might 'help' during the procedure or hospital visit.
- Read books with your child about going to the doctor or hospital.
- Role-play with a doll or stuffed toy to help prepare your child. Your child can pretend the doll or stuffed toy is going to the doctor and can give the doll a checkup, listen to its heart, or even give the doll an injection. Playing doctor is a great way to

prepare and teach your child about medical sounds, smells, and sights. Play gives children a sense of control and a way to work out and understand their feelings.

- Use a doll or stuffed toy to provide a safe way to talk to your child about her feelings and what will occur.
- Ask your child if she wants to bring the doll or toy to the doctor or hospital.

If your child goes to the hospital, she will feel better learning about the hospital and getting ready for the new experiences. The 'clingy' infant arrives around 10 months of age, and parents know when they see it. Suddenly, leaving the child's line of sight causes the little one great distress—thanks in part to the child's undeveloped sense of time and lack of experience with a parent's absence. Sometimes during stressful situations, separation from parents is more difficult and distress lasts for a longer time. Don't leave your child without telling her that you will be back soon.

Fortunately, separation anxiety passes with time. It's a normal stage of development for most children, usually ending by the last half of the second year. As the toddler learns that parents keep coming back after they leave, the fear subsides and the child's confidence builds. It's getting from here to there that can make for some trying moments, and often some tender ones as well.

As a child grows, those fears change. The fears of body changes, pain, appearance, and privacy deepen as the child gets older. Many hospitals offer a special program with hands-on activities for children, where they can see and explore real medical equipment. Ask your child's doctor for this information. Pre-admission and pre-operative programs are usually offered by the Child Life department at your hospital or through the Department of Pediatrics. For a hospital visit, you can pack some special things to have from home. Most children pack a few favorite things like pajamas, books, games, or a special toy. Some children like to bring pictures from home or their own blanket or pillow. Some tests and procedures may hurt in the hospital. Use the techniques on this website to help your child during difficult times. Use the hospital checklist on this website to help you get ready for a hospital stay. Ask to speak to a child life specialist or a nurse. She will help your child during her hospitalization.

2. Comforting Positions (Infancy and Up)

You are the best source of comfort for your child! Hold your infant or young child. Have your infant/child sit on your lap (chest to chest, sideways, or back to chest). This will help your child stay calm, feel in control and be comforted. You can practice hugging! Holding your infant in an upright position or having your child sit on your lap will help her relax. When a child lies on her back, she feels vulnerable. Physical touch provides security and warmth. Touching includes stroking, swaddling, holding, rocking, and cuddling. Once infants learn to sit up, they are so proud of this milestone that the act of making an infant or child lie down may result in her crying or her struggling to get up. School-age children sometimes like to hold their parent's hand, and teenagers should be given the choice of what they want to do.

3. Positive Reinforcement (6 Months and Up)

Lavish your child with praise! Praise your child for helping and staying still. Praise your child for having finished the procedure even if she cries. Remember that crying is a way of coping for some children. Bring small rewards such as stickers and other treats.

4. Distraction (6 Months and Up)

If your child wants to watch the procedure, let her! If not, help your child focus on something other than the procedure. Read a pop-up book or storybook; sing a song; focus on a soothing, diversional object; look at photographs and talk to your child about them; blow on a pinwheel; recite familiar nursery rhymes; blow bubbles; practice counting or saying the alphabet. Older children may enjoy playing with electronic games, a computer tablet, or listening to music with earphones. Before the visit, help your child create a list of things she would like to use as a distraction. Bring some toys with you.

5. Deep Breathing (School-Age and Up)

Deep breathing will help your child to relax and slow her heart rate. Help your child get into a comfortable position. Tell your child to breathe in deeply through her nose, count to three and blow out through her mouth. Encourage your child throughout the procedure. Breathe with your child, and breathe slowly! Use explanations your child will understand when explaining the breathing (for example, take a deep breath in like you are smelling flowers, count to three, and blow out slowly as if you were blowing out lots of birthday candles). Use a pinwheel, breathe in, count to three and then blow on the pinwheel. Pinwheels are fun to watch and help your child relax. Blowing bubbles always helps with deep breathing.

6. Guided Imagery (School-Age and Up)

Help your child see a picture in her mind of something or someone that she likes. Children do not have to close their eyes (many are afraid of 'sneak attacks'), but it is helpful. Combine imagery with deep breathing. In a soothing voice, tell your child a story. Some things children like to imagine are stories of stars, rainbows, snowflakes, butterflies, animals, flowers, the beach, or their favorite places. You could place your child on a magic carpet that flies over rivers, mountains, and lakes and help her to visualize this in her mind.

7. Positive Self-Talk (Preschool and Up)

This technique is used prior to a painful procedure and should be ongoing. Encourage your child to replace negative thoughts with positive ones. This technique relies on a self-fulfilling prophecy. For example, help your child to stop thoughts like "I can't do this" or "This is going to hurt." Help her to replace negative thoughts with comments like "This might hurt a little, but I will feel better soon" or "I know I can do it!" Tell your child what a good job she is doing. Support and encouragement during the procedure will help your children feel more comfortable.

8. Relaxation (School-Age and Up)

Help your child to relax her body so that she will feel more comfortable. Have her lie down and get comfy. Now, have her close her eyes and begin to relax her body as you talk. Ask her to wiggle her toes and feet and then let them relax. Next have your child squeeze her eyes tight and then let them relax. Tell your child to squeeze her whole body tight and let it relax and be floppy like a rag doll. This is fun to do and helps her learn to relax. When you visit the doctor, your child can pretend to be floppy in a sitting position. Your child can also squeeze and release a tension ball.

Coping Techniques and Materials by Age

Infants

Parental presence
Distractions (6 months +)
Comforting positions
Rapid rocking and patting
Sucking
Singing
Music.

Toddlers

Parental presence
Distractions (i.e., photographs, comforting positions)
Pop-up book, pinwheel, magic wand
Music
Spinning toy, bubble blowing
Rocking
Singing.

Preschoolers

Parental presence
Distractions (i.e., pop-up book)
Comforting positions
Magic wand, use photograph
Singing
Spinning toy, bubble blowing
Music
Imagery (i.e., favorite story or favorite place)
Deep breathing (i.e., breathe in, count to three and pretend to blow out candles on a birthday cake, or blow on a pinwheel).

School-Age

Parental presence (as needed)
Distractions (i.e., books, spinning toy)

Singing
Pinwheel, magic wand, or an iPad
Music (supervised by a child life specialist or parent), bubble blowing
Relaxation (i.e., rag doll, tension ball)
Imagery (i.e., favorite place or favorite thing)
Deep breathing (i.e., breathe in, count to three and pretend to blow out candles on a birthday cake, or blow on a pinwheel).

Books About Going to the Doctor for Young Children

Berenstain, S., & Berenstain, J. (1981). *The Berenstain Bears go to the doctor.* New York: Random House.
Brazelton, T.B. (1987). *Going to the doctor.* Reading, MA: Addison-Wesley/Lawrence.
Civardi, A., & Cartwright, S. (1988, 1999). *Going to the doctor.* London: Usborne.
Markoff, H. (2000). *What to expect when you go to the doctor.* New York: HarperCollins.
Zoehfeld, K.W. (1999). *Pooh plays doctor.* US: Disney Press.

Books About Going to the Hospital for Young Children

Bemelman, L. (1977). *Madeline.* New York: Puffin.
Civardi, A., & Cartwright, S. (1987, 1992). *Going to the hospital.* London: Usborne.
Hautzig, D. (1985). *A visit to the Sesame Street Hospital.* Westminster, MD: Random House.
Jennings, S. (2000). *Franklin goes to the hospital.* Toronto, CA: Kids Can Press LTD.
Rey, M., & Rey, H.A. (1966). *Curious George goes to the hospital.* New York: Houghton Mifflin Co.
Rogers, F. (1999). *Going to the hospital.* Topeka, KS: Econo-Clad Book.
Wood, J.R. (2009). *What will I see? And who are those people wearing funny clothes?* Bloomington, IN: Author House.

SUGGESTED READING FOR PARENTS

Books About Child Development, Parenting, Child Life, Child Psychology, Childhood Pain, Hospitalization, and Coping Techniques

Achterberg, J. (1985). *Imagery in healing.* Boston, MA: New Science Library.
Boston Children's Hospital. (1987). *The new child health encyclopedia: The complete guide for parents.* New York: Delacorte Press/Lawrence.
Bowlby, J. (1969–1980). *Attachment and loss* (3 vols.). New York: Basic Books.
Brazelton, T.B. (1984). *To listen to a child.* Reading, MA: Addison Wesley/Lawrence.
Brazelton, T.B. (1985). *Working and caring.* Reading, MA: Addison Wesley/Lawrence.
Brazelton, T.B. (1992). *Touchpoints.* Reading, MA: Perseus Books.
Epstein, G. (1989). *Healing visualizations: Creative health through imagery.* New York: Bantam Books.
Erickson, E. (1950). *Childhood and society.* New York: Norton.
Freiberg, S. (1959). *The magic years.* New York: Scribner's.

Galinsky, E. (1987). *The six stages of parenthood*. Reading, MA: Addison-Wesley/Lawrence.

Krieger, D. (1983). *Accepting your power to heal: The practice of therapeutic touch*. Santa Fe, NM: Bear.

Kuttner, L. (1996, 2008). *A child in pain: How to help, what to do*. Vancouver, BC: Hartley and Marks.

Leach, P. (1983). *Babyhood*. New York: Knopf.

Loewy, J. V., MacGregor, B., Richards, K., & Rodriguez, J. (1997). *Music therapy and pediatric pain*. Cherry Hill, NJ: Jeffrey Books.

McGrath, P. (1990). *Pain in children: Nature, assessment and treatment*. New York: Guilford Press.

McMahon, L. (1992). *The handbook of play therapy*. London: Routledge.

Murdock, M. (1987). *Spinning inwards*. Boston, MA: Shambhala.

Murkoff, H. (2012). *What to expect the first year*. New York: HarperCollins.

Petrillo, M., & Sanger, S. (1980). *Emotional care of hospitalized children*. Philadelphia: J. B. Lippincott.

PROFESSIONAL REFERENCES AND RESOURCES

Books and Journal Articles

Child Life Council. (2009). *Anthology of Child Life focus (1999–2009): Child Life Council Bulletin Newsletter*.

Gaynard, L., Wolfer, J., Goldberger, J., Thompson, R., Redburn, L., & Laidley, L. (1998). *Psychosocial care of children in hospitals: A clinical practice manual*. Rockville, MD: Child Life Council (now Association of Child Life Professionals).

Loewy, J. (1999). Music therapy: Significant helper in healing, soothing children. *AAP News*, *1*(12), 29–32.

Meyer, D. J., & Vadasy, P. F. (2008). *Sibshops: Workshops for siblings of children with special needs* (rev. ed.). Baltimore, MD: Brookes.

Plank, E. N. (1959). *Working with children in hospitals: A guide for the professional team*. London: Tavistock.

Stephens, B. K., Barkey, M. E., & Hall, H. R. (1999). Techniques to comfort children during stressful procedures. *Advances in Mind-body Medicine*, *15*(1), 49–60.

Thompson, R. (Ed.). (2009). *The handbook of child life: A guide for pediatric psychosocial care*. Springfield, IL: Charles C. Thomas.

WEBSITE ARTICLES

Nemours Foundation. Doctor visits. KidsHealth.org. Retrieved September 20, 2017, from: www.kidshealth.org/parent/system/doctor/dr_visits.html#cat173

PBS Parents. Talking with kids about health. Retrieved June 30, 2017 from: www.pbs.org/parents/talkingwithkids/health/doctor_before.html

ADDITIONAL RESOURCES BY PATRICIA WEINER

Home With Your Baby
http://mommybites.com/col1/baby/home-baby

Suggested Reading for Children and Parents About Going to the Doctor or Hospital
http://mommybites.com/col1/baby/suggested-reading-for-children-and-parents-about-going-to-the-doctor-or-hospital

Preparing for Your Child's Medical Visits: Comforting Techniques
http://mommybites.com/col1/baby/preparing-for-your-child%E2%80%99s-medical-visits-comforting-techniques

Preparing for Your Child's Medical Visits: Important Tips
http://mommybites.com/col1/baby/preparing-for-your-childs-medical-visits-important-tips

A Child with Chronic Illness Goes to School
http://mommybites.com/col1/preschool/child-chronic-illness-school

Play is Critical to Healthy Brain Development
http://mommybites.com/newyork/03/21/play-critical-healthy-brain-development

Tips for Parents of Children with Special Needs
http://mommybites.com/newyork/05/06/tips-for-parents-of-children-with-special-needs

Educational Planning for Children with Special Health Care Needs
http://mommybites.com/newyork/03/08/educational-planning-children-special-care-needs

Traumatic Brain Injury and Orthopedic Impairments
http://mommybites.com/newyork/02/01/traumatic-brain-injury

Children with Chronic Health Issues
http://mommybites.com/newyork/01/11/chronic-health-issues

Afterword

What a grand adventure through the worlds of Medical Play Therapy and Child Life this has been. And what a privilege it has been for me to work with such dedicated and passionate teachers, researchers, and healers. While the cumulative experiences of the contributors to this volume span decades and generations, theories and ideologies, settings and locales, their commitment to the singular mission of helping children, teens, and families in medical need binds them. Whether working with the parents of children on a routine well visit, a frightened child wrestling with a chronic health challenge, or the family of a teen soon to breathe her last breath, these talented and dedicated clinicians have demonstrated the significance and power of play to teach, heal, and prepare children, teens, and their caretakers for perilous and often unchartered journeys into the painful recesses of life and death.

It was during my senior year of college that I was first introduced to Child Life while engaged in my psychology internship at Maimonides Medical Center in Brooklyn, New York. There, a little girl that I called Naomi was battling the ravages of what was then called failure to thrive syndrome. She was as enthralled with my shiny keys as I was with that fascinating play-space in which we connected and from which I moved on into a career as a psychologist, and eventually play therapist. Since that pivotal experience, I have worked in various playrooms with several children struggling to make sense of their medical burdens; a 7-year-old forced to contend with demands placed upon her and her parents by epidermolysis bullosa; a 9-year-old confused by the incursion of cancer into the lives of her mother and grandmother; a 4-year-old facing what would surely be a confusing and painful surgical procedure with psychological and physical ramifications that would surely follow him well into adulthood and parenthood.

And there at the center of my work with these and many other children, teens, and families, whether in playrooms, classrooms, or my own life . . . has been the life-giving, healing, and inescapable power of play.

Thank you for being part of this journey with us.

Lawrence C. Rubin

Index

Page numbers for figures are in *italics*, and page numbers for tables are in **bold**.